Teaching in the Age of Medical Technology

Dachel Martínez Asanza
National School of Public Health, Cuba & University of Medical Sciences of Havana, Cuba

IGI Global
Scientific Publishing
Publishing Tomorrow's Research Today

Vice President of Editorial	Melissa Wagner
Director of Acquisitions	Mikaela Felty
Director of Book Development	Jocelynn Hessler
Production Manager	Mike Brehm
Cover Design	Jose Rosado

Published in the United States of America by
IGI Global Scientific Publishing
701 East Chocolate Avenue
Hershey, PA, 17033, USA
Tel: 717-533-8845
Fax: 717-533-7115
Website: https://www.igi-global.com E-mail: cust@igi-global.com

Library of Congress Cataloging-in-Publication Data

LCCN: 2025012912 (CIP Data Pending)
ISBN13: 9798337315195
Isbn13Softcover: 9798337315201
EISBN13: 9798337315218

British Cataloguing in Publication Data
A Cataloguing in Publication record for this book is available from the British Library.

Table of Contents

Foreword xii

Preface xiv

Chapter 1
The Impact of Technology on Teaching and Clinical Practice in Dentistry: An Update 1
Dachel Martínez Asanza, National School of Public Health (ENSAP), Havana Medical Sciences University, Cuba
Farida Mouloudj, University of Medea, Algeria
Murtala Ismail Adaka, Bayero University, Nigeria
Adania Siva Guanche Martínez, University of Medical Sciences of Havana, Cuba
Adrián Álvarez Pérez, Havana Medical Sciences University, Cuba

Chapter 2
Improving Technology Literacy in Health Professional Education 33
Chunfang Zhou, University of Southern Denmark, Denmark
Anna Marie Lassen, University College Northern Denmark, Denmark

Chapter 3
Opportunities and Challenges of AI-Driven Transformation in Medical Education 63
Flaka Hoti, University of Gjakova "Fehmi Agani", Kosovo
Kamel Mouloudj, University of Medea, Algeria
Doruntina Kabashi, Main Family Medicine Center in Peja, Kosovo
Hasime Arif Bacaj Terziqi, University of Gjakova "Fehmi Agani", Kosovo
Antigona Ukëhaxhaj, University of Gjakova "Fehmi Agani", Kosovo & National Institute of Public Health, Kosovo

Chapter 4
AI for Personalized Learning in Medical Education 91
Hayatullah Niazai, Ahmad Shah Abdali Medical College, Afghanistan
Wali Khan Monib, Shaikh Zayed University, Afghanistan

Chapter 5
Teaching Medicine With Generative Artificial Intelligence (GenAI): A Review of Practices, Pitfalls, and Possibilities in Medical Education 123
Manuel B. Garcia, FEU Institute of Technology, Philippines
Raquel Simões de Almeida, Polytechnic of Porto, Portugal
Dharel P. Acut, Cebu Technological University, Philippines
Rui Pedro Pereira de Almeida, University of Algarve, Portugal
Precious S. Garcia, Jose Rizal University, Philippines
Eleonora Stefani, University of Padova, Italy

Chapter 6
Impact of Wearable Technology on Medical Education 157
Pandimurugan Vellaisamy, Acharya University, Karakul, Uzbekistan
Sajeer Karattil, University of Technology and Applied Sciences, Oman
Mohammed Mubarak Mohammed Al Araimi, University of Technology and Applied Sciences, Oman
V. Rajaram, SRM Institute of Science and Technology, India
B. Balakiruthiga, SRM Institute of Science and Technology, India
Angayarkanni S. A., SRM Institute of Science and Technology, India
Baiju B. V., Vellore Institute of Technology, India

Chapter 7
Mobile Learning in Medical Education 195
Pudasaini Pramila, Life Skills Education, Nepal
Ioannis Adamopoulos, School of Public Health, University of West Attica, Greece
Alisha Rijal, Yeti Health Science Academy, Nepal

Chapter 8
3D Printing Revolutionizing Rural Dental Care: Empowering Healthier Smiles.. 227
Mariya Dimitrova, Department of Prosthetic Dentistry, Faculty of Dental Medicine, Medical University of Plovdiv, Bulgaria

Chapter 9
Ethical Considerations in Using Technology for Medical Education: Ethics in Medical Education 279
Ioannis Adamopoulos, School of Public Health, University of West Attica, Greece
Pramila Thapa, Life Skills Education, Nepal
Niki Syrou, University of Thessaly, Greece

Compilation of References 315

About The Contributors 395

Index 405

Detailed Table of Contents

Foreword xii

Preface xiv

Chapter 1
The Impact of Technology on Teaching and Clinical Practice in Dentistry: An Update 1
Dachel Martínez Asanza, National School of Public Health (ENSAP), Havana Medical Sciences University, Cuba
Farida Mouloudj, University of Medea, Algeria
Murtala Ismail Adaka, Bayero University, Nigeria
Adania Siva Guanche Martínez, University of Medical Sciences of Havana, Cuba
Adrián Álvarez Pérez, Havana Medical Sciences University, Cuba

Dental education is experiencing a considerable transformation across emerging technologies. This chapter presents a narrative review around the impact of virtual simulators, teledentistry, 3D printing, artificial intelligence, virtual and augmented reality on dental training. It was analyzed 17 articles published between 2020 and 2024 in PubMed, SciELO, and Google Scholar. The results revealed that simulators offer safe practice environments, teledentistry facilitates remote care and 3D printing with AI enhances personalized prosthetics and diagnosis. In addition, virtual and augmented reality are bringing the surgical precision to new levels. While there are still hurdles to overcome, such as figuring out how to weave these technologies into the curriculum, training the faculty, protecting data, and making sure everyone has equal access. This overview illustrates an immense progress and challenges in the digital transformation of dental education.

Chapter 2
Improving Technology Literacy in Health Professional Education 33
Chunfang Zhou, University of Southern Denmark, Denmark
Anna Marie Lassen, University College Northern Denmark, Denmark

This chapter explores how technology literacy in health professional education can be improved through Reflective Practice-Based Learning (RPL). Two research questions are asked: 1) How can we deepen our theoretical understanding of Reflective Practice-Based Learning (RPL) as a pedagogy for fostering technology literacy? and 2) How can we enhance technology literacy in health professional education through the practical application of RPL? To answer these questions, this chapter integrates theoretical perspectives on technology literacy, learning, knowledge, and health professional education into a unified framework. This also includes a case description focused on the practical implementation of a RPL-based course. The findings highlight the theoretical and practical significance of RPL in advancing technology literacy education and driving pedagogical innovation in teaching and learning in the age of medical technology for the future.

Chapter 3
Opportunities and Challenges of AI-Driven Transformation in Medical Education 63
Flaka Hoti, University of Gjakova "Fehmi Agani", Kosovo
Kamel Mouloudj, University of Medea, Algeria
Doruntina Kabashi, Main Family Medicine Center in Peja, Kosovo
Hasime Arif Bacaj Terziqi, University of Gjakova "Fehmi Agani", Kosovo
Antigona Ukëhaxhaj, University of Gjakova "Fehmi Agani", Kosovo & National Institute of Public Health, Kosovo

The integration of artificial intelligence (AI) and digital technologies is reshaping the landscape of medical education. This chapter explores how AI enhances clinical reasoning, personalizes learning pathways, and supports the digital transformation of teaching and assessment. Drawing on a narrative review of recent literature, the chapter identifies both the opportunities and challenges associated with implementing AI in medical curricula. Particular attention is given to institutional resistance, ethical and data privacy concerns, infrastructural constraints, and the lack of faculty training. Recommendations are offered for educators, institutions, policymakers, and technology developers to facilitate responsible and effective adoption. By addressing these barriers and fostering collaboration across sectors, AI can serve as a powerful catalyst for innovation in medical education. The chapter concludes by emphasizing the need for ongoing investment, ethical oversight, and educator empowerment to ensure that AI contributes meaningfully to the development of future healthcare.

Chapter 4
AI for Personalized Learning in Medical Education 91
Hayatullah Niazai, Ahmad Shah Abdali Medical College, Afghanistan
Wali Khan Monib, Shaikh Zayed University, Afghanistan

Personalized learning involves tailoring learning experiences to individual learners' needs, preferences, and progress. However, ensuring personalized learning remains a challenging task. Artificial intelligence (AI) usage can be an opportunity to enhance personalized learning. This chapter explores AI role in enhancing personalized learning in medical education. The chapter covers content development, AI-assisted tutoring, adaptive case-based learning, automated assessments, immediate feedback, and clinical decision-making in personalized medical education. It further discusses AI in conducting literature reviews and knowledge synthesis in medical education. Moreover, it provides insights into AI risks and ethical considerations in medical education, including potential bias, data privacy, accuracy and reliability challenges, and over-reliance on this technology. It emphasizes the need to promote AI literacy among medical learners, offering insights into effective AI-assisted personalized learning in medical education.

Chapter 5
Teaching Medicine With Generative Artificial Intelligence (GenAI): A Review of Practices, Pitfalls, and Possibilities in Medical Education 123
Manuel B. Garcia, FEU Institute of Technology, Philippines
Raquel Simões de Almeida, Polytechnic of Porto, Portugal
Dharel P. Acut, Cebu Technological University, Philippines
Rui Pedro Pereira de Almeida, University of Algarve, Portugal
Precious S. Garcia, Jose Rizal University, Philippines
Eleonora Stefani, University of Padova, Italy

Once confined to science fiction and speculative futures, generative artificial intelligence (GenAI) has swiftly entered the lecture halls of modern medical education. Despite its expanding use, a synthesis of its implementation, limitations, and educational value remains underexplored. This review aims to critically examine current applications, identify pedagogical pitfalls, and delineate future trajectories for GenAI in medical training. Key innovations include AI-driven content generation tailored to curricular benchmarks, automated assessments with real-time diagnostic feedback, and immersive virtual patient simulations replicating complex pathophysiologies. Additional advances span multilingual knowledge translation, anatomically precise surgical training environments, and adaptive learning systems powered by intelligent tutoring frameworks. As discussed herein, GenAI holds transformative potential for advancing clinical competence in an evolving medical landscape—provided its integration is evidence-based, ethically sound, and educationally coherent.

Chapter 6
Impact of Wearable Technology on Medical Education 157
Pandimurugan Vellaisamy, Acharya University, Karakul, Uzbekistan
Sajeer Karattil, University of Technology and Applied Sciences, Oman
Mohammed Mubarak Mohammed Al Araimi, University of Technology and Applied Sciences, Oman
V. Rajaram, SRM Institute of Science and Technology, India
B. Balakiruthiga, SRM Institute of Science and Technology, India
Angayarkanni S. A., SRM Institute of Science and Technology, India
Baiju B. V., Vellore Institute of Technology, India

Health Information Technology (HIT) along with the Internet of Medical Things (IoMT) employs wearable technology to monitor diseases through its capability to prevent medical mistakes from occurring. The devices track vital signs which medical professionals use for precise treatment decisions through real-time data transmission. IoT-driven medical devices improve telehealth service delivery as well as enhance patient monitoring functions. Virtual and augmented reality powers educational wearables to assist medical student surgical training as well as human anatomy education. Research professionals obtain immediate biological feedback through their diagnostic work and clinical preparation. Wearable technology enhances healthcare operations through its support of educational initiatives and research activities which lead to better medical discoveries today and in upcoming years.

Chapter 7
Mobile Learning in Medical Education 195
Pudasaini Pramila, Life Skills Education, Nepal
Ioannis Adamopoulos, School of Public Health, University of West Attica, Greece
Alisha Rijal, Yeti Health Science Academy, Nepal

Mobile learning (mLearning) is revolutionizing medical education with its flexibility, accessibility, and interactive features. This chapter identifies gaps in integrating mLearning into curricula, focusing on challenges like digital distractions, usability, and cost. Using PRISMA 2020 guidelines, it reviews literature from Scopus, Medline, PubMed, and Web of Science. Findings highlight benefits like enhanced engagement and clinical reasoning through gamified tools but note challenges like high costs and limited patient interaction. Recommendations include blended learning, collaboration, and theories like SDT and CLT to boost motivation and efficiency. The chapter emphasizes further research to optimize mLearning for improved global healthcare education.

Chapter 8
3D Printing Revolutionizing Rural Dental Care: Empowering Healthier Smiles........ 227
Mariya Dimitrova, Department of Prosthetic Dentistry, Faculty of Dental Medicine, Medical University of Plovdiv, Bulgaria

3D printing, or additive manufacturing, is transforming dentistry by enabling precise, affordable, and localized production of dental devices. Using a layer-by-layer process with materials like resins and metals, it creates prosthetics, orthodontic devices, and surgical guides, improving workflows and patient care. In rural areas, where economic and infrastructure barriers limit access to specialized dental care, 3D printing offers a revolutionary solution. By enabling on-site production of custom devices, it reduces costs, shortens treatment times, and bridges the gap between rural and urban healthcare. Successful cases in India, Sub-Saharan Africa, and Southeast Asia highlight its potential to empower local providers and improve accessibility. However, challenges like high startup costs, limited materials, and training requirements hinder broader adoption. Future advancements, including AI integration and improved materials, could overcome these barriers.3D printing promises equitable, high-quality dental care by decentralizing production and improving access.

Chapter 9
Ethical Considerations in Using Technology for Medical Education: Ethics in Medical Education........ 279
Ioannis Adamopoulos, School of Public Health, University of West Attica, Greece
Pramila Thapa, Life Skills Education, Nepal
Niki Syrou, University of Thessaly, Greece

Background: Medical education is integrating technology, including artificial intelligence, but ethical concerns remain. Objective: This study aims to enhance the role of ethics in medicine, focusing on the integration of human intelligence, particularly social and emotional intelligence, for ethical decision-making in medical education. Methods: The study uses a scoping review design to examine and explore key approaches to ethical considerations in using technology for medical education. Results: The data synthesis process identifies themes concerning behavior changes, technology acceptance, digital distraction, and AI mobile learning. Technology integration in medical education has led to significant advancements in assessment, learning, and professional development. Conclusions: Using Technology for Medical Education has enhanced learning outcomes, provided creative teaching methods, and increased resource access. The digitalization of medical education has led to the development of clinical skills and increased access to resources.

Compilation of References 315

About The Contributors 395

Index 405

Foreword

In recent years, the convergence of medicine and technology has accelerated beyond what many of us could have imagined just a decade ago. The evolution of educational practices within medical and dental training is no longer a matter of incremental adaptation—it is a paradigm shift. From artificial intelligence to wearable devices, from mobile learning to 3D printing, technology is reshaping not just how we teach but how we think about what it means to learn in the healthcare professions.

Teaching in the Age of Medical Technology arrives at a crucial moment in this transformation. This book offers an insightful, evidence-informed, and multidisciplinary examination of how technology is being deployed to reimagine medical education. It is refreshing in its scope and depth, addressing not only the innovations themselves but also the pedagogical, ethical, and institutional contexts that determine their success or failure.

The breadth of this volume is one of its greatest strengths. The chapters take the reader on a journey from high-tech simulations in dental training to the use of Reflective Practice-Based Learning for cultivating digital literacy. Several chapters engage critically with the promises and pitfalls of artificial intelligence—including its role in personalized learning and generative content creation—while others explore the practical applications of wearable devices and mobile learning tools. Particularly commendable is the book's attention to equity, such as in its discussion of 3D printing's potential to transform dental care in rural and underserved communities.

This collection does not shy away from complexity. It is honest about the barriers—whether institutional resistance, ethical concerns, or faculty preparedness—and yet remains optimistic about the future. It rightly calls for interdisciplinary collaboration, continuous educator development, and ethical safeguards, offering practical guidance while inspiring readers to act.

For medical educators, curriculum developers, institutional leaders, and even policymakers, this book will serve as a valuable resource. It offers not only theoretical frameworks but actionable strategies grounded in real-world case studies and scholarly research.

Above all, Teaching in the Age of Medical Technology reminds us that the ultimate goal of innovation is not technology for its own sake but better learning, better care, and better outcomes for patients. I commend the editors and contributors for assembling a volume that is both visionary and grounded, ambitious and accessible.

This book deserves to be read widely and discussed deeply. It is a significant contribution to the ongoing evolution of health professions education.

Indira Gómez Capote
Havana Dental School, Cuba

Preface

In the ever-evolving landscape of healthcare and higher education, the integration of technology into medical education is no longer a speculative endeavor—it is a pressing necessity. As digital innovations continue to advance at a rapid pace, the way we teach, learn, and practice medicine is being fundamentally reimagined. Teaching in the Age of Medical Technology is both a timely and comprehensive response to this evolution. This edited volume captures the diversity, complexity, and potential of technology-enhanced medical education in the 21st century.

OVERVIEW OF THE SUBJECT MATTER

Medical education has traditionally relied on face-to-face instruction, textbooks, and cadaver-based training. While these foundational practices remain valuable, they are increasingly being supplemented—and in many cases replaced—by new technological tools that offer unprecedented interactivity, accessibility, and personalization. From artificial intelligence and mobile learning to virtual reality, wearable devices, and 3D printing, today's medical educators are faced with a wealth of tools that can enhance both teaching and clinical training.

This book explores how these technologies are being used, adapted, and evaluated in diverse contexts of medical and dental education. It examines both the transformative opportunities and the practical challenges that come with digital integration. By bringing together experts and educators across disciplines, the volume offers a balanced perspective that emphasizes pedagogical rigor, technological literacy, ethical considerations, and future preparedness.

The Role of Technology in Today's Medical Education Landscape

The COVID-19 pandemic accelerated the adoption of digital platforms in education, but the shift toward technology had already been underway for more than a decade. What makes this moment unique is not only the pace of innovation but the scale at which new tools are being embedded into curricula and clinical settings. For educators, this raises important questions about how best to train the next generation of doctors, dentists, nurses, and allied health professionals.

In this context, medical education is tasked with adapting to a world in which knowledge is more accessible, patient data more abundant, and simulation technologies more sophisticated. At the same time, ethical concerns, faculty training, curriculum redesign, and equitable access remain as important as ever. This book does not seek to offer simple answers, but rather provides a multifaceted exploration of these developments—through theoretical insights, practical frameworks, and global case studies.

Intended Audience

This book is intended for a wide and interdisciplinary audience. It is especially valuable for:

- Medical, dental, and nursing educators seeking innovative teaching methods.
- Curriculum developers and instructional designers working in health professions education.
- Health sciences students and residents interested in technology-enhanced learning.
- Policymakers, deans, and academic leaders planning digital transformation in educational institutions.
- Technologists, ed-tech developers, and AI researchers engaged in the healthcare sector.

Whether one is implementing a new learning management system, considering the ethical implications of AI, or exploring the potential of 3D printing in underserved communities, this volume offers essential insights and practical guidance.

CHAPTER DESCRIPTIONS

Chapter 1: The Impact of Technology on Teaching and Clinical Practice in Dentistry: An Update

This chapter offers a comprehensive narrative review of emerging technologies that are transforming dental education. Drawing from 17 peer-reviewed articles, the authors explore the impact of virtual simulators, teledentistry, 3D printing, artificial intelligence, and augmented/virtual reality. These tools are shown to enhance student safety, enable remote diagnosis, and improve surgical precision. However, the chapter also highlights challenges in faculty training, data privacy, and curriculum integration—underscoring the need for thoughtful and inclusive digital strategies.

Chapter 2: Improving Technology Literacy in Health Professional Education

Focusing on Reflective Practice-Based Learning (RPL), this chapter introduces a pedagogical model to enhance technology literacy among health professionals. The authors propose a theoretical framework that integrates concepts of knowledge acquisition, reflection, and digital fluency. Through a detailed case study, the chapter demonstrates how RPL can be effectively implemented in classroom settings, fostering critical thinking and lifelong learning. It calls for a shift from content-heavy curricula to learner-centered, reflective models that better align with the demands of the digital age.

Chapter 3: Opportunities and Challenges of AI-Driven Transformation in Medical Education

This chapter delves into the dual nature of artificial intelligence in medical education. On one hand, AI offers promising tools for personalizing learning, enhancing clinical reasoning, and transforming assessment. On the other hand, it introduces ethical dilemmas, institutional resistance, and data privacy risks. Drawing on current literature, the authors offer strategic recommendations for managing these tensions. The chapter underscores that successful AI adoption requires multi-stakeholder collaboration, ongoing educator training, and a strong ethical framework.

Chapter 4: AI for Personalized Learning in Medical Education

This chapter explores how AI can support personalized medical learning through adaptive case-based instruction, intelligent tutoring systems, and automated assessments. It highlights specific applications such as content curation, clinical decision-making tools, and real-time feedback mechanisms. While emphasizing the potential for improved outcomes, the authors also raise concerns about data accuracy, learner dependence, and algorithmic bias. The chapter concludes by calling for comprehensive AI literacy initiatives to prepare educators and students alike.

Chapter 5: Teaching Medicine with Generative Artificial Intelligence (GenAI): A Review of Practices, Pitfalls, and Possibilities

This timely chapter investigates how generative AI is shaping medical training. Applications range from AI-generated teaching materials to immersive virtual patient simulations and multilingual instructional tools. The authors offer a critical review of current practices, noting both pedagogical innovations and limitations. As GenAI continues to evolve, the chapter emphasizes the importance of aligning technological tools with educational outcomes, promoting responsible usage, and ensuring inclusivity in AI-driven learning environments.

Chapter 6: Impact of Wearable Technology on Medical Education

Wearable devices powered by the Internet of Medical Things (IoMT) are providing new ways to monitor patient vitals, deliver real-time feedback, and support remote diagnostics. This chapter examines how wearables are being used to enhance surgical training, human anatomy instruction, and telehealth education. It discusses the educational benefits of integrating augmented and virtual reality into wearable platforms, while also addressing data management and user engagement. The chapter positions wearable technology as a vital tool for experiential learning and continuous professional development.

Chapter 7: Mobile Learning in Medical Education

Through a systematic literature review, this chapter evaluates the potential and limitations of mobile learning (mLearning) in medical education. It discusses the benefits of mobile apps, gamified content, and asynchronous learning, while also identifying barriers such as digital fatigue, access inequality, and cost. Grounded in

Self-Determination Theory and Cognitive Load Theory, the chapter proposes a blended learning framework that maximizes motivation and efficiency. It calls for continued research and institutional support to scale mLearning in diverse global contexts.

Chapter 8: 3D Printing Revolutionizing Rural Dental Care

Focusing on rural and underserved populations, this chapter explores how 3D printing is democratizing access to dental care. By enabling the on-site production of prosthetics and surgical guides, 3D printing reduces treatment delays and costs. Case studies from India, Africa, and Southeast Asia illustrate the transformative impact of this technology. Yet, the chapter also identifies challenges, including high setup costs and limited technical expertise. It advocates for targeted investments and AI-integrated 3D printing systems to bridge gaps in global oral healthcare.

Chapter 9: Ethical Considerations in Using Technology for Medical Education

As digital technologies permeate medical education, ethical concerns become more prominent. This chapter synthesizes literature on behavioral change, digital distraction, and AI governance. It explores how social and emotional intelligence can guide ethical decision-making in tech-enhanced learning environments. The authors emphasize that while digitalization has expanded access and innovation, it must be accompanied by ethical guidelines that uphold professionalism, equity, and human dignity in educational practice.

CONCLUSION: THE BOOK'S IMPACT AND CONTRIBUTION

Teaching in the Age of Medical Technology is more than a collection of topical essays—it is a blueprint for navigating the challenges and possibilities of a new educational frontier. The volume brings together empirical evidence, pedagogical strategies, and global insights to offer a multifaceted view of digital transformation in medical and dental education.

By addressing the intersections of technology, pedagogy, and ethics, this book equips readers with the knowledge and tools needed to shape the future of health professions education. It champions a forward-thinking approach that respects foundational principles while embracing innovation. As medical education continues to evolve, the themes and strategies discussed in this volume will remain critical to ensuring quality, equity, and excellence in teaching and learning.

We are grateful to the contributors who have shared their expertise and vision, and we hope this book will inspire dialogue, innovation, and sustained improvement in how we educate the healthcare workforce of tomorrow.

Dachel Martínez Asanza

Chapter 1

The Impact of Technology on Teaching and Clinical Practice in Dentistry: An Update

Dachel Martínez Asanza
https://orcid.org/0000-0002-1830-7137
National School of Public Health (ENSAP), Havana Medical Sciences University, Cuba

Farida Mouloudj
https://orcid.org/0009-0005-2759-9708
University of Medea, Algeria

Murtala Ismail Adaka
https://orcid.org/0000-0003-4298-1970
Bayero University, Nigeria

Adania Siva Guanche Martínez
University of Medical Sciences of Havana, Cuba

Adrián Álvarez Pérez
https://orcid.org/0009-0001-3079-5858
Havana Medical Sciences University, Cuba

ABSTRACT

Dental education is experiencing a considerable transformation across emerging

DOI: 10.4018/979-8-3373-1519-5.ch001

technologies. This chapter presents a narrative review around the impact of virtual simulators, teledentistry, 3D printing, artificial intelligence, virtual and augmented reality on dental training. It was analyzed 17 articles published between 2020 and 2024 in PubMed, SciELO, and Google Scholar. The results revealed that simulators offer safe practice environments, teledentistry facilitates remote care and 3D printing with AI enhances personalized prosthetics and diagnosis. In addition, virtual and augmented reality are bringing the surgical precision to new levels. While there are still hurdles to overcome, such as figuring out how to weave these technologies into the curriculum, training the faculty, protecting data, and making sure everyone has equal access. This overview illustrates an immense progress and challenges in the digital transformation of dental education.

INTRODUCTION

The 2030 Agenda for Sustainable Development underscores inclusive, equitable, and quality education as a source of societal progress, combined with permanent learning opportunities for all individuals. (Economic Commission for Latin America and the Caribbean [CEPAL], 2018). Martínez-Asanza et al. (2018) posit that this vision reflects a collective commitment to fostering equitable societies where holistic development hinges on universal access to educational resources across life stages.

Building on this worldwide effort, the World Health Organization's (WHO, 2021) digital health plan promotes flexible technologies as things everyone can use, emphasizing fairness and equal access to healthcare for all. While this approach helps fill in the gaps in the system by using new ideas, but it also brings up certain risks. This includes spreading false information to patients, cybersecurity threats, weaknesses in teledentistry platforms, and tricky ethical questions in around using data for diagnoses. In this context, the WHO, rooted in international treaties, ensures that as healthcare, including dentistry, embraces the digital age, it prioritizes patient safety and upholds human dignity.

Nowadays, healthcare professional training faces a serious challenge: ensuring educational programs not only address societal requirements but also keep pace with rapidly evolving technological advancements (Artaza et al., 2020; Hays et al., 2020; Madfa et al., 2023; Radwan et al., 2023; Lin et al., 2023; Thurzo et al., 2023; Spielman, 2024). For dental education, this involves tackling workforce shortages and disparities in access to oral healthcare, while integrating cutting-edge tools like virtual reality (VR) simulators for cavity preparation and AI-powered diagnostic systems into training.

Valcárcel-Izquierdo and Díaz-Díaz (2019) argue that medical education sciences focus on cultivating human resources within and for the healthcare sector. Additionally, Martínez-Asanza (2021) accentuates the significance of bridging theoretical knowledge with practical experience in dental training, warranting it aligns as closely as possible with the real-world contexts where graduates will eventually practice.

The COVID-19 pandemic acted as a catalyst for rapid adoption of digital technologies. For instance virtual reality case libraries and teledentistry platforms transcended traditional training limitations, enabling dental students in resource-constrained settings to refine procedural precision remotely (Costa et al., 2021; Tiol-Carrillo, 2021; Escobar-Taipe, 2023).

Concurrently, advancements like intraoral scanners, digital radiography, and chairside CAD/CAM systems have redefined clinical workflows, reducing margin error in restorations by up to 70% and enabling same-day prosthetic solutions (Gracco et al., 2023; Gawali et al., 2024). These tools, however, demand curricular overhauls to ensure graduates master both technical competencies and adaptive problem-solving skills (Silva-Velasco, 2023; Vera-Carrasco, 2024). This chapter addresses two pivotal questions: (1) What recent technological advancements are reshaping dental education and clinical practice? (2) How do these innovations influence pedagogical methodologies, clinical outcomes, and equitable patient care?

The objective of this chapter is a narrative review of evidence from 2020-2024, highlighting how dentistry's digital transformation reshapes both education and practice, while critically evaluating gaps accessibility, educator preparedness, and patient-centered outcomes.

BACKGROUND

Modern technological advancements have considerably renovated dental education and clinical practice, redesigning both knowledge delivery and the development of clinical skills (Escobar-Taipe, 2023). As pointed out by Haleem et al. (2022) and Elundu et al. (2024), the use of digital tools, cutting-edge simulations, and creative educational resources has revamped teaching methods and transformed the way students interact with real-life clinical situations.

Although these advancements, substantial challenges remain (Mouloudj et al., 2025). One main concern, underlined by researchers like Martínez-Asanza (2018), Mhlongo et al. (2023), Michel-Villarreal et al. (2023), Gkrimpizi et al. (2023), and Mpuangnan (2024), is the hesitance of certain educators and practitioners to embrace new educational frameworks and technologies. This kind of resistance can really affect how effective training programs and hinder the acquisition of essential competencies by students.

Another pressing issue is the need to keep up with the rapid evolution of dental technologies and scientific breakthroughs. As noted by DaSilva et al. (2022) and Sirko & Shi (2024), advancements like AI-driven diagnostics and biomimetic materials demand ongoing professional development. Martínez-Asanza (2025) emphasizes that the constant introduction of new techniques and treatments requires a commitment to lifelong learning to uphold high standards in patient care.

This condition calls for updating the academic curriculum and making concerted efforts to create a culture of continuous education among dental professionals. Tackling these challenges calls for a team effort that brings together everyone involved: clinicians, policymakers, educators, and community members. It's crucial to form strategic partnerships and create open channels for sharing knowledge. This approach ensures that training programs align with workforce demands and comply with evidence-based care standards.

MAIN FOCUS OF THE CHAPTER

Issues, Controversies, Problems

The incorporation of technology into practice and education within the dental field has raised a notable debate concerning its accessibility, efficiency, ethics, and the preservation of essential skills. As advanced innovations get introduced, dental training is increasingly being modified through the use of virtual reality (VR) and artificial intelligence (AI) (Alqahtani, 2024, & Jha Kukreja & Kukreja, 2025). For example, Lin et al. (2024) state that VR simulators aid with helping students master intricate skills, such as restoration or surgery, by providing a safe environment where they can develop their skills through immersive practice.

While technology advances is arguably beneficial, there is still some concern regarding the long-term consequences on clinical competence and dexterity. Innovations such as 3D intraoral scanners and CAD/CAM systems have enhanced efficiency in the human-operated prosthetic design process, which diminishes the margin for error (Usman et al., 2024; Alqahtani, 2024). Some detractors, however, warn about the risks involved with excessive automation. They claim that reliance on algorithms to accomplish tasks as radiograph interpretation can weaken a clinician's evaluator and critical thinking skills. Moreover, the stiff financial demands that come with adopting this technology may widen the disparity gap between well-endowed and financially-strapped institutions.

Ethical considerations pose even deeper dynamics to the landscape. Concerns like data privacy in teledentistry and patient distrust of the "impersonal" nature of treatment rendered by machines underscore the consequences of ignoring careful planning and integration. While older techniques like teaching using life-sized mannequins and analog radiographs foster practical skills mastery, current advances facilitate the convergence of disciplines, including engineering and dentistry, through digital workflows. Martínez-Asanza et al., (2024a) argues that many issues, including the existence of incompatible digital silos and constant need for reskilling, underscore a principle: technology must enhance human work, not replace expertise.

At last, the aim is to balance precision and accessibility, while maintaining the kind, patient-focused dental care that characterizes the profession. By redressing inequities, protecting clinical autonomy, and cultivating morally responsible adoption, the field can manage the task of embracing, while also preserving, the duality of its mission: to advance technological progress and to protect its foundation of moral values.

Definition and Scope of Innovative Technologies in Dental Education and Clinical Practice

At the present time, dentistry is experiencing an outstanding transformation, thanks to a diversity of digital tools, methods, and systems that are set to change both education and clinical practice for the better. As pointed out by DaSilva et al. (2022), Martínez-Asanza (2024b), Martínez Asanza et al. (2024c) and Sirko and Shi (2024), these innovations are all about improving patient care and enriching the learning experience for future dental professionals.

These technologies include applications that influence scientific and technological developments to boost oral health. They make health promotion and disease prevention more efficient, permit for precise diagnoses, and enable effective treatments and rehabilitation, all while guaranteeing that patients receive ongoing support (Carvalho & Zanatta, 2024). The range of examples is impressive, from digital education platforms and training simulations to artificial intelligence, CAD/CAM systems, augmented and virtual reality, and telehealth consultations.

By embracing these innovations, dental education and clinical practice are moving towards more personalized, efficient, and evidence-based methods. This shift is expected to significantly improve both the training of students and the outcomes for patients.

BENEFITS OF INTEGRATING TECHNOLOGIES IN DENTAL EDUCATION AND CLINICAL PRACTICE

As underscored by Mun et al. (2025), the dental curriculum functions as a dynamic and evolving framework considered to equip future professionals with the scientific knowledge, technical skills, clinical competencies, and ethical values essential to meet the ever-evolving demands of modern healthcare. The incorporation of emerging technologies is indispensable to this mission. García-Ancira and Treviño-Cubero (2020) further point out that aligning graduate competencies with societal expectations fosters the development of dentists who are not only clinically adept but also adaptable and socially accountable practitioners.

Technological Integration in Clinical Practice

Enhanced Diagnostics and Treatment Precision

The integration of intraoral scanners and CAD/CAM technologies has transformed diagnostic and restorative workflows by enabling the generation of highly accurate digital models and personalized treatment solutions (Tiol-Carrillo, 2021; Jurado et al., 2021; Fukuhara-Nakama et al., 2023; Martínez-Asanza et al., 2024b). These digital tools not only reduce dependence on traditional impressions but also enhance patient comfort and streamline communication between clinics and laboratories.

Patient-Centered Care

According to Jun et al. (2025), digital treatment planning software permits patients to visualize the expected outcomes, thereby facilitating informed decision-making and enhancing satisfaction. Moreover, digital data management and stringent sterilization protocols help to raise safety and hygiene standards.

Efficiency and Communication

Digital workflows streamline procedures, reducing chair time and minimizing errors. Cloud-based platforms enable real-time collaboration among dental teams, supporting more integrated and responsive care (Alfallaj et al., 2023).

Technological Advancements in Dental Education

Flexible Learning Environments

Digital platforms, including virtual simulations and interactive modules, provide students with 24/7 access to educational resources, bridging gaps in traditional instruction and supporting self-paced learning (Silva-Velasco, 2023; Vera-Carrasco, 2024; Zitzmann et al., 2020; Escobar-Taipe et al., 2023).

Competency-Driven Pedagogy

Incorporating information and communication technologies (ICTs) into curricula promotes active learning, critical thinking, and hands-on virtual training (Casola-Rivera, 2020; Díaz-Lozada et al., 2022; Yazdanpanahi et al., 2022). Research-driven innovation ensures alignment with existing clinical advancements (Macanchí-Pico et al., 2020; Palacios-Núñez et al., 2021; Tripathi et al., 2024).

Ethical and Adaptive Skill Development

Technology not only improves technical mastery but also supports the development of ethical reasoning and adaptability, essential for navigating complex clinical scenarios (Gal et al., 2021; Thurzo et al., 2023). In brief, technology has redefined modern dentistry by merging efficiency, safety, and personalization in patient care, while simultaneously transforming educational methodologies. The integration of digital tools prepares graduates to excel as technically proficient, ethically grounded, and socially responsive professionals. This interaction between innovation and pedagogy ensures that dentistry remains at the vanguard of healthcare evolution, equipped to address both present and future challenges.

METHODOLOGY

This narrative review addresses key research questions related to technological advancements in academic training and clinical practices in dentistry. The formulated research questions are as follows: (1) What recent technological advancements are reshaping dental education and clinical practice? (2) How do these innovations influence pedagogical methodologies, clinical outcomes, and equitable patient care?

Article Selection

This review employed a systematic approach to literature selection, guided by the PRISMA (Preferred Reporting Items for Systematic Reviews and Meta-Analyses) framework(Page et al., 2021). While narrative reviews typically allow greater flexibility, we adapted PRISMA principles to enhace transparency in documenting our search and inclusion process.

Our search targeted peer-reviewed articles published between January 2020 to December 2024 in English and Spanish sourced from PubMed, Scielo, and Google Scholar. To ensure methodological rigor, the strategy combined core terms related to dental education with keywords reflecting technological innovations. These keywords included *"dental education", "curriculum", "dentistry", "educational technology", "simulation training", "teledentistry", "3D printing", "artificial intelligence", "virtual reality",* and *"augmented reality".* Boolean operators (AND/OR) were applied to refine results, prioritizing studies that explicitly explored the integration of digital tools or emerging technologies into dental pedagogy or clinical training.

Studies were excluded if they didn't explicitly focus on technology-driven educational interventions, lacked relevance to dental training, or were purely descriptive without evaluative data. The selection process aligned with criteria from *the Scale for the Assessment of Narrative Review Articles* (SANRA; Baethge et al., 2019), emphasizing clarity of purpose, practical utility, and critical analysis of included sources.

This approach balanced the structured reproducibility of systematic reviews with the contextual depth characteristics of narrative syntheses, ensuring a focused yet comprehensive exploration of modern advancements in dental education.

Literature Analysis

A word cloud (see Fig. 1) was generated using WordArt based on the abstracts of the 17 included articles to identify central concepts that guided thematic synthesis. This word cloud allowed visualization of the most relevant topics and their frequency in the reviewed literature, facilitating the identification of patterns and trends in technological advancements in dentistry.

Figure 1. Word Cloud [Proposed by the authors, results using Edit word art - Wordart. com (2025). https://wordart.com/create

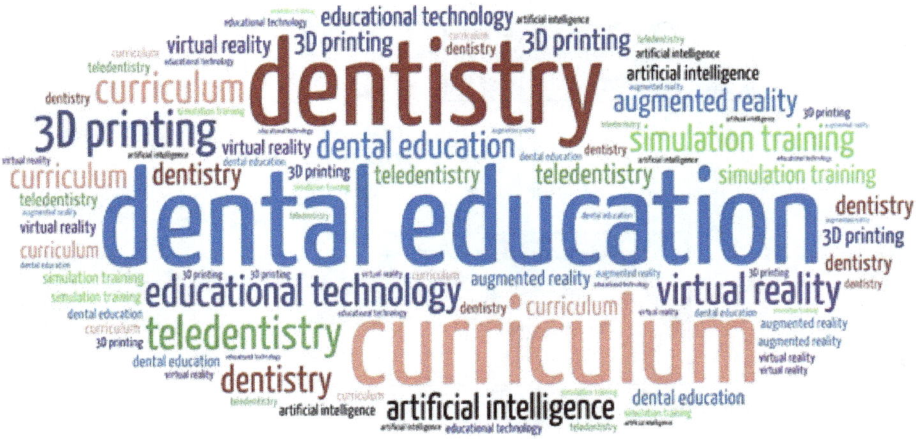

Inclusion and Exclusion Criteria

The key criteria for including studies were met when references to technological advancements in academic training and clinical dental practices appeared in the title or abstract. The collected data encompassed various types of publications, such as review articles, mini-reviews, brief communications, discussions, and short surveys. Subsequently, the abstracts of the remaining articles were assessed. The analysis focused on works that specifically emphasized the significance of technological advancements used in study curricula, both in theory and practice of dental education (articles addressing the teaching of dental practices using modern technologies).

Case reports, position papers, book chapters, non-peer-reviewed articles, and ongoing studies were excluded, as well as studies that did not focus on both theoretical and practical dental education.

The Rayyan platform was used to automatically eliminate duplicates and assess the titles and abstracts of the collected articles. This narrative review synthesizes the latest literature concerning the possible applications of technology in teaching and clinical practice in dentistry.

After conducting the search, a total of 77 articles were retrieved, including 59 from SciELO, 11 from PubMed and 7 from Google Scholar. Figure 2 shows the flowchart representing the search process. By applying additional selection criteria, the initial group of articles was significantly narrowed down to 17, which were chosen as the final sample for the study.

Figure 2. PRISMA flow chart showing the inclusion and exclusion criteria

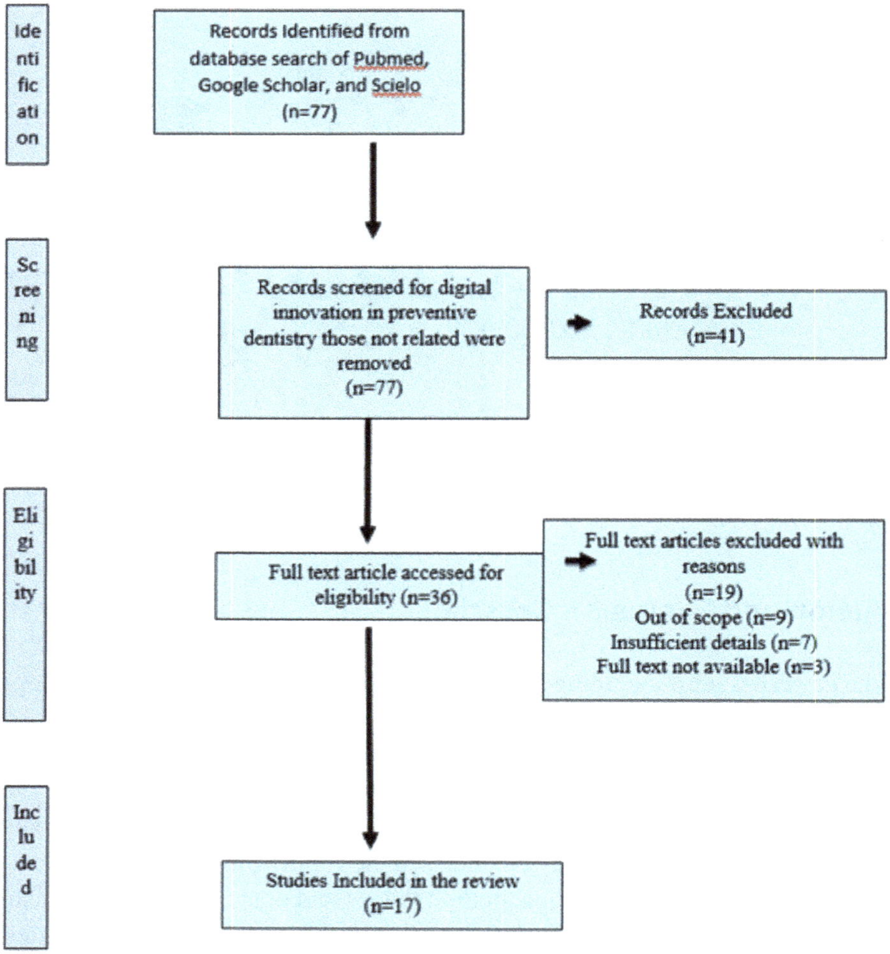

Data Collection

Data extracted and collected from the included articles are detailed in Table 1 and organized according to the following parameters: authors, publication year, journal name, article title, key relevant findings, and aim.

Table 1. Overview of the research included in this review, organized according to the following factors: authors, publication year, journal name, article title, key relevant findings, and aim

First author, year, *Journal*	**Article title**	**Key relevant findings**	**Aim**
Schlenz et al. (2020) *BMC Oral Health*	Undergraduate dental students' perspective on the implementation of digital dentistry in the preclinical curriculum: a questionnaire survey	Students appreciated digital integration in teaching for engagement but favored instructor feedback. Over 90% anticipated using intraoral scanners in their future practice. Despite technical challenges, digital tools provide a valuable complement to traditional manual skills training.	To assess the students' perspective on the implementation with a questionnaire survey.
Zitzmann et al. (2020) *International Journal of Environmental Research and Public Health*	Digital Undergraduate Education in Dentistry: A Systematic Review	Digitalization has significant potential to transform dental education, enhancing preparation for future dentists. Interactive e-learning and 24/7 access will improve the educational experience, while augmented and virtual reality technologies are expected to play a crucial role in shaping the future of dental training.	To investigate current penetration and educational quality enhancements from digitalization in the dental curriculum.
Costa et al. (2021) *Odovtos International Journal of Dental Sciences*	Digital technology in dental education during COVID-19 pandemic: worldwide experience of professors and students	Professors and students faced challenges adapting to digital technologies for distance learning during COVID-19 isolation. Factors like gender, age, location, and university type influenced their experiences. Preferred technologies, especially among Latin American and Brazilian educators and students, could be integrated into face-to-face activities to enhance future dental education.	To assess the use and experience with digital communication tools among dentistry professors and students to adapt to distance learning during the Covid-19 pandemic.
Jurado et al. (2021) *Journal of Oral Sciences*	Successful development and implementation of a digital dentistry curriculum at US dental school	A U.S. dental school faced challenges integrating new technology into traditional restorative procedures. To address this, a CAD/CAM division was established to introduce digital dentistry concepts to students and faculty, enhancing their exposure to modern dental practices.	To describe methods that were adopted to improve acceptance and increase the productivity of chair side CAD/CAM restorations for both students and faculty at the dental school in US

continued on following page

Table 1. Continued

First author, year, *Journal*	**Article title**	**Key relevant findings**	**Aim**
Yazdanpanahi et al. (2022) *Acta medica Iranica*	Investigating the application of new technologies in dental education: A systematic review	Technology offers many opportunities for teaching and learning solutions. Therefore, dental schools should use technology to support clinical and theoretical education. Digital assessment gadgets in restorative dentistry and dentures allow students to evaluate their performance in real time without direct surveillance.	To investigate the application of new technologies in dental education
Thurzo et al. (2023). *Education Sciences*	Impact of Artificial Intelligence on Dental Education: A Review and Guide for Curriculum Update	AI is transforming dental education by enhancing diagnostics, treatment planning, and patient communication. However, educators often lack the skills to assess AI applications. Curriculum updates are necessary to integrate AI effectively, addressing ethical and legal concerns for responsible implementation.	To provide an up-to-date overview of the upcoming changes and a brief analysis of the influential advancements in the use of AI in dental education since 2020
Erdilek et al. (2023) *Dent Med Probl*	Digitalization era of dental education: A systematic review	Augmented Reality (AR) and Virtual Reality (VR) technologies enhance medical visualization and feedback, improving skill acquisition in dental education. Digital simulations develop clinical competencies, bridging theory and practice, and fostering personalized learning experiences.	To evaluate the use of augmented and virtual reality in pre-clinical dental education.
Fukuhara-Nakama et al. (2023) *Revista Estomatológica Herediana*	Introduction of CAD-CAM technology in dental education: a student and teacher perspectives	57.9% of students and 37.5% of educators suggest that CAD-CAM instruction should commence in the third year. Training sessions were beneficial, and the technology is preferred for fixed prosthetics. Both groups hold a positive perception regarding its introduction in dental clinical courses.	To describe the student and teacher's perceptions of the process of introducing CAD-CAM technology in dental education

continued on following page

Table 1. Continued

First author, year, *Journal*	**Article title**	**Key relevant findings**	**Aim**
Escobar-Taipe et al. (2023) *Revista Facultad de Odontología Universidad de Antioquia*	Digitalization in dental education	Digitalization in dentistry is crucial for student training, enhancing skills with advanced tools. Blended learning is most effective, combining digital and traditional methods. However, exclusive virtual learning, as during COVID-19, led to dissatisfaction due to limited hands-on experience.	To describe digitalization in dental training, the technological tools used and the students´ perception of digital education in dentistry
Alfallaj et al. (2023) *International Journal of Environmental Research and Public Health*	The Status of Digital Dental Technology Implementation in the Saudi Dental Schools' Curriculum: A National Cross-Sectional Survey for Healthcare Digitization	This national study revealed that digital dental technologies (DDT) are not fully integrated into Saudi Arabian dental curricula and patient care. No link was found between funding sources and DDT implementation. Saudi dental schools must prioritize DDT adoption to align with Vision 2030 and graduate dentists proficient in digital care.	To assess the adoption of digital dental technologies in Saudi Arabian undergraduate dental education and evaluate the influence of dental schools' funding sources on the integration of these technologies.
Nassani et al. (2024) *Dentistry Journal*	The Impact of Technology Teaching in the Dental Predoctoral Curriculum on Students Perception of Digital Dentistry	The presence of technology in practice and in educational academic environments significantly improved students' interest and perception of their knowledge and skill.	To assess dental students' perceptions of digital technologies by exposing them to a preclinical simulation exercise of scanning, designing, and manufacturing a computer-aided provisional fixed dental restoration.
Tripathiet al. (2024) *Journal of Oral Biology and Craniofacial Research*	Developing an instructional module of "digital dentistry" for undergraduate prosthodontics curriculum	Thematic analysis of focus groups revealed both theoretical and practical aspects of digital dentistry learning. A module was developed using a modified Delphi technique. The module can be implemented in dental institutes based on available resources and infrastructure, addressing the need for structured digital dentistry education.	To prepare a module on "Digital Dentistry", which can be used to sensitize dental undergraduate students during their final year Prosthodontics curriculum.

continued on following page

Table 1. Continued

First author, year, *Journal*	**Article title**	**Key relevant findings**	**Aim**
Liu et al. (2024) *Journal of Dental Sciences*	Analysis of approved dental teaching projects in the teaching practice research program in 8 dental schools of Taiwan from 2018 to 2023	Between 2018 and 2023, 24 dental teaching projects were approved, with digital dentistry and innovative teaching models emerging as the leading research topics. Despite increasing interest, dental education research remains underrepresented in Taiwanese dental schools, with a mean approval rate of 2.9% over six years.	To analyze dental teaching projects conducted under this program from 2018 to 2023.
Syedet al. (2024) *PloS One*	Comparison of virtual clinical scenario and role play in learning oral pathology among dental students	Dental students exposed to role play significantly outperformed those using virtual clinical scenarios in post-test scores ($P = 0.04$). Role play received higher feedback across multiple aspects ($P < 0.05$), emerging as the preferred method for enhancing learning in oral pathology. Both techniques improved diagnostic skills, but role play demonstrated superior educational impact.	To compare usefulness of virtual clinical scenario and role play in learning oral pathology among second-year dental students.
Lin et al. (2024) *Journal of Dental Sciences*	The use of augmented reality (AR) and virtual reality (VR) in dental surgery education and practice: A narrative review	Augmented reality (AR) and virtual reality (VR) enhance dental surgery precision and training. AR improves surgical outcomes, while VR boosts skill retention. Despite high costs and integration challenges, future developments aim to enhance realism and personalize learning experiences.	To analyze current utilities, limitations, and future potentials of AR and VR in dental surgery education.

continued on following page

Table 1. Continued

First author, year, *Journal*	**Article title**	**Key relevant findings**	**Aim**
Daud et al. (2024) *BMC Oral Health*	The impact of virtual reality haptic simulators in pre-clinical restorative dentistry: a qualitative enquiry into dental students' perceptions	Virtual reality haptic simulators (VRHS) play a vital role in modern dental education, offering innovative solutions for training and evaluation. However, students emphasize the need for enhanced realism and immersive learning experiences. Dental educators should carefully sequence VRHS integration into curricula to optimize learning outcomes and align with evolving pedagogical strategies.	To delve deep into undergraduates' dental students' perceptions related to the impact of VRHS in pre-clinical restorative dentistry.
Robson et al. (2024) *International journal of computerized dentistry*	A systematic review of methodology for the creation of virtual 3D models for use in dental education and a narrative review	There are no specific studies on the creation of dental 3D models. This research summarizes common techniques for fabricating 3D models in dentistry. The field is rapidly evolving with software updates and new programs, highlighting the need to further explore educational applications.	To answer the focused research question, "What software techniques are used in the creation of digital 3D models for use in dental education?"

DISCUSSION

Digitalization has patent a turning point in dental education, as reflected in the 17 articles reviewed in this study. Overall, students view the integration of digital technologies positively. Schlenz et al. (2020) and Nassani et al. (2024) note that introducing tools such as intraoral scanners and CAD/CAM systems augments students' motivation and their sense of competence, with many believing these resources will be essential in their future clinical practice. Nevertheless, there remains a preference for direct instructor feedback over digital alternatives, indicating that technology should serve as a complement rather than a replacement for traditional teaching.

Furthermore, both the systematic review by Zitzmann et al. (2020) and the work of Yazdanpanahi et al. (2022) agree that digitalization has the potential to revolutionize dental training by enabling more interactive, flexible, and personalized educational experiences. Tools such as augmented reality (AR) and virtual reality (VR), as reported by Erdilek et al. (2023) and Lin et al. (2024), enhance anatomical visualization, support the development of clinical skills, and improve precision in surgical procedures. However, high costs and challenges associated to curriculum integration continue to limit widespread adoption, and students, as highlighted by Daud et al. (2024), are calling for more realistic and immersive experiences within these simulations.

The COVID-19 pandemic, according to Costa et al. (2021) and Escobar-Taipe et al. (2023), accelerated the adoption of digital platforms and distance learning. While virtual instruction allowed academic continuity, both students and faculty faced adaptation challenges and expressed dissatisfaction with the lack of hands-on experience, underscoring the importance of hybrid models that blend digital resources with in-person activities (Mouloudj et al., 2025).

Regarding curriculum implementation, Jurado et al. (2021) and Tripathi et al. (2024) demonstrate that developing structured modules and specialized divisions in digital dentistry facilitates the acceptance and mastery of new technologies among both students and educators. Fukuhara-Nakama et al. (2023) emphasizes that both groups consider it appropriate to introduce CAD/CAM training during intermediate stages of the curriculum, and they particularly appreciate its inclusion in the area of fixed prosthodontics.

Internationally, the integration of digital technologies varies considerably. Al-fallaj et al. (2023) show that in Saudi Arabia, the adoption of digital technologies in dental curricula is limited and depends more on institutional commitment and alignment with national policies than on available funding. In Taiwan, according to Liu et al. (2024), although interest in digitalization and innovative teaching models is growing, educational research remains scarce, which hinders the generation of robust evidence to guide innovation.

AI is emerging as a transformative factor, optimizing diagnosis, treatment planning, and patient communication (Thurzo et al., 2023). However, a gap remains in faculty training to evaluate and implement these tools, as well as a need to address the ethical and legal aspects associated with their use.

On another front, the development of digital 3D models and digital assessment in dentistry is advancing rapidly, though standardization and solid evidence regarding their educational impact are still lacking (Robson et al., 2024). Yazdanpanahi et al. (2022) points out that technology enables students to assess their performance in real time and independently, which may foster self-assessment and autonomous learning.

It is also worth noting that while virtual tools contribute to learning, traditional methods such as role play can offer distinct advantages in specific areas, such as the teaching of oral pathology (Syed et al., 2024). This suggests that pedagogical innovation should consider the nature of the competencies to be developed and not rely exclusively on technology.

At the authors' discretion, digitalization symbolizes an exceptional opportunity to modernize dental education, but its application must be strategic, taking into account investment in infrastructure, faculty training, curricular updates, and an appropriate balance between traditional and digital methods. Only in this way will they be able to prepare future dentists to tackle the challenges and seize the opportunities of a constantly evolving profession.

CHALLENGES AND ETHICAL CONSIDERATIONS IN ADOPTING DIGITAL INNOVATIONS FOR DENTAL EDUCATION AND PRACTICE

The successful implementation of digital health tools in dentistry requires more than technical proficiency; it demands a holistic strategy that balances innovation with core human values. While technologies such as AI, VR, and 3D imaging hold the potential to revolutionize dental education and clinical care, their integration must prioritize patient well-being, equity, and sustainability. As emphasized by the World Health Organization (2021), digital solutions should empower individuals, foster trust, and adapt to local contexts, rather than exacerbate existing disparities.

Bridging the Cost and Access Gap

The initial investment required for advanced tools-such as intraoral scanners and CAD/CAM systems-can be prohibitive, particularly for smaller institutions and underserved regions. Alfallaj et al. (2023) highlight that the adoption of digital dental technologies remains limited in certain contexts, not solely due to funding, but also because of institutional priorities and policy alignment. Collaborative resource-sharing and tiered pricing models may help ensure that technology becomes a standard component of equitable care, rather than a luxury accessible only to well-resourced settings.

Safeguarding Patient Data in a Digital World

The transition from paper records to cloud-based systems introduces new challenges in data privacy and security. Practices must implement robust encryption and regular cybersecurity audits to maintain patient trust. Thurzo et al. (2023) emphasize the importance of transparency, ensuring patients understand how their data may be used in AI training and providing them the right to opt out without penalty.

Balancing Algorithms and Clinical Judgment

AI-driven diagnostics can enhance accuracy and efficiency, but should not supplant clinical expertise. As noted by Schlenz et al. (2020) and Thurzo et al. (2023), students and educators value digital tools as complements to, rather than replacements for, traditional training and instructor feedback. Developers must also audit AI systems for potential biases, particularly regarding underrepresented populations, to prevent misdiagnosis and ensure ethical use.

Preserving the Human Touch in Technology-Driven Care

While digital solutions can improve precision and workflow, maintaining empathy and patient-centered care remains essential. Escobar-Taipe et al. (2023) found that exclusive reliance on virtual learning led to dissatisfaction among students, underscoring the need for blended approaches that combine technological innovation with hands-on experience and human interaction.

Preparing Educators and Clinicians for the Digital Shift

The effective adoption of digital innovations depends on continuous faculty development and structured curricular integration. Jurado et al. (2021) and Tripathi et al. (2024) demonstrate that dedicated training and hybrid curricula-combining digital and traditional techniques-are critical for equipping both students and educators with the necessary competencies. Ongoing support for experienced clinicians is also vital to facilitate smooth transitions and prevent workflow disruptions.

The Path Forward: Technology as a Force for Good

Digital innovation in dentistry is not about replacing foundational skills, but about enhancing care while upholding the profession's core ethical values. By addressing cost barriers, safeguarding data, and maintaining the centrality of human connection, the dental field can harness technology responsibly. As Chérrez-Ojeda et al. (2020) and Naik et al. (2022) remind us, the future of dentistry will be shaped not only by technological advances, but also by professionals who apply them with wisdom, compassion, and a commitment to equity.

SOLUTIONS AND RECOMMENDATIONS

Modern dentistry confronts a pressing dilemma: incorporating cutting-edge technologies while conserving foundational clinical expertise and avoiding the exacerbation of healthcare disparities. Innovations such as AI-driven diagnostic algorithms and haptic-enhanced virtual simulators offer unprecedented precision and efficiency.

However, their adoption demands deliberate, equity-centered approaches that uphold ethical standards, ensure universal access, and foster interdisciplinary partnerships. The following proposals outline actionable pathways to harmonize technological progress with the irreplaceable human elements of care, guided by insights from Lin et al. (2024) and Najeeb & Islam (2025).

Hybrid Education for Comprehensive Learning

Research by Schlenz et al. (2020), Zitzmann et al. (2020), and Escobar-Taipe et al. (2023) highlights the efficacy of blended learning models in dental education. VR simulators and digital platforms enable students to refine clinical skills in risk-free, customizable environments while receiving real-time performance analytics (Fu et al., 2024). That said, these technologies must *augment*, not replace, traditional hands-on training with mannequins and live patient interactions, which are irreplaceable for cultivating manual precision and tactile judgment.

To satisfactorily prepare graduates for contemporary collaborative practice, curricula should combine interprofessional education through shared modules with allied health disciplines. Accentuating areas such as 3D imaging and AI-assisted diagnostics can provide a cohesive framework, enabling teams to effectively manage multidisciplinary care with enhanced technical proficiency and clear role delineation (Poblete et al., 2020; Winterhalter et al., 2024).

AI as Clinical Support, Not Substitution

AI has demonstrated utility in areas such as radiographic analysis and early caries detection (Thurzo et al., 2023). Nevertheless, its use should be limited to a supportive role, with clinicians retaining final responsibility for diagnoses and treatment plans. To prevent overreliance on technology, mandatory certification programs in emerging tools-such as intraoral scanners and CAD/CAM systems-are recommended (Jurado et al., 2021; Fukuhara-Nakama et al., 2023). Such training ensures that professionals master both technical operation and critical interpretation, preserving clinical judgment.

Democratizing Technology

Addressing the technological gap between affluent and underserved regions requires collaborative solutions. Alfallaj et al. (2023) highlight disparities in the integration of digital dental technologies, independent of funding sources. Partnerships among universities, government agencies, and industry can help subsidize equipment and expand access to up-to-date educational resources. Open-source platforms and teledentistry initiatives (Kanani et al., 2024; Martínez-Asanza, 2025) are vital for reaching rural communities and supporting remote consultations. Standardizing care protocols and prioritizing vulnerable populations will help ensure that innovation does not deepen inequalities.

Ethics and Data Security in the Digital Era

Protecting patient data is paramount as digital records and AI applications become more prevalent. Robust electronic health records with advanced encryption, explicit informed consent for data use, and regular external audits of diagnostic algorithms are essential to maintain transparency and fairness (Thurzo et al., 2023). These practices build trust and safeguard patient rights in an increasingly digital environment.

Universal Standards for Integration

Interoperability between devices and software is crucial for optimizing workflows and minimizing technical errors. The adoption of universal standards, such as DICOM for imaging, facilitates collaboration among specialists and ensures compatibility across platforms (Benoit et al., 2022; Gurupur, 2024).

Humanizing the Patient Experience

While technology can enhance communication and treatment planning, it must not detract from the human connection at the core of dental care. Interactive 3D models and patient-facing apps can improve understanding and engagement, but should always be balanced with empathetic, in-person interactions (Escobar-Taipe et al., 2023). Dentists should act as "tech translators," demystifying digital tools and involving patients in shared decision-making.

In summary, the future of dentistry lies not in choosing between technology and tradition, but in ethically and inclusively integrating both. By following evidence-based recommendations and fostering ongoing collaboration among stakeholders, the profession can harness the transformative potential of innovation while preserving its humanistic essence.

LIMITATIONS AND FUTURE RESEARCH DIRECTIONS

The integration of technology into dental education and practice represents a significant milestone for the profession, bringing notable advancements but also presenting critical challenges. As highlighted by Gracco et al. (2023) and Spielman (2024), key limitations include the need for sustained investment in faculty training and the persistent technological and economic disparities that hinder equitable access to advanced tools such as CAD/CAM systems and robotics (Annamma et al., 2024). Studies such as Alfallaj et al. (2023) further reveal that these disparities are not solely dependent on funding, but also on institutional priorities and policy alignment.

Another limitation is the variable acceptance and readiness among educators and students to adopt innovative technologies. Schlenz et al. (2020) and Fukuhara-Nakama et al. (2023) report that while students generally view digital tools positively, there remains a strong preference for traditional instructor feedback and hands-on experience. Exclusive reliance on virtual learning, as observed during the COVID-19 pandemic, led to dissatisfaction due to limited clinical exposure (Escobar-Taipe et al., 2023).

Future research should prioritize the evaluation of hybrid educational models that effectively combine digital and traditional methods (Escobar-Taipe et al., 2023; Zitzmann et al., 2020). Establishing international standards for technology integration and fostering collaborations between academia and industry are essential to support under-resourced regions (AlGerafi et al., 2023). Additionally, long-term studies are needed to assess the impact of emerging technologies-such as artificial intelligence and virtual reality-on clinical outcomes, skill acquisition, and patient satisfaction (Santamato et al., 2024; Thorat et al., 2024; Alqutaibi et al., 2024; Lin et al., 2024).

Addressing these challenges requires a comprehensive approach that includes sustainable infrastructure investment, continuous faculty development, and regulatory frameworks that balance innovation with ethical and legal considerations (Thurzo et al., 2023). Successful integration experiences in countries like Germany and Japan underscore the importance of reducing economic disparities and promoting international collaboration to ensure that technological advancements benefit all dental communities (Khatoon & Velidand, 2025).

CONCLUSION

The integration of innovative technologies into dental education and clinical practice marks a pivotal transformation in the profession, delivering substantial improvements in precision, efficiency, and quality of care (DaSilva et al., 2022).

Advanced tools such as VR, AR, and haptic simulators have enriched preclinical training by enabling students to practice complex procedures in safe, controlled environments (Daud et al., 2024). Similarly, the adoption of CAD/CAM systems and intraoral scanners has enhanced the accuracy of prosthetic fabrication and dental restorations, reducing treatment times and improving clinical outcomes (Molina et al., 2023; Gawali et al., 2024).

Teledentistry has expanded access to remote dental services, particularly benefiting underserved populations (Kanani et al., 2024; Martínez-Asanza, 2025). However, challenges remain, including insufficient infrastructure, resource disparities, and the need for robust implementation strategies (Zamiri & Esmaeili, 2024; Sato et al., 2025). Effective integration of these technologies requires ongoing faculty development and the establishment of international standards to ensure interoperability, safety, and equitable adoption (Benoit et al., 2022; Gurupur, 2024).

Leading countries are increasingly incorporating technological innovations into dental curricula, as recommended by global organizations, to better prepare future professionals for contemporary clinical challenges. Strengthening partnerships between academic institutions and technology companies will be essential for fostering innovation and facilitating knowledge exchange.

Despite the transformative impact of technology, it is imperative to address persistent barriers and promote equitable integration across both clinical practice and academic settings. Future research should focus on the continuous evaluation of emerging technologies to further enhance the quality of dental education and patient care worldwide.

In summary, the ongoing fusion of innovation and dentistry is reshaping all aspects of the profession-from the classroom to the clinic. By embracing technological advancements while addressing systemic barriers, the dental community can ensure equitable access to high-quality education and care, ultimately advancing global oral health outcomes.

ACKNOWLEDGMENT

This research received no specific grant from any funding agency in the public, commercial, or not-for profit sectors.

REFERENCES

Alfallaj, H. A., Afrashtehfar, K. I., Asiri, A. K., Almasoud, F. S., Alnaqa, G. H., & Al-Angari, N. S. (2023). The Status of Digital Dental Technology Implementation in the Saudi Dental Schools' Curriculum: A National Cross-Sectional Survey for Healthcare Digitization. *International Journal of Environmental Research and Public Health*, *20*(1), 321. DOI: 10.3390/ijerph20010321 PMID: 36612639

AlGerafi, M. A. M., Zhou, Y., Oubibi, M., & Wijaya, T. T. (2023). Unlocking the Potential: A Comprehensive Evaluation of Augmented Reality and Virtual Reality in Education. *Electronics (Basel)*, *12*(18), 3953. DOI: 10.3390/electronics12183953

Alqahtani, S. A. H. (2024). Enhancing dental practice. Cutting-edge digital innovations. *Brazilian Journal of Oral Sciences*, *23*, e0244785. https://dpi.org/10.20396/bjos.v23i00.8674785. DOI: 10.20396/bjos.v23i00.8674785

Alqutaibi, A. Y., Hamadallah, H. H., Oqbi, H. F., Almuzaini, S. A., & Borzangy, S. (2024). Current applications and future perspective of virtual reality in dental education and practice in Saudi Arabia: A scoping review. *The Saudi Dental Journal*, *36*(11), 1406–1416. DOI: 10.1016/j.sdentj.2024.09.007 PMID: 39619710

Annamma, L. M., Varma, S. R., Abuttayem, H., Prasad, P., Azim, S. A., Odah, R., George, B. T., Nair, C., & Karobari, M. I. (2024). Current challenges in dental education- a scoping review. *BMC Medical Education*, *24*(1), 1523. DOI: 10.1186/s12909-024-06545-1 PMID: 39716191

Artaza, O., Santacruz, J., Girard, J. E., Alvarez, D., Barria, S., Tetelboin, C., Tomasina, F., & Medina, A. (2020). Formación de recursos humanos para la salud universal: Acciones estratégicas desde las instituciones académicas. *Revista Panamericana de Salud Pública = Pan American Journal of Public Health*, *44*(e83), 1. Advance online publication. DOI: 10.26633/RPSP.2020.83 PMID: 32733545

Baethge, C., Goldbeck-Wood, S., & Mertens, S. (2019). SANRA—A scale for the quality assessment of narrative review articles. *Research Integrity and Peer Review*, *4*(1), 5. DOI: 10.1186/s41073-019-0064-8 PMID: 30962953

Benoit, B., Frédéric, B., & Jean-Charles, D. (2022). Current state of dental informatics in the field of health information systems: A scoping review. *BMC Oral Health*, *22*(1), 131. DOI: 10.1186/s12903-022-02163-9 PMID: 35439988

Bonny, T., Al Nassan, W., Obaideen, K., Al Mallahi, M. N., Mohammad, Y., & El-Damanhoury, H. M. (2023). Contemporary Role and Applications of Artificial Intelligence in Dentistry. *F1000 Research*, *12*, 1179. DOI: 10.12688/f1000research.140204.1 PMID: 37942018

Carvalho, L. F. C. S., & Zanatta, R. F. (2024). Editorial: Technological innovation for improved prevention and diagnosis of oral disease. *Frontiers in Oral Health*, *5*(1481890), 1481890. Advance online publication. DOI: 10.3389/froh.2024.1481890 PMID: 39355782

Casola— Rivera, W. (2020). El papel de la didáctica en los proceso de enseñanza y aprendizaje universitarios. *Comunicación (Cartago)*, *29*(1), 38–51. DOI: 10.18845/rc.v29i11-2020.5258

CEPAL. (2018). *La Agenda 2030 y los Objetivos de Desarrollo Sostenible: una oportunidad para América Latina y el Caribe*. https://repositorio.cepal.org/bitstream/handle/11362/40155/24/S1801141_es.pdf

Chérrez-Ojeda, I., Vera, C., Vanegas, E., Gallardo, J. C., Felix, M., Espinoza-Fuentes, F., Chedraui, P., Gavilanes, A. W. D., & Mata, V. L. (2020). The use of information and communication technologies in Latin American dentists: A cross-sectional study from Ecuador. *BMC Oral Health*, *20*(1), 146. DOI: 10.1186/s12903-020-01137-z PMID: 32429887

Comisión Económica para América Latina y el Caribe. CEPAL. (2018). La Agenda 2030 y los Objetivos de Desarrollo Sostenible: una oportunidad para América Latina y el Caribe. Disponible en: https://repositorio.cepal.org/bitstream/handle/11362/40155/24/S1801141_es.pdf

Costa, E. D., Brasil, D. M., Santaella, G. M., Cascante-Sequeira, D., Ludovichetti, F. S., & Freitas, D. Q. (2021). Digital technology in dental education during COVID-19 pandemic: Worldwide experience of professors and students. *Odovtos*, *23*(3), 179–208. DOI: 10.15517/ijds.2021.47770

DaSilva, A.F., Robinson, M.A., Shi, W., & McCauley, L.K. (2022). The Forefront of Dentistry Promising Tech-Innovations and New Treatments. *JDR clinical and translational research*, 7(1-suppl), 16S-24S. https://doi.org/DOI: 10.1177/23800844221116850

Daud, A., Matoug-Elwerfelli, M., Khalid, A., & Ali, K. (2024). The impact of virtual reality haptic simulators in pre-clinical restorative dentistry: A qualitative enquiry into dental students' perceptions. *BMC Oral Health*, *24*(1), 988. DOI: 10.1186/s12903-024-04704-w PMID: 39180025

Díaz Lozada, J. A., & de la Rúa Batistapau, M. (2022). Uso de las TIC en la preparación docente de profesores en condiciones de distanciamiento social. Mendive. *Review of Education*, *20*(1), 172–182.

Elundu, C., Amaechi, D. C., Okatta, A. U., Amaechi, E. C., Elundu, T. C., Ezeh, C. P., & Elundu, I. D. (2024). The impact of Simulation-based training in medical education. *Revista de Medicina (São Paulo)*, *103*(27), e38813. DOI: 10.1097/MD.0000000000038813 PMID: 38968472

Erdilek, D., Gümüştaş, B., & Güray Efes, B. (2023). Digitalization era of dental education: A systematic review. *Dental and Medical Problems*, *60*(3), 513–525. DOI: 10.17219/dmp/156804 PMID: 37747703

Escobar-Taipe, A. M., Rivera-Marcatinco, M., Veliz-Vicharra, S., & Mattos-Vela, M. A. (2023). La digitalización en la formación odontológica. *Revista de la Facultad de Odontología Universidad de Antioquia*, *35*(1), 62–75. DOI: 10.17533/udea.rfo.v35n1a5

Fu, Y., Chu, F., Lu, X., Wang, C., Xiao, N., Jiang, J., Zheng, J., & Jiang, H. (2024). Assessment and evaluation of online education and virtual simulation technology in dental education: A cross-sectional survey. *BMC Medical Education*, *24*(1), 191. DOI: 10.1186/s12909-024-05171-1 PMID: 38403582

Fukuhara-Nakama, M., Chávez-Alayo, P., Flores-Mas, R., Fernández-Jacinto, L., Castilla-Camacho, M., Maldonado-Mendoza, M., & Loechle-Verde, O. (2023). Introducción de la tecnología CAD-CAM en la educación dental: Una mirada desde los estudiantes y los docentes. *Revista Estomatológica Herediana*, *33*(4), 372–376. DOI: 10.20453/reh.v33i4.5123

García-Ancira, C., & Treviño-Cubero, A. (2020). Las competencias universitarias y el perfil de egreso. *RevistaEstudios del desarrollo social: Cuba y América Latina*, 8 (1). http://scielo.sld.cu/scielo.php?script=sci_arttext&pid=S12308-013220200003&lng=es&tlng=es

Gawali, N., Shah, P. P., Gowdar, I. M., Bhavsar, K. A., Giri, D., & Laddha, R. (2024). The Evolution of Digital Dentistry: A Comprehensive Review. *Journal of Pharmacy & Bioallied Sciences*, *16*(Suppl 3), S1920–S1922. DOI: 10.4103/jpbs.jpbs_11_24 PMID: 39346228

Gkrimpizi, T., Peristeras, V., & Magnisalis, I. (2023). Classification of barriers to digital transformation in higher education institutions: Systematic literature review. *Education Sciences*, *13*(7), 746. DOI: 10.3390/educsci13070746

Gracco, A., De Stefani, A., & Bruno, G. (2023). Influence of New Technology in Dental Care: A Public Health Perspective. *International Journal of Environmental Research and Public Health*, *20*(7), 5364. DOI: 10.3390/ijerph20075364 PMID: 37047978

Gurupur, V. P., Vu, G., Mayya, V., & King, C. (2024). The Need for Standards in Evaluating the Quality of Electronic Health Records and Dental Records: A Narrative Review. *Big Data and Cognitive Computing*, *8*(12), 168. DOI: 10.3390/bdcc8120168

Haleem, A., Javaid, M. A., & Suman, R. (2022). Understanding the role of digital technologies in education: A review. *Sustainable Operations and Computers*, *3*, 275–285. DOI: 10.1016/j.susoc.2022.05.004

Hays, R. B., Ramani, S., & Hassell, A. (2020). Healthcare systems and the sciences of health professional education. *Advances in Health Sciences Education : Theory and Practice*, *25*(5), 1149–1162. DOI: 10.1007/s10459-020-10010-1 PMID: 33206272

Hsu, M. S., Yeh, C. L., Cheng, S. J., & Lin, C. P. (2025). Integrating digital technologies in dental technician education: A comparative study of national examination in Asian countries. *Journal of Dental Sciences*, *20*(1), 28–35. DOI: 10.1016/j.jds.2024.10.017 PMID: 39873091

Jha Kukreja, B., & Kukreja, P. (2025). Integration of Artificial Intelligence in Dentistry: A Systematic Review of Educational and Clinical Implications. *Cureus*, *17*(2), e79350. DOI: 10.7759/cureus.79350 PMID: 40125123

Jun, M.-K., Kim, J.-W., & Ku, H.-M. (2025). Three-dimensional printing in dentistry: A scoping review of clinical applications, advantages, and current limitations. *Oral*, *5*(2), 24. DOI: 10.3390/oral5020024

Jurado, C. A., Tsujimoto, A., Punj, A., Aida, N., Miyazaki, M., & Watanabe, H. (2021). Successful of development and implementation of a digital dentistry curriculum at US dental School. *Journal of Oral Science*, *63*(4), 358–360. DOI: 10.2334/josnusd.21-0070 PMID: 34497245

Kanani, H., Khubchandani, M., Dangore-Khasbage, S., & Pandey, R. (2024). Teledentistry: A Comprehensive Review and Its Application in Pediatric Dental Care. *Cureus*, *16*(1), e52685. DOI: 10.7759/cureus.52685 PMID: 38384649

Khatoon, U. T., & Velidandi, A. (2025). An Overview on the Role of Government Initiatives in Nanotechnology Innovation for Sustainable Economic Development and Research Progress. *Sustainability (Basel)*, *17*(3), 1250. DOI: 10.3390/su17031250

Lin, G. S. S., Goh, S. M., & Halil, M. H. M. (2023). Unravelling the impact of dental workforce training and education programmes on policy evolution: Mixed-method study protocol. *Health Research Policy and Systems*, *21*(95), 95. Advance online publication. DOI: 10.1186/s12961-023-01048-9 PMID: 37700266

Lin, P.-Y., Chen, T.-C., Lin, C.-J., Huang, C.-C., Tsai, Y.-H., Tsai, Y.-L., & Wang, C.-Y. (2024). The use of augmented reality (AR) and virtual reality (VR) in dental surgery education and practice: A narrative review. *Journal of Dental Sciences*, *19*(Suppl 2), S91–S101. DOI: 10.1016/j.jds.2024.10.011 PMID: 39807259

Liu, C.-M., Su, N.-Y., Chen, Y.-T., Chiang, C.-P., & Yu, C.-H. (2024). Analysis of approved dental teaching projects in the teaching practice research program in 8 dental schools of Taiwan from 2018 to 2023. *Journal of Dental Sciences*, *19*(2), 1083–1086. DOI: 10.1016/j.jds.2024.01.021 PMID: 38618124

Macanchí-Pico, M. L., Orozco-Castillo, B. M., & Campoverde-Encalada, M. A. (2020). Innovación educativa, pedagógica y didáctica. Concepciones para la práctica en la educación superior. *Revista Universidad y Sociedad*, *12*(1), 396-403. http://scielo.sld.cu/scielo.php?script=sci_arttext&pid=S2218-36202020000100396&lng=es&tlng=es

Madfa, A. A., Al-Ibrahim, I. K., Alshammary, F. L., Alharbi, S. M., & Alharbi, B. B. (2023). An audit of Saudi dental students' opinions and attitudes toward digital dentistry. *The Open Dentistry Journal*, *17*(1), e18742106276082. Advance online publication. DOI: 10.2174/0118742106276082231123053341

Martínez- Asanza. D. (Ed.). (2024a). *Transforming Dental Health in Rural Communities: Digital Dentistry*. IGI Global. https://doi.org/DOI: 10.4018/979-8-3693-7165-7

Martínez- Asanza. D. (Ed.). (2024b). *Leveraging Digital Technology for Preventive Dentistry*. IGI Global. https://doi.org/DOI: 10.4018/979-8-3693-3872-8

Martínez- Asanza. D., Rojas Herrera, I. A., Njoku, A. U., Reyes Puig, A. C., Mouloudj, F., Capote, I. G., & Maupome, G. (2024c). Study Plans and Programs Supporting Geriatric Dentistry Teaching in Cuba: An Update. In D. Martínez Asanza (Ed.), *Geriatric Dentistry in the Age of Digital Technology* (pp. 174-191). IGI Global. https://doi.org/DOI: 10.4018/979-8-3693-0260-6.ch007

Martínez- Asanza. D. (Ed.). (2024d). *Geriatric Dentistry in the Age of Digital Technology*. IGI Global. https://doi.org/DOI: 10.4018/979-8-3693-0260-6

Martínez Asanza, D. (2018). ¿Enseñanza tradicional en el siglo XXI? *Revista Neuronum, 4*(1), 99–106. http://eduneuro.com/revista/index.php/revistaneuronum/article/view/108/98

Martínez-Asanza, D. (2021). La visita a la familia en la carrera de Estomatología: una estructura didáctica [thesis]. La Habana: Universidad de Ciencias Médicas de La Habana. https://tesis.sld.cu/index.php?P=FullRecord&ID=1812

Martínez-Asanza, D. (2025). Emerging Trends and Future Perspectives in Digital Dentistry for Rural Areas: An Update. D. Asanza (Ed.), *Transforming Dental Health in Rural Communities: Digital Dentistry* (pp. 1-20). IGI Global. https://doi.org/DOI: 10.4018/979-8-3693-7165-7.ch001

Martínez-Asanza, D., Rojas-Herrera, I. A., Mouloudj, K., Garrido-Amable, O., & Muzzamil, M. (2024e). Impact of Digital Innovations in Preventive Dentistry: A Narrative Review. In Asanza, D. (Ed.), *Leveraging Digital Technology for Preventive Dentistry* (pp. 55–84). IGI Global., DOI: 10.4018/979-8-3693-3872-8.ch003

Mhlongo, S., Mbatha, K., Ramatsetse, B., & Dlamini, R. (2023). Challenges, opportunities, and prospects of adopting and using smart digital technologies in learning environments: An iterative review. *Heliyon*, *9*(6), e16348. DOI: 10.1016/j.heliyon.2023.e16348 PMID: 37274691

Michel-Villarreal, R., Vilalta-Perdomo, E., Salinas-Navarro, D. E., Thierry-Aguilera, R., & Gerardou, F. S. (2023). Challenges and opportunities of Generative AI for Higher education as explained by ChatGPT. *Education Sciences*, *13*(9), 856. DOI: 10.3390/educsci13090856

Molina, W. P. C., Caisaguano, J. W. R., & Núñez, M. A. R. (2023). Utilidad de la tecnología CAD/CAM en la fabricación de prótesis dentales. *Medisur*, *21*(6), 1305–1311. http://scielo.sld.cu/scielo.php?script=sci_arttext&pid=S1727-897X2023000601305&lng=es&tlng=es

Mouloudj, F., Aljaeed, S. A., & Asanza, D. M. (2025). Understanding Students' Intentions to Use AI for English Language Learning. In Ali, M., Anwar, M., Fazal, S., & Ayyaz, S. (Eds.), *AI Applications for English Language Learning* (pp. 157–178). IGI Global., DOI: 10.4018/979-8-3693-9077-1.ch007

Mouloudj, K. LE, V. L., Bouarar, A., Bouarar, A. C., Martínez-Asanza, D., & Srivastava, M. (2024). Adopting Artificial Intelligence in Healthcare: A Narrative Review. In S. Teixeira & J. Remondes (Eds.). *The Use of Artificial Intelligence in Digital Marketing: Competitive Strategies and Tactics* (pp. 1-20). IGI Global. https://doi.org/DOI: 10.4018/978-1-6684-9324-3.ch001

Mpuangnan, K. N. (2024). Teacher preparedness and professional development needs for successful technology integration in teacher education. *Cogent Education*, *11*(1), 2408837. Advance online publication. DOI: 10.1080/2331186X.2024.2408837

Mun, M., Byrne, S., Shaw, L., & Lyons, K. (2025). Digital dentists: A curriculum for the 21st century. *JMIR Medical Education*, *11*(1), e54153. DOI: 10.2196/54153 PMID: 39789757

Naik, N., Hameed, B. M. Z., Shetty, D. K., Swain, D., Shah, M., Paul, R., Aggarwal, K., Ibrahim, S., Patil, V., Smriti, K., Shetty, S., Rai, B. P., Chlosta, P., & Somani, B. K. (2022). Legal and ethical consideration in Artificial Intelligence in healthcare: Who takes responsibility? *Frontiers in Surgery*, *9*, 862322. DOI: 10.3389/fsurg.2022.862322 PMID: 35360424

Najeeb, M., & Islam, S. (2025). Artificial intelligence (AI) in restorative dentistry: Current trends and future prospects. *BMC Oral Health*, *25*(1), 592. DOI: 10.1186/s12903-025-05989-1 PMID: 40251567

Nassani, L. M., Bencharit, S., Schumacher, F., Lu, W.-E., Resende, R., & Fernandes, G. V. O. (2024). The Impact of Technology Teaching in the Dental Predoctoral Curriculum on Students' Perception of Digital Dentistry. *Dentistry Journal*, *12*(3), 75. DOI: 10.3390/dj12030075 PMID: 38534299

Page, , McKenzie, J. E., Bossuyt, P. M., Boutron, I., Hoffmann, T. C., Mulrow, C. D., Shamseer, L., Tetzlaff, J. M., Akl, E. A., Brennan, S. E., Chou, R., Glanville, J., Grimshaw, J. M., Hróbjartsson, A., Lalu, M. M., Li, T., Loder, E. W., Mayo-Wilson, E., McDonald, S., & Alonso-Fernández, S. (2021). Declaración PRISMA 2020: Una guía actualizada para la publicación de revisiones sistemáticas. *Revista Española de Cardiología*, *74*(9), 790–799. DOI: 10.1016/j.recesp.2021.06.016 PMID: 34446261

Palacios-Núñez, M. L., Toribio-López, A., & Deroncele-Acosta, A. (2021). Innovación educativa en el desarrollo de aprendizajes relevantes: una revisión sistemática de literatura. *Revista Universidad y Sociedad, 13*(5), 134-145.http://scielo.sld.cu/scielo.php?script=sci_arttext&pid=S2218-36202021000500134&lng=es&tlng=es

Poblete, P., McAleer, S., & Mason, A. G. (2020). 3D Technology Development and Dental Education: What Topics Are Best Suited for 3D Learning Resources? *Dentistry Journal*, *8*(3), 95. DOI: 10.3390/dj8030095 PMID: 32882795

Radwan, H. A., Alsharif, A. T., Alsharif, M. T., Aloufi, M. R., & Alshammari, B. S. (2023). Digital technologies in dentistry in Saudi Arabia: Perceptions, practices and Challenges. *Digital Health*, *9*, 2055207631197095. DOI: 10.1177/20552076231197095 PMID: 37662673

Robson, J., Rung, A., McCusker, M., Grant, G., & George, R. (2024). A systematic review of methodology for the creation of virtual 3D models for use in dental education and a narrative review. *International Journal of Computerized Dentistry, 27*(4), 337–343. DOI: 10.3290/j.ijcd.b4224867 PMID: 37477083

Santamato, V., Tricase, C., Faccilongo, N., Iacoviello, M., & Marengo, A. (2024). Exploring the Impact of Artificial Intelligence on Healthcare Management: A Combined Systematic Review and Machine-Learning Approach. *Applied Sciences (Basel, Switzerland), 14*(22), 10144. DOI: 10.3390/app142210144

Sato, S. N., Condes Moreno, E., Rubio-Zarapuz, A., Dalamitros, A. A., Yañez-Sepulveda, R., Tornero-Aguilera, J. F., & Clemente-Suárez, V. J. (2024). Navigating the New Normal: Adapting Online and Distance Learning in the Post-Pandemic Era. *Education Sciences, 14*(1), 19. DOI: 10.3390/educsci14010019

Schlenz, M. A., Michel, K., Wegner, K., Schmidt, A., Rehmann, P., & Wöstmann, B. (2020). Undergraduate dental students' perspective on the implementation of digital dentistry in the preclinical curriculum: A questionnaire survey. *BMC Oral Health, 20*(1), 78. DOI: 10.1186/s12903-020-01071-0 PMID: 32188456

Silva-Velasco, E., López-Aballe, M., & Mayedo-Núñez, Y. (2023). La Educación Médica y su papel en la formación clínica de los estudiantes de Medicina. *Luz, 22*(3), 150-160. http://scielo.sld.cu/scielo.php?script=sci_arttext&pid=S1814-151X2023000300150&lng=es&tlng=es

Sirko, J., & Shi, W. (2024). Disruptive innovation events in dentistry. *JADA Foundational Science, 3*(100036), 100036. DOI: 10.1016/j.jfscie.2024.100036 PMID: 39384257

Spielman, A. I. (2024). Dental education and practice: Past, present, and future trends. *Frontiers in Oral Health, 5*, 1368121. DOI: 10.3389/froh.2024.1368121 PMID: 38694791

Syed, S. A., Sheikh, M., Syed, F. A., Atif, S., Iqbal, A., & Zeeshan, G. (2024). Comparison of virtual clinical scenario and role play in learning oral pathology among dental students. *PLoS One, 19*(7), e0306712. DOI: 10.1371/journal.pone.0306712 PMID: 38976658

Thurzo, A., Strunga, M., Urban, R., Surovková, J., & Afrashtehfar, K. I. (2023). Impact of Artificial Intelligence on Dental Education: A Review and Guide for Curriculum Update. *Education Sciences, 13*(2), 150. DOI: 10.3390/educsci13020150

Tiol-Carrillo, A. (2021). Aplicación de las tecnologías en la educación en odontología durante la pandemia por COVID-19. *Revista ADM, 78*(3), 155–161. DOI: 10.35366/100073

Tripathi, S., Manoharan, P. S., & Nagda, S. (2024). Developing an instructional module of "digital dentistry" for undergraduate prosthodontics curriculum. *Journal of Oral Biology and Craniofacial Research, 14*(1), 44–48. DOI: 10.1016/j.jobcr.2023.12.001 PMID: 38188908

Usman, M. (2024). Integration of Three-Dimensional Scanning and Computer-Aided Design/ Computer-Aided Manufacturing (CAD//CAM) Technology in Routine Prosthodontic Practice: A Cross-Sectional Study in Kerala. *Cureus, 16*(12), e76409. DOI: 10.7759/cureus.76409 PMID: 39867077

Valcárcel-Izquierdo, N., & Díaz-Díaz, A. A. (2019). *Epistemología de las Ciencias de la Educación Médica*. Universidad de Ciencias Médicas de La Habana., http://bvs.sld.cu/libros/epistemologia_ciencias_educacion_medica/epistemologia_ciencias_educacion.pdf

Vera-Carrasco, O. (2024). La educación médica en principios éticos, bioéticos, deontológicos, valores y actitudes. *Revista Médica La Paz, 30*(2), 63-68. http://www.scielo.org.bo/scielo.php?script=sci_arttext&pid=S1726-89582024000200063&lng=es&tlng=es

Winterhalter, L., Kofler, F., Ströbele, D. A., Othman, A., & von See, C. (2024). AI-Assisted Diagnostics in Dentistry: An Eye-Tracking Study on User Behavior. *Journal of Clinical and Experimental Dentistry, 16*(5), e547–e555. DOI: 10.4317/jced.61491 PMID: 38988762

World Health Organization. (2021). Global strategy on digital health 2020-2025. https://www.who.int/docs/default-source/documents/gs4hdaa2a9f352b0445bafbc79ca799dce4d.pdf

Yazdanpanahi, F., Shahi, M., & Davaridolatabadi, N. (2022). Investigating the application of new technologies in dental education: A systematic review. *Acta Medica Iranica*. Advance online publication. DOI: 10.18502/acta.v60i8.10830

Zamiri, M., & Esmaeili, A. (2024). Methods and Technologies for Supporting Knowledge Sharing within Learning Communities: A Systematic Literature Review. *Administrative Sciences, 14*(1), 17. DOI: 10.3390/admsci14010017

Zitzmann, N. U., Matthisson, L., Ohla, H., & Joda, T. (2020). Digital Undergraduate Education in Dentistry: A Systematic Review. *International Journal of Environmental Research and Public Health*, *17*(9), 3269. DOI: 10.3390/ijerph17093269 PMID: 32392877

KEY TERMS AND DEFINITIONS

3D Printing: This technology creates physical models from digital designs, making it incredibly useful for designing prosthetics and personalized anatomical models in dental education.

Artificial Intelligence (AI): These systems mimic human intelligence to assist with tasks like diagnosis, treatment planning, and personalized learning in dentistry.

Augmented Reality (AR): This overlays digital information onto the real world, enabling real-time simulations and visualizations of dental procedures.

Computer-Aided Design/ Computer-Aided Manufacturing (CAD/CAM): This stands for computer-aided design and manufacturing, which allows for the precise and efficient creation of dental restorations and prosthetics.

Dental Clinical Practice: This encompasses the clinical, diagnostic, and therapeutic activities that dental professionals perform in patient care.

Dental Education: This is a structured training program that combines theory, clinical practice, and ongoing learning to prepare future dentists.

Educational Technology: These are the digital tools and interactive methods that really boost teaching and learning in the field of dentistry.

Simulation Training: This involves using simulators and virtual scenarios to safely practice clinical skills in a controlled setting.

Teledentistry: This refers to providing dental services remotely through digital technologies, which helps improve access and training for patients and professionals alike.

Virtual Reality (VR): These are immersive digital environments that allow for interactive practice and visualization of dental procedures.

Chapter 2
Improving Technology Literacy in Health Professional Education

Chunfang Zhou
https://orcid.org/0000-0003-4994-0207
University of Southern Denmark, Denmark

Anna Marie Lassen
https://orcid.org/0000-0003-4197-6336
University College Northern Denmark, Denmark

ABSTRACT

This chapter explores how technology literacy in health professional education can be improved through Reflective Practice-Based Learning (RPL). Two research questions are asked: 1) How can we deepen our theoretical understanding of Reflective Practice-Based Learning (RPL) as a pedagogy for fostering technology literacy? and 2) How can we enhance technology literacy in health professional education through the practical application of RPL? To answer these questions, this chapter integrates theoretical perspectives on technology literacy, learning, knowledge, and health professional education into a unified framework. This also includes a case description focused on the practical implementation of a RPL-based course. The findings highlight the theoretical and practical significance of RPL in advancing technology literacy education and driving pedagogical innovation in teaching and learning in the age of medical technology for the future.

DOI: 10.4018/979-8-3373-1519-5.ch002

INTRODUCTION

The use of new technologies has increasingly been recognized as a crucial means to enhance the quality of healthcare and health services in general. The medical and health sectors have benefited from various technology solutions and services that improve efficiency, facilitate disease prevention, and empower patients (Zhou & Lassen, 2024). From Electronic Health Records (EHRs) to advanced diagnostic tools powered by artificial intelligence, these innovations have reshaped the way healthcare is delivered. For instance, wearable devices and mobile health applications now enable real-time health monitoring (Guillodo et al., 2020), while telemedicine has broken geographical barriers, ensuring that patients in remote areas have access to quality care (Tierney et al., 2024).

Health professionals play a pivotal role in this ecosystem (Moudatsou et al., 2020). They serve as the critical link connecting people with technology, information, and knowledge. Their ability to interpret complex data from these technologies and translate it into actionable insights is indispensable (Dash et al., 2019). Moreover, healthcare providers not only adopt new tools but also act as educators and advocates, empowering patients to leverage technology for self-care and informed decision-making (Bastable et al., 2019). As the integration of digital tools continues to grow, the demand for technologically proficient health professionals who can navigate this evolving landscape becomes more evident (Locsin, 2017). Therefore, beyond being caregivers, health professionals act as communicators, educators, team members, managers, leaders, and policymakers (Frenk et al., 2010).

However, the adoption of these technologies also brings challenges, such as the need for specialized training (Shachak et al., 2024), addressing ethical concerns (Tocin et al., 2023), and ensuring data privacy and security (Zhou & Lassen, 2024). Developing strategies to equip healthcare providers with the necessary skills and fostering a culture of trust and adaptability will be essential for maximizing the potential of technology in healthcare. Thus, while technology enhances the reach and effectiveness of health services, the human element remains irreplaceable, highlighting the importance of a balanced, human-centric approach to innovation (Rožanec et al., 2023; Grover et al., 2024). The technology skills required by health professionals extend beyond understanding of how these tools function (Zhou & Lassen, 2024). They also encompass abilities such as instructing patients in their use and collaborating with engineers to resolve technology-related issues in professional practice (Conard, 2019; Dunn & Hazzard, 2019).

Parallel to these challenges in healthcare practice, education reforms have gained momentum. Education innovation is crucial to foster technology literacy in healthcare professional education, as it enables the integration of new digital tools, methodologies, and collaborative learning models (Zhou & Lassen, 2024).

To meet the evolving demands of healthcare, curricula must be designed to not only teach technical skills but also promote critical thinking, adaptability, and ethical decision-making in the use of technology (Konttila et al., 2019). These points drive this chapter to focus on improving technology literacy in health professional education and exploring a case study on Reflective Practice-Based Learning (RPL) at the University of Northern Denmark (UCN).

A BRIEF LITERATURE REVIEW AND RESEARCH QUESTIONS

What can we learn from recent research on technology literacy development in health professional education? A brief literature review reveals a growing focus on various innovative educational approaches. Those approaches such as simulation-based learning, blended learning environments, problem-based learning, and real-world problem-solving, can provide healthcare students with the hands-on experience and context-driven understanding necessary to navigate complex technology-driven healthcare settings (Zhou & Lassen, 2024). These innovations ensure that students are prepared to effectively use emerging technologies in patient care and contribute to the continuous transformation of healthcare practices. As Frenk and his colleagues (2010) pointed out, the acceleration of knowledge flows, technological advancements, and the migration of both professionals and patients necessitate a redesign of professional health education. Professional health education institutions have expanded their traditional role as formal learning environments, where students typically acquire knowledge through lectures or library resources. These institutions now incorporate innovative learning approaches that transcend the classroom and create opportunities to bridge theory and professional practice (Zhou & Lassen, 2024). Such changes have inspired educators to re-evaluate the meaning of professional education and explore new methods of teaching and learning (Lassen & Kjærgaard, 2022).

Building on these considerations, this chapter explores how technology literacy in health professional education can be improved through an innovative pedagogy method of RPL. It aims to address two questions:

1) How can we deepen our theoretical understanding of RPL as a pedagogy for fostering technology literacy? And
2) How can RPL be applied in practice to improve technology literacy in health professional education?

To answer these questions, the chapter firstly develops a theoretical framework that bridges research on technology literacy, learning, knowledge, and health professional education. This framework emphasizes that technology literacy development should be viewed as a situational phenomenon. It highlights how RPL creates favorable conditions for health professional students to engage in learning activities through knowledge exchanges between tacit and explicit models in professional practice, which is a critical factor in improving technology literacy. Secondly, the chapter provides a case as an example based on one of the authors' teaching experiences. It describes how a course was implemented within an RPL environment at the University College of Northern Denmark (UCN). The case focuses on a two-week interdisciplinary elective course, 'Technology in the Present and Future', designed for physiotherapy and occupational therapy students. It shows how students participated in and learned from the course, shedding light on how RPL can enable young health professionals to apply knowledge in professional practice. It also discusses how practice-oriented teaching and reflective learning activities motivate students to improve their technology literacy in diverse contexts of technology implementation.

IMPROVING TECHNOLOGY LITERACY THROUGH REFLECTIVE PRACTICE-BASED LEARNING (RPL)

How can we deepen our theoretical understanding of RPL as an effective pedagogy for fostering technology literacy? This research question guides the development of a new theoretical framework that integrates studies on technology literacy, learning, knowledge, and health professional education. In the following sections, we first highlight the critical need for technology literacy in health professional practice. We then discuss how the development of technology literacy can be supported through a model of knowledge exchange. This model emphasizes the dynamic interplay between tacit and explicit knowledge in professional contexts. Building on this foundation, we explore how RPL can create a supportive learning environment that promotes the development of technology literacy among health professional students. These ideas provide the structure for the subsequent discussion.

Technology Literacy in Health Professional Practice

Traditionally, 'literacy' has been defined as the ability to read, write, speak, and listen in ways that support effective communication and help individuals make sense of the world (Judson, 2009). It is considered a macro-skill that, once mastered, can be applied to an infinite range of information. Recent studies (Moore, 2010) have broadened the definition of literacy to encompass domains beyond reading and writing, describing it as mastery or competence in a specific area. For example, various types of literacy such as digital literacy, numeracy, media literacy, cultural literacy and Al literacy, etc (Zhou, Petri & Bhattacharyya, 2025). Literacy evolves with societal changes and technological advancements, shaping how individuals engage with the world. It empowers people to make informed decisions, participate meaningfully in society, and access opportunities for personal and professional growth. In an increasingly complex, interconnected world, the scope of literacy continues to expand, reflecting the diverse skills needed to thrive in contemporary life (Zhou & Lassen, 2024). Therefore, literacy development occurs not only in schools but also in everyday life, playing a fundamental role in students' ability to learn in educational settings and contribute meaningfully to society (Barton & Lennon, 2020).

In the 21st century, technology literacy has emerged as a vital skill. Narrowly defined, technology literacy refers to the ability to use computers and other technologies to enhance learning, productivity, and performance (Moore, 2010; Zhou et al., 2025). In a broader sense, it includes the capacity to use technology effectively for accessing, evaluating, integrating, creating, and communicating information, thereby supporting the learning process through problem-solving and critical thinking (Estes, 2017). Moore (2010) identifies three levels of technology literacy: 1) Identifying technologies relevant to a task, 2) Understanding how to use the technology and navigate its interface, and 3) Grasping the inner workings or structure of the technology. Thus, technology literacy should not be viewed as an isolated set of skills but rather as a strategic enabler for achieving broader learning objectives (Moore, 2010; Zhou et al., 2025). Its interdisciplinary nature further highlights the importance of thinking broadly across disciplines. As Bugliarello (2016) argues, technological literacy encompasses the ability to use technological tools to understand how technology can address individual and societal problems. It also involves recognizing the processes involved in designing tools, modifying nature, and understanding the limitations, possibilities, and consequences of technological advancements.

The need for technology literacy and digital skills among health professionals has been widely recognized (European Health Parliament, 2016). This encompasses not only technical skills, such as operating devices or software, but also the capacity to analyze how technology influences society, solve problems using digital tools, and make informed decisions about its application. In healthcare, technology literacy is vital for leveraging digital innovations like electronic health records, AI-powered diagnostics, and telemedicine to enhance patient care and improve health outcomes. Health professionals are expected to be proficient in using e-health and mHealth solutions effectively, responsibly, and ethically, with the patients' best interests as the focal point (Zhou & Lassen, 2024). Physicians, nurses, physiotherapists, occupational therapists, dentists, pharmacists, and midwives are required to possess a range of skills, including communication, data analysis, computer literacy, medical device compatibility, data protection, mobile applications, cloud storage, internet use, and smart device operation to read, understand, and share information. Additionally, non-clinical and administrative staff need competencies in project management, communication, computer literacy, information security, and clinical software usage. IT professionals in healthcare must possess expertise in data privacy, information security, ethics, software engineering, and database development. These diverse skill sets underscore the interdisciplinary demands of technology literacy in health sectors (Zhou & Lassen, 2024).

Technology Literacy and Knowledge

The literature emphasizes the role of knowledge in the development of technology literacy (Ingerman & Collier-Reed, 2011). As Levande (2003) suggested, the relationship between knowledge and technology literacy is deeply interconnected. Technology literacy encompasses the capability to interact with technology and apply technological knowledge. This enables individuals to access, apply, and critically engage with knowledge through digital tools and platforms, transforming how information is acquired, shared, and utilized. In turn, knowledge informs the effective use of technology by providing the conceptual and contextual understanding needed to navigate and evaluate technological innovations. Together, they empower individuals to adapt to evolving technologies, solve complex problems, and make informed decisions in dynamic environments like healthcare and education. Achieving technology literacy involves both knowledge and active awareness of technology - understanding how it is used, how it works, and how it transforms practice (Moore, 2010). These points highlight the importance of linking our understanding of technology literacy with both tacit and explicit knowledge (Zhou, 2012):

- Tacit knowledge: Practical, action-oriented knowledge or 'know-how' acquired through personal experience and practice. It is seldom expressed openly and often resembles intuition.
- Explicit knowledge: Academic knowledge or 'know-what' that is articulated in formal language, typically documented in print or electronic media. It is often based on established work processes and relies on a people-to-documents approach.

The two knowledge models have been widely discussed in various contexts of professional practice and organizations. Explicit knowledge is formal, structured, and easily articulated or documented. It includes information that can be written down, codified, and shared systematically through manuals, protocols, guidelines, textbooks, or digital databases. For instance, clinical guidelines for treating specific diseases, research studies, diagnostic protocols, and patient care workflows are examples of explicit knowledge. In healthcare, explicit knowledge is essential for standardizing practices, ensuring consistency, and promoting evidence-based care; it serves as the foundation for medical education and policy-making, ensuring that healthcare practices align with the latest research and standards. In contrast, tacit knowledge is personal, experiential, and difficult to articulate or formalize. It is rooted in individual intuition, experience, judgement, and context. Tacit knowledge often manifests in the ability to recognize subtle patient cues, manage complex or ambiguous cases, or adapt treatments to patient needs. For example, a seasoned nurse might notice subtle changes in a patient's demeanor that signal early signs of distress, or a surgeon might adjust their technique based on the feel of tissues during an operation. Tacit knowledge develops through hands-on practice, mentorship, and years of experience. However, because tacit knowledge is not easily codified, it can be challenging to capture and transfer. It is often shared through informal interactions, such as shadowing, storytelling, or collaborative problem-solving, where junior health professionals learn from their more experienced colleagues.

In healthcare practice, understanding the distinction between tacit knowledge and explicit knowledge is crucial for fostering effective collaboration, decision-making, and knowledge transfer among health professionals (Zhou & Lassen, 2024). While explicit knowledge provides the foundation for standardized practices, tacit knowledge enables adaptability, creativity, and personalized care. For example, a clinician may follow explicit guidelines to diagnose a condition but rely on tacit knowledge to navigate uncertainties or tailor treatments to a patient's cultural and social context. Bridging the gap between tacit and explicit knowledge is critical for effective healthcare practice. This can be achieved through reflective practices, fostering mentorship and peer learning, encouraging interdisciplinary collaboration, and leveraging technology to capture and share experiential insights. For instance, simulation-based training can help codify tacit knowledge into explicit learning materials, while debriefing sessions after medical procedures allow practitioners to reflect and share their experiences. In addition to tacit and explicit knowledge, two levels of knowledge - individual and collective knowledge - are also emphasized. As Zhou (2012) observed, shaping new knowledge requires an understanding of existing knowledge and opportunities to engage with it, thereby enabling its transformation into new insights. In professional practice, collective intelligence is increasingly recognized as a valuable tool. It relies on communication, coordination, cooperation, and conversation, facilitated through links, exchanges, and messages.

Accordingly, we view professional practice as a complex, thoughtful, and intentional process of integrating problem-solving and specialized knowledge to achieve meaningful outcomes (Wenger, 1998). Professional practice is not simply about applying established knowledge, but rather about continuously adapting and evolving based on emerging challenges, technological advancements, and changing contexts. This integration of problem-solving and specialized knowledge involves a dynamic process of reflection, action, and adaptation, where professionals draw upon their expertise while also responding to new information and situations in real time. The goal is not just the application of predefined solutions, but the creation of innovative, contextually relevant approaches that lead to positive, impactful outcomes. Through transformative learning, personality-integrated knowledge is developed, enabling associations across all subjectively relevant contexts (Illeris, 2007). This emphasizes the need for individuals to undergo deep shifts in perspective that allow them to connect and apply knowledge in ways that are personally meaningful and professionally effective. This type of learning goes beyond simple knowledge acquisition, fostering a more holistic understanding that integrates cognitive, emotional, and social dimensions (Illeris, 2007). Personality-integrated knowledge is crucial in this process, as it recognizes that learners bring their individual experiences, values, and identities into their professional practices, which shapes how they process and apply new knowledge (Wenger, 1998). It is through these personalized connections that individuals can adapt their learning to different professional environments and problems, ensuring their responses are both innovative and context-sensitive (Zhou, et al., 2025).

The integration of problem-solving and knowledge takes place both within the mind of an individual and among participants in groups. This dual process reflects the social nature of professional practice, where individuals collaborate with others to share, test, and refine ideas (Zhou, 2012). Professional expertise is not only constructed internally through individual learning but also through interactions with colleagues, mentors, and other stakeholders. Group dynamics, collective decision-making, and collaborative problem-solving enable the synthesis of diverse perspectives and approaches, which ultimately enriches the decision-making process and enhances the overall quality of outcomes (Zhou, 2012). This collaborative aspect of learning underscores the importance of communities of practice, where knowledge is co-created and distributed across individuals and groups, fostering an environment of shared growth and innovation (Wenger, 1998). Therefore, participants must not only remain informed about emerging technologies but also stay aware of knowledge and skills from other domains (Zhou et al., 2025). In an increasingly interconnected world, professional practice requires the ability to integrate insights from multiple disciplines, as challenges are often multifaceted and require diverse expertise (Zhou & Lassen, 2024). Healthcare professionals, for example, must not only keep up with the latest medical technologies but also stay informed about advances in areas such as data science, ethics, and social dynamics (Dash et al., 2019). The ability to bridge knowledge from different domains enables professionals to develop more comprehensive solutions and to better anticipate and address the complexities they encounter in practice. This interdisciplinary awareness is key to foster innovation and adaptability, ensuring that professionals are equipped to handle the demands of a rapidly changing world and to make informed, ethical decisions in their work (Illeris, 2007).

These points underscore that the development of technology literacy often arises from the interplay between tacit and explicit knowledge and between individual and collective knowledge. Acquiring new technological knowledge is inherently tied to interactions between individuals and their contexts (Zhou & Lassen, 2024). Technology literacy development is thus a situational phenomenon centered on interactions with technology. As Young, Cole, and Denton (2002) highlight, the concept of technology literacy embodies what it means to have knowledge of a particular situation. This involves the interplay of socialization, externalization, combination, and internalization, as represented in the model proposed by Nonaka and Takeuchi (1998) (Figure 1).

Figure 1. Model of Knowledge according to Nonaka and Takeuchi (1998)

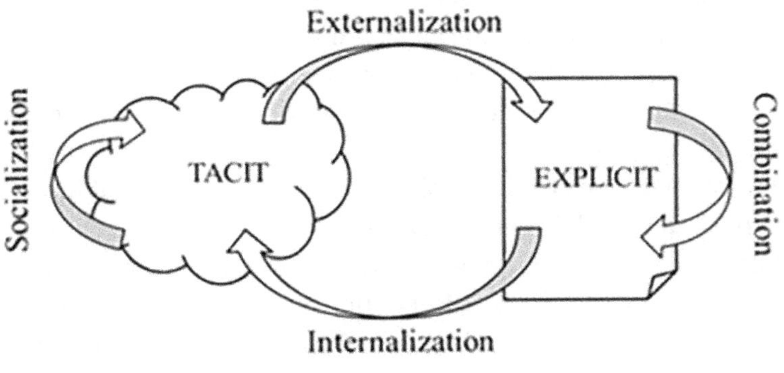

Inspired by this model, we conceptualize technology literacy as comprising elements of knowledge, personal engagement, and social engagement. These elements provide the foundation for developing technology literacy and applying these competencies to solve problems within a focused process (Ingerman & Collier-Reed, 2011). A crucial enabler of the interaction between different models and forms of knowledge is communication skills. As Hardinata, Suchyadi, and Wulandari (2021) suggested, communication is a vital skill for building social relationships and engaging with the environment through various media channels. Effective and successful communication facilitates the transformation of tacit knowledge into explicit knowledge and enables the sharing of individual knowledge within collective practices. In collaborative contexts, participants build on one another's ideas to develop shared understandings that exceed what any individual participant could achieve alone. This process requires critical and constructive negotiation of each participant's suggestions. Well-founded arguments and counterarguments must be presented, critically evaluated, and refined through collective dialogue. This collaborative dynamic encourages all participants in a particular technological context to work together, leveraging technologies or addressing technology-related challenges (Zhou & Lassen, 2024).

Theories on Reflective Practice-Based Learning (RPL)

The knowledge model described above suggests that the approach of RPL can provide a supportive learning environment for developing health professional students' technology literacy. According to Horn and her colleagues (2020), RPL is a complex concept encompassing three terms: 'reflective', 'practice', and 'learning'. These terms are rooted in social learning theories, which emphasize a) knowledge as being constructed through interaction rather than rote memorization, and b) learning as being developed more through person-environment interactions and collaborative processes than through individual cognitive processes (Zhou & Lassen, 2024). From a social perspective to teaching and learning, pedagogical designs facilitating literacy and competency development emphasize key concepts such as interaction, practice, experience, reflection, learning-in-context, and active engagement (Zhou et al., 2025).

In general education, reflection typically refers to critical thinking that enables individuals to take action (Wahlgren et al., 2002). In professional settings, reflection involves learning to act in specific ways within professional practice and justifying the motivations behind these actions. Reflection is thus socially contextualized, contributing to both learning and qualified actions (Schön, 1983). According to Wenger (1998), learning arises from the dynamic interplay between social competence and personal experience - a two-way relationship between individuals and the social learning systems they inhabit. As Zhou (2012) notes, learning is fundamentally situated, occurring when a disruption in routine prompts the learner to reflect on a situation, solve a problem, share an idea, or seek understanding. This type of learning happens serendipitously in various contexts: at work, when routine methods fail; at home, through reflective conversations; or at play, while mastering a new activity. In this sense, RPL encourages students' reflection by setting learning goals pursued through engaging activities, assessed formatively to facilitate reflective learning experiences and the mutual sharing of experiences (Gnaur et al., 2015).

RPL emphasizes practice-oriented teaching and learning, engaging students in deeper learning through diverse situational contexts. Students apply theoretical knowledge or course material to real-life situations or novel problem-solving contexts

(Faust & Paulson, 1998). A social perspective on learning asserts that learning cannot be separated from practice (Horn et al., 2020). Wenger (1998) integrates key components in his social theory of learning to characterize social participation as a process of learning and knowing. These components include a) Meaning - the pursuit of understanding and significance, b) Practice - shared historical and social resources, frameworks, and perspectives that sustain mutual engagement in a community, c) Community - the social context that facilitates interaction and collaboration, and d) Identity - how learning shapes the individual's sense of self. Practice involves learners' reflection on their experiences, knowledge, and inquiries to enhance their ability to intervene, interpret, and act effectively (Zhou, 2012). Reflective practices link feeling, thinking, and doing, enabling individuals to improve their effectiveness by developing new insights (Robbins & Dunn, 2019; Rolfe & Freshwater, 2020). Lave and Wenger (1991) also emphasize the importance of the relationships among practitioners, their practice, and the broader social and economic contexts of their communities in shaping practical knowledge.

The principles of RPL are grounded in the interconnected concepts of experience, thinking, and action (Horn et al., 2020). These principles align with Kolb's (1984) experiential learning theory, which defines learning as the process through which knowledge is created by transforming experience. Kolb's model depicts two dialectically related modes of grasping experience - Concrete Experience (CE) and Abstract Conceptualization (AC) - and two dialectically related modes of transforming experience - Reflective Observation (RO) and Active Experimentation (AE) (See Figure 2).

Figure 2. Experiential Learning Cycle by Kolb (1984)

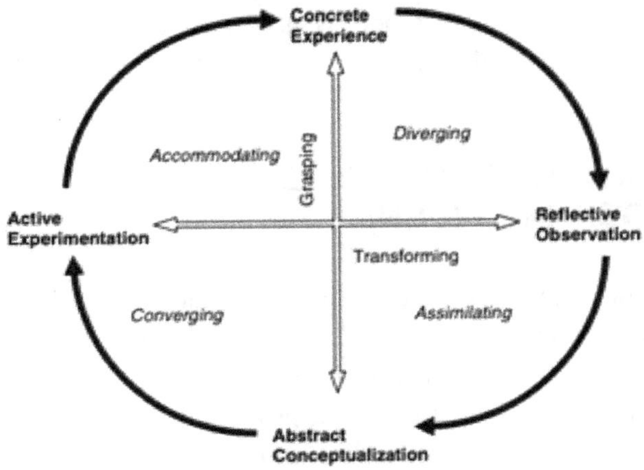

From Figure 2, we observe that experiential learning is a process of constructing knowledge through a creative tension among the four learning modes, responsive to contextual demands. This process is depicted as an idealized learning cycle or spiral, where the learner engages in experiencing, reflecting, thinking, and acting in a recursive manner, adapting to the learning situation and content (Kolb & Kolb, 2008). Concrete experiences form the foundation for observations and reflections, which are then assimilated and distilled into abstract concepts. These concepts guide new implications for action, which can be actively tested and used to create further experiences (Kolb & Kolb, 2008). Through this iterative learning cycle, knowledge is continuously derived from and tested against the learner's experiences. As Wahlgren et al. (2020) describe, experiences represent a specific and complex relationship between the individual and the broader world, in which the individual and their environment mutually influence one another. Experiential learning involves direct engagement with real-world phenomena that form the focus of learning. This engagement transcends mere cognition, incorporating a holistic interaction with the environment (Horn et al., 2020).

Building on these theoretical understandings, we propose that RPL is an effective pedagogy that provides a supportive learning environment for health professional students to enhance their technology literacy. As Horn et al. (2020) suggest, the key concepts of learning in RPL are implemented through a broad framework of activities and actions. These include theoretical lessons, clinical teaching, learning activities, internships, project writing, casework, guidance sessions, facilitation, and laboratory work. To connect these ideas to the relationship between technology literacy and knowledge, it is important to highlight that RPL fosters diverse knowledge exchanges and interactions - socialization, externalization, combination, and internalization. Beyond the development of technology literacy, RPL also offers students opportunities to cultivate other essential skills and attributes, such as communication, interdisciplinary thinking, professional identities, and ethical awareness.

A CASE AT UNIVERSITY COLLEGE OF NORTHERN DENMARK (UCN)

In practice, how can we organize teaching activities inspired by the theoretical discussion? This section provides a detailed case that addresses the second research question in this chapter. The case demonstrates how a course was developed to enhance technology literacy among health professional students at UCN. It also exemplifies how theoretical understanding can be deepened through the detailed description of a course process, answering the questions of 'what', 'how', and 'why' the teaching practice was designed and implemented. The following sections first introduce the methodology and background of the case, leading to a discussion on how RPL principles were implemented at UCN. We explore how students developed technology literacy through practical experiences, gained knowledge from a user perspective, and were motivated to explore new applications of technology in their professional domains. These details showcase our efforts to apply RPL principles to teaching practices, highlighting the alignment between theory and practice in fostering technology literacy.

A Case as an Example

As Dowling and Cooney (2012) suggested, designing a research project requires selecting a method that best aligns with the research question while leveraging the researchers' own knowledge and experience of the phenomenon to achieve credibility. This chapter presents a case that illustrates how RPL facilitates technology literacy development among health professional students.

We highlight that a case study can offer a detailed, real-world examination of a specific situation, providing deep insights into complex issues, practices, or processes. According to Freebody (2003), educational practices and experiences are often characterized by uncertainty, complexity, messiness, and fleeting properties, which call for distinctive research approaches to description, understanding, and explanation. This highlights the need for nuanced methodologies that capture the dynamic and often unpredictable nature of educational environments. The goal of a case study is to establish an inquiry through which both researchers and educators can reflect on specific instances of educational practice, facilitating a deeper understanding of how teaching and learning unfold in real-life contexts.

In such cases, teachers are always teaching subjects matter to specific learners, in unique settings, and under conditions that shape and influence teaching and learning practices. These conditions are not merely 'background' variables but integral, lived dimensions of each teaching-learning event. For example, the social, cultural, and institutional factors surrounding a classroom can significantly impact the methods and effectiveness of instruction. Case studies capture these dimensions by focusing on the interplay between teacher decisions, student responses, and the broader context. This approach encourages a holistic view, allowing for the identification of patterns, challenges, and successes that may not be immediately evident through more controlled or generalized research methods.

Case studies emphasize the significance of time and place, reflecting a commitment to the importance of localized experiences. By focusing on specific instances within a particular context, they allow researchers to explore how different variables interact and influence outcomes, thus revealing rich, context-specific insights. Moreover, they serve as a means of conducting and disseminating research to influence practice and refine theoretical approaches to understanding practice (Zhou & Lassen, 2024). This makes case studies an invaluable tool for both theorists and practitioners, as they provide actionable insights that can inform and improve real-world practices, while also contributing to the evolution of theory and pedagogy in the field.

In line with these points, this chapter highlights a case that connects the theoretical framework with practice within the specific context of RPL at UCN. One of the authors draws upon her teaching experience as the basis for describing the case, offering insights into the process of course development. Rather than collecting empirical data from students, the case is presented by transforming the author's participatory experiences - design, development, observation, and reflection - into a research resource. Thus, the findings are shared through a narrative approach, rooted in the educator's subjective experience. The researcher adopts multiple roles, including educator and participant, within the RPL environment. In this participatory framework, objectivity is not the gold standard; instead, critical subjectivity and reflexivity are emphasized (Zhou & Lassen, 2024). The following sections provide a detailed report of the author's experiences, offering a reflective account of the case study.

Brief Background of the Case

UCN offers a two-week interdisciplinary elective course for physiotherapy and occupational therapy students. The course is designed to equip students with the skills to address healthcare tasks in a professional context, reflecting the growing use of healthcare and welfare technology solutions in interactions with patients and other citizens.

The primary objective of the elective is to enhance students' ability to understand, analyse, and evaluate technological solutions, methods, and potential applications. Another key aim is to improve their competencies in managing and implementing these technological solutions through close collaboration with practice. Reflective learning in practice serves as the foundation for student collaboration with industry and healthcare practitioners during the two weeks. Students engage with real-world problems posed by health professionals and technology developers from practice. External speakers, including citizens and employees, are invited to provide practical perspectives through introductory sessions. Students tackle these problems using knowledge and skills derived from theories, observations, interviews, and practice testing. The lectures are partially relocated from UCN to the Centre for Welfare Technology, where both advanced technology and dedicated classrooms are available. The curriculum is structured around practice-oriented teaching and learning activities, drawing inspiration from fundamental principles, methods, and techniques of reflective practice-oriented learning (Lassen & Andersen, 2021).

The Implementation of RPL

The case reflects how an elective course is designed based on the fundamental principles of RPL. The elective, titled 'Technology in the Present and Future', aims to address both current healthcare and welfare technology tasks and future technology demands in a constantly evolving health sector. The two-week course is designed for third-semester physiotherapy and occupational therapy students, who finished their first-year study, and who have developed a monodisciplinary focus on understanding their occupation and its identity. Students who choose this elective have a special interest in technology and seek to gain qualifications and skills beyond the basic curriculum.

The goal of the course is to provide students with the foundational qualifications needed for future roles involving the implementation and application of welfare and healthcare technology, such as a consultant for welfare technology in a municipality. The course covers interdisciplinary technologies used across professions, including nursing, physiotherapy, occupational therapy, teaching, and nursing aid. These technologies include virtual training systems, wash and dry toilets, feeding robots, and virtual reality equipment designed to train patients with physical and psychological disabilities. From an organizational perspective, the purpose of these technologies is to enhance the physical and psychological work environments for healthcare professionals, improve care and rehabilitation quality for citizens/patients, and optimize resource use in municipalities and regions (Lassen & Andersen, 2021).

The course is structured so that students work in groups to create evaluation reports on one of health and welfare technologies. They collaborate with the Centre for Welfare Technology to select these technologies and have opportunities to test them. The evaluation report is structured according to the Welfare Technology Assessment (VTV), which covers the following areas: 1) technology (area of application, efficiency, and risk assessment), 2) citizen/patient (psychological, physical, and social aspects), 3) organization (structural, personal, and environmental aspects), and 4) economy (national, operating, and maintenance costs). Ethics is a fifth consideration, where students must explore the ethical implications of the technology. At the end of the course, students present the most significant perspectives and create a video demonstrating the technology's use for employees and/or citizens as the ultimate users (Lassen & Andersen, 2021). The course structure is designed to facilitate learning through 'reflection over/in/with practice, coupled with theoretical analysis and practical synthesis', which is the essence of RPL. While working on the evaluation report, students are encouraged to critically reflect on the potential of technology applications in the Danish healthcare system. This reflective process encourages students to refine their reasoning based on the various dimensions of the evaluation. Their conclusions integrate both theoretical and practical aspects and provide a comprehensive executive summary and recommendations.

The course follows a chronological order designed around RPL's key concepts: experience, thinking, and action. In the first week, the focus is on creating broad experiences with technology, particularly the technologies selected by each group. These experiences include theoretical lectures from external and internal speakers, focusing on the dimensions that will be addressed in the evaluation report. Additionally, the students visit the Centre for Welfare Technology to engage in hands-on testing and discussions with consultants. As students gain experience, reflective thinking is facilitated, connecting knowledge from lectures to their hands-on technology testing (Lassen & Andersen, 2021).

Thinking leads to the first part of the evaluation report, which involves defining the problem and determining how empirical knowledge and research will be gathered. Facilitated by supervisors and Centre for Welfare Technology consultants, students begin to reflect on appropriate search terms and relevant informants to contact. The second week provides more space for reflection on practice as students work on their evaluation report and prepare for their verbal presentations. A second visit to the Centre for Welfare Technology allows students to record a brief demonstration video of the technology, which will be included in their final presentation. These recordings and presentations require pre-reflection on the information needed by the intended recipients of their evaluation reports.

In summary, the course aligns with RPL's core principles: 1) Students' own experiences are included in the teaching, 2) The course allows for adequate interruptions, and 3) The course is designed as an exploration. The course is continuously adapted and developed based on student feedback and evaluations (Lassen & Andersen, 202; Zhou & Lassen, 2024).

Teaching for Real Experiences

The students are eager for hands-on experimentation and testing of the chosen technologies. They need to touch, try, and experience the technologies firsthand. At this stage in their education, the students have limited experience with using health and welfare technologies, particularly in the context of working as healthcare professionals. They have not yet had extended training periods where they could interact with technology or collaborate with other groups. Their curiosity about technological advancements in healthcare is a key reason for choosing this elective, and they require in-depth study to understand the technology and its diverse applications. As outlined in the first fundamental principle of RPL, students' own experiences are integrated into the learning process. This is achieved by giving students the opportunity to test technologies during both an introductory and follow-up visit to the Centre for Welfare Technology, followed by reflection and supplementary exercises. This is described in more detail below.

The primary focus in the first week of the elective is on creating experiences for the students through an all-day visit to the Centre for Welfare Technology. During this visit, students have opportunities to try out various health and welfare technologies, gaining an in-depth understanding of the technology they are evaluating for their report. The teaching occurs at both UCN and the Centre for Welfare Technology. When the students need to test a specific technology, the sessions take place at the Centre. Additionally, students can arrange with the centre to work in groups if they feel this approach better suits their learning style. The teaching is designed to provide students with concrete situations where they engage with the technology, facilitating experiential learning. Reflection questions are posed during the testing process to deepen their understanding: Which citizen/patient groups would benefit from the technology? What are the scalability and adaptability aspects of the technology? How do professional work practices integrate with the technology? These different experiences form the foundation for defining a relevant problem that the students will focus on while working on their evaluation report. The work that follows is rooted in experience-based learning, where students apply theoretical knowledge to their own specific technology and problem definition. The process is not purely inductive, as students are given the report dimensions to guide their work, which frames the final summary (Lassen & Andersen, 2021).

In the second week, students further explore the technology during a return visit to the Centre for Welfare Technology. The objective of this visit is to produce an introductory video, in which students present the technology's various applications, limitations, and a practical demonstration. This video will be part of their verbal presentation on the last day of the course. For example, students might produce a video demonstrating how to adjust and operate an eating robot for use for young residents with physical, psychological, or developmental disabilities. The video would serve as an instructional tool for pedagogues and social healthcare workers who support the residents in using the technology. Through this process, students not only learn to communicate their findings but also reflect on their previous experiences from the first visit to the Centre. These reflections are used to plan the recordings, ensuring they are relevant to the intended audience. The return visit also allows students to experiment further with the technology, after having had time to reflect on their earlier experiences (Lassen & Andersen, 2021).

In addition to gathering empirical knowledge through interviews or literature searches, students are encouraged to focus on their own experiences with the technology. They are asked to document their reflections for each of the various dimensions of the evaluation report. This approach underscores the value of experience-based knowledge, motivating students to engage in an inductive learning process (Lassen & Andersen, 2021).

Knowledge on User Experiences

The students seek insight into the users' own experiences with technology, including how users perceive the introduction, implementation, and everyday use of technology. While students test the technology themselves, they do not fully understand its impact on the users' surroundings, how it helps maintain their everyday life, or how it affects their social relationships. They lack long-term experience with technology that might reveal other possibilities and limitations beyond what can be observed during short testing and assessment sessions (Lassen & Andersen, 2021). To address this gap, the students need first-hand accounts from actual users who rely on technology in their daily lives.

To accommodate this need, lectures are planned with appropriate interruptions, as recommended by the second fundamental principle of RPL. These interruptions are structured to promote reflective thinking about the use of technology, how it is taught, and how the students, as future professionals, can support users in integrating this technology into their lives. User visits are arranged in both the first and second week to provide the students with valuable real-world perspectives on technology use. These visits serve as important disturbances that support the reflective process, which is further integrated into the students' evaluation reports. The role of user visits as a means of providing appropriate interruptions is described in the following lines (Lassen & Andersen, 2021).

The lectures are scheduled with continual interruptions through various introductory presentations and user visits. The purpose of these interruptions is to introduce new knowledge and diverse perspectives -both theoretical and practical - on the technology. The first user visit takes place on the first day of the elective and features a volunteer from an elderly people's association who shares personal experiences of using technology and assisting older individuals in using a PC and other everyday devices. The volunteer is in their mid-80s, and their presence and stories challenge the students' preconceptions about elderly people's abilities with technology. This visit provides students with fresh perspectives on the possibilities and challenges of using technology with senior citizens. The visit is consistently well-received in course evaluations, and students frequently request more opportunities to hear from users with similar experiences (Lassen & Andersen, 2021).

The second user visit offers new insights into how technology can help sustain social relationships and communication with family and friends in school and institutional settings. It also highlights human dependence on technology and the role of professionals in analyzing, adjusting, and adapting technology for different individual needs. For this visit, students are required to prepare questions for a parent of a child with cerebral palsy, who has both verbal and physical disabilities. As part of their preparation, the students view a video showing how the child and family use of technology to communicate in everyday life. During the visit, students are responsible for controlling the session and asking investigative questions that will help them identify both the visible and more subtle challenges and possibilities of the technology. This visit places students in a situation where they need to improvise or rely on their own experiences with technology to communicate with the child. This visit offers students both perceptual and emotional experiences, as well as reflections on the real challenges and contextual settings users face. These experiences provide valuable insights beyond those gained from the students' own technology testing. The goal is to help students understand that user experiences are often highly personal and context specific. For professionals, it is crucial to have a deep understanding of specific specialist fields to analyse and assess the applicability of technology in various situations. These insights lead to further reflections on the technology being evaluated in the report, such as considering which patient groups may benefit from the technology and in what settings it can be most effectively used (Lassen & Andersen, 2021).

Exploring New Working Areas with Technology

The students have requested more insights into potential future roles and responsibilities related to the practical testing, implementation, and evaluation of health and welfare technological solutions. This suggests that they struggle with transferring what they've learned in the elective subject to their understanding of the roles that physiotherapists and occupational therapists might assume after graduation. Working with health and welfare technology is a specialized field that is only touched upon briefly in their basic education. Therefore, it's essential during the elective subject to clarify the connection between the course content and potential future job positions (Lassen & Andersen, 2021).

The third fundamental principle in RPL - 'education is organized as exploration' - serves as an inspiration. This principle is realized by simulating a role as technology consultants for an imaginary municipality. In this simulation, the students are tasked with constructing an evaluation report on a selected technology. The goal is for the students to create meaning from the learning experience and apply that meaning to the simulated employment scenario. They will research the technology from various perspectives, as outlined in the diverse dimensions of the evaluation report (Lassen & Andersen, 2021).

Before the start of the elective, students receive a welcome letter and a letter of employment. This provides them with a clear understanding of the assignments they will undertake as technology consultants during the course. The letter outlines the municipality's expectations for their work in the upcoming years, as well as the specific assignments for the next two weeks. It specifies that the students must submit an evaluation report on a particular welfare technology after completing the course. This allows students to know what is expected of them from the outset and clarifies the product they must deliver by the end of the elective. These expectations are based on real-world assignments developed in cooperation with industry practice. The entire course is structured as an exploration, where meaning is created and collapsed throughout the two weeks, a process that is introduced to students both initially and during the course. The first exploration involves working as technology consultants in a municipality, where the students will receive an overall introduction to the evaluation report they must prepare, along with a verbal instruction video. The evaluation report is intended for municipal decision-makers, and its purpose is not to draw conclusions but to summarize the potential applications of the technology from different perspectives. Through testing, data collection, and discussions, students engage in the process of creating a new understanding of the technology, which they then communicate to decision-makers. The elective course is planned as an abductive learning process, where the knowledge gained by the students is presented as if they were real technology consultants in the municipality, though they will receive guidance and lectures throughout the process (Lassen & Andersen, 2021).

A key element of organizing the lectures as an exploration is facilitating students' work with technology from multiple perspectives. Introductory presentations, based on the five dimensions of the evaluation report, enable students to apply their knowledge and information to the selected technology. For example, when evaluating the use of wash-and-dry toilets in nursing homes, students consider various viewpoints. From a citizen perspective, such technology may increase independence by enabling individuals to visit the toilet unaided. From an economic perspective, it could save time for nursing staff. However, from an employee perspective, some may argue against their use, as assisting with toilet visits can provide valuable opportunities for staff to observe issues like decubitus ulcers (Lassen & Andersen, 2021).

The teaching is designed as an employment simulation, offering both insight and confidence in fulfilling assignments as technology consultants with the competencies and skill sets acquired as healthcare professionals. These professionals are in high demand for interdisciplinary roles working with health and welfare technology. To emphasize the value of their work in practice, the students' final evaluation reports will be published and made publicly available at the Centre for Welfare Technology in collaboration with the design education program at UCN (Lassen & Andersen, 2021).

DISCUSSION

Innovative Pedagogical Design for Technology Literacy

This chapter makes an important theoretical contribution by linking our understanding of technology literacy to theories of knowledge in professional practice. The dialogues between different knowledge models can be understood as situated activities that drive knowledge transformation through processes of socialization, externalization, combination, and internalization (Zhou, 2012). These processes, as articulated by Nonaka and Takeuchi (1995), emphasize the dynamic and iterative nature of knowledge creation, where individuals and groups interact to produce, share, and refine their understanding in real-world contexts. In the context of technology literacy, this transformation is critical as it reflects how individuals adapt and apply new technological knowledge within professional practices, such as in healthcare or education. Technology literacy is not merely about acquiring technical skills but also about understanding how these skills integrate with professional knowledge and influence decision-making processes (Judson, 2010).

Technology literacy education demands the design of pedagogies that create appropriate conditions for facilitating interactions and conversations between different knowledge models (Zhou et al., 2025). These pedagogies should be designed to promote an environment where students are actively engaged in the learning process, exploring the connections between theoretical knowledge and practical application. The challenge is to craft educational strategies that do not merely focus on the transmission of knowledge but encourage the co-construction of knowledge between students, educators, and technological tools (Illeries, 2007). By fostering these interactions, educators can help students navigate complex technological landscapes and develop critical thinking and problem-solving skills that are essential for professional practice (Zhou, 2012). The pedagogies implemented should motivate students' learning experiences within a participatory framework, ensuring that learning is not just an individual process but a collective one. Learning, in this sense, becomes a collaborative venture where students are encouraged to share their ideas, challenge each other's perspectives, and co-create new understanding (Wenger, 1998). This approach highlights the importance of social learning and knowledge exchange within educational settings, reflecting the idea that true learning often occurs in dynamic, interactive environments (Horn et al., 2020). By adopting participatory pedagogies, educators can ensure that students not only acquire technology literacy but also engage in the ongoing process of knowledge production that mirrors the collaborative nature of professional practice (Zhou & Lassen, 2024).

Developing Technology Literacy for Students in RPL

As the case study described, RPL offers health professional students a supportive learning environment for technology literacy development. RPL, as an approach to acknowledging and integrating learners' previous experiences, positions students as active agents in their own educational journeys. From the case study, we learn that RPL positions professional students at the center of the process of technology literacy development. In this model, students are not passive recipients of information; rather, they take an active role in producing knowledge and meaning, bringing their expertise, experiences, and ideas into the learning environment (Zhou, 2012). This student-centered approach ensures that learning is grounded in real-world contexts, allowing students to see the relevance and applicability of their new knowledge. In this approach, students are given the opportunity to actively engage with technology contexts in meaningful ways, offering them immediate hands-on experiences (Zhou & Lassen, 2024). These experiences help students feel more in control of their own learning journey in technology knowledge, as they are directly involved in experimenting with and applying new technologies. This approach also allows them to test their understanding and refine their skills through practical, authentic experiences (Faust & Paulson, 1998; Estes, 2017). Furthermore, RPL offers opportunities for students to present themselves through individual study tasks or collaborative group activities. The combination of individual and collective tasks ensures that students can personalize their learning while also benefiting from the perspectives and knowledge of their peers.

In other words, as students learn new technology knowledge, they make new connections between ideas and create meaning from them in practice, thereby constructing their own knowledge. This active learning process is essential for technology literacy, as it encourages students to not only acquire technical skills but also to integrate them into their professional practices. The experience involves not only what students learn from practice but also their individual and collective reflections on those experiences as sources of understanding (Schön, 1983; 1987). These reflections allow students to critically examine their learning, assess their progress, and refine their skills, ensuring that the knowledge they develop is deeply rooted in both theory and practice (Zhou et al., 2025). Through this iterative process, students become more adept at navigating the complexities of technology in their professional contexts, making them more prepared for the evolving demands of their fields (Estes, 2017).

From the case study, we also learn that collaboration between UCN and the Centre for Welfare Technology plays a key role in motivating students to apply theories to practice. This highlights that the successful implementation of RPL and the development of health professional students' technology literacy require the active involvement of professional education institutions in practice within professional communities (Wenger, 1998). Such communities can serve as networks of mutual relationships that engage diverse stakeholders - such as universities, industries, enterprises, and governments - to collaborate and provide multiple channels of resources for teaching and learning (Horn et al., 2020). The advantage of enabling occupational therapy and physiotherapy students to work together on a practical case involving technology, and to have hands-on experience with the technology itself, is that it allows them to incorporate both tacit and explicit knowledge. In such situations, students are challenged by their peers to articulate their implicit knowledge. Moreover, students engage in collective learning when they investigate and test technology together in groups. By working with a specific technology, the technology becomes a shared interest, allowing students to focus more on the opportunities and challenges it presents, rather than prioritizing their respective professions.

CONCLUSION

The development and advancement of technology directly affect the quality and effectiveness of healthcare in professional practice, which underscores the importance of improving technology literacy in health professional education. The practice of technology is inherently complex, involving many interdisciplinary problems that must be solved. Technology can be seen as the practical implementation of solutions to problems, but it is also connected to the non-technological dimensions of reality. These include diverse factors such as will, drive, motive, aspiration, intention, and choice, all of which aim to satisfy basic biological needs or pursue efficiency. This perspective reflects the fact that the development of technology literacy requires students to gain knowledge in both 'know-what' and 'know-how', with an emphasis on the interaction of knowledge at both individual and collective levels. The model of RPL has significant implications for enhancing technology literacy education for the future, as health professional students should be given numerous opportunities to acquire technology knowledge, understand the diverse contextual factors involved in the creation and development of technologies, and explore the impacts of technologies on individuals, environments, and society. This leads us to recommend that in order to strengthen health professional education and training in technology literacy, it is essential to promote interdisciplinary collaboration and integrate hands-on activities, reflections and authentic learning experiences with various medical technologies and digital tools. It is also important to emphasize creative problem-solving skills, critical thinking, ethical concerns, and capabilities of data interpretation. All these points highlight how a human-centered design approach can empower health professionals to engage responsibly and effectively with emerging technologies in clinical practice.

REFERENCES

Barton, G., & Lennon, S. (2020). Literacy. In *Teaching Middle Years* (pp. 115–132). Routledge. DOI: 10.4324/9781003117780-9

Bastable, S. B., Sopczyk, D., Gramet, P., & Jacobs, K. (2019). *Health professional as educator: principles of teaching and learning: principles of teaching and learning*. Jones & Bartlett Learning.

Bugliarello, G. (2000). Reflections on technological literacy. *Bulletin of Science, Technology & Society*, *20*(2), 83–89. DOI: 10.1177/027046760002000201

Conard, S. (2019). Best practices in digital health literacy. *International Journal of Cardiology*, *292*, 277–279. DOI: 10.1016/j.ijcard.2019.05.070 PMID: 31230937

Dash, S., Shakyawar, S. K., Sharma, M., & Kaushik, S. (2019). Big data in healthcare: Management, analysis and future prospects. *Journal of Big Data*, *6*(1), 1–25. DOI: 10.1186/s40537-019-0217-0

Dowling, M., & Cooney, A. (2012). Research approaches related to phenomenology: Negotiating a complex landscape. *Nurse Researcher*, *20*(2), 21–27. DOI: 10.7748/nr2012.11.20.2.21.c9440 PMID: 23316534

Dunn, P., & Hazzard, E. (2019). Technology approaches to digital health literacy. *International Journal of Cardiology*, *293*, 294–296. DOI: 10.1016/j.ijcard.2019.06.039 PMID: 31350037

Estes, J. S. (2017). Teacher preparation programs and learner-centred, technology-integrated instruction. In *Handbook of Research on Learner-centred Pedagogy in Teacher Education and Professional Development* (pp. 85–103). IGI Global. DOI: 10.4018/978-1-5225-0892-2.ch005

European Health Parliament. (2016). *Digital Skills for Health Professionals*. https://www.healthparliament.eu/wp-content/uploads/2017/09/Digital-skills-for-health-professionals.pdf

Faust, J. L., & Paulson, D. R. (1998). Active learning in the college classroom. *Journal on Excellence in College Teaching*, *9*(2), 3–24.

Freebody, P. (2003). *Qualitative Research in Education: Interaction and Practice*. SAGE Publications. DOI: 10.4135/9781849209670

Frenk, J., Chen, L., Bhutta, Z. A., Cohen, J., Crisp, N., Evans, T., Fineberg, H., Garcia, P., Ke, Y., Kelley, P., Kistnasamy, B., Meleis, A., Naylor, D., Pablos-Mendez, A., Reddy, S., Scrimshaw, S., Sepulveda, J., Serwadda, D., & Zurayk, H. (2010). Health professionals for a new century: Transforming education to strengthen health systems in an interdependent world. *Lancet*, *376*(9756), 1923–1958. DOI: 10.1016/S0140-6736(10)61854-5 PMID: 21112623

Gnaur, D., Svidt, K., & Thygesen, M. K. (2015). Developing students' collaborative skills in interdisciplinary learning environments. *International Journal of Engineering Education*, *31*(1B), 257–266.

Grover, V., & Balusamy, B. MK, N., Anand, V., & Milanova, M. (Eds.). (2024). *Approaches to Human-centered AI in Healthcare*. IGI Global.

Guillodo, E., Lemey, C., Simonnet, M., Walter, M., Baca-García, E., Masetti, V., Moga, S., Larsen, M., Ropars, J., & Berrouiguet, S. (2020). Clinical applications of mobile health wearable–based sleep monitoring: Systematic review. *JMIR mHealth and uHealth*, *8*(4), e10733. DOI: 10.2196/10733 PMID: 32234707

Hardinata, S., Suchyadi, Y., & Wulandari, D. (2021). Strengthening technological literacy in junior high school teachers in the industrial revolution era 4.0. *Journal of Humanities and Social Studies*, *5*(3), 330–335.

Horn, L. H., Jensen, C. G., Kjærgaard, T., Lukassen, B., Sørensen, I. M., Valbak-Andersen, C., & Bund-gaard, S. B. (2020). *White Paper on Reflective Practice-Based Learning*. University College of Northern Denmark.

Illers, K. (2007). *How We Learn: Learning and Non-Learning in School and Beyond*. Routledge. DOI: 10.4324/9780203939895

Ingerman, Å., & Collier-Reed, B. (2011). Technological literacy reconsidered: A model for enactment. *International Journal of Technology and Design Education*, *21*(2), 137–148. DOI: 10.1007/s10798-009-9108-6

Judson, E. (2010). Improving technology literacy: Does it open doors to traditional content? *Educational Technology Research and Development*, *58*(3), 271–284. DOI: 10.1007/s11423-009-9135-8

Kolb, A. Y., & Kolb, D. A. (2009). Experiential learning theory: a dynamic, holistic approach to management learning, education and development. In Armstrong, S. J., & Fukami, C. V. (Eds.), *The SAGE Handbook of Management Learning, Education and Development* (pp. 42–68). SAGE Publishing. DOI: 10.4135/9780857021038.n3

Kolb, D. A. (1984). *Experiential Learning: Experience as the Source of Learning and Development*. Prentice-Hall, Inc.

Konttila, J., Siira, H., Kyngäs, H., Lahtinen, M., Elo, S., Kääriäinen, M., Kaakinen, P., Oikarinen, A., Yamakawa, M., Fukui, S., Utsumi, M., Higami, Y., Higuchi, A., & Mikkonen, K. (2019). Healthcare professionals' competence in digitalisation: A systematic review. *Journal of Clinical Nursing*, *28*(5-6), 745–761. DOI: 10.1111/jocn.14710 PMID: 30376199

Lassen, A. M., & Andersen, M. F. (2021). Valgfagsudvikling på to sundhedsuddannelser. I L. H. Horn, P. M. Pedersen, & M. Georgsen (red.), *Teori og Praksis i Professionsdidaktik: En Bog om Refleksiv Praksislæring* (pp. 171-182). Aalborg Universitetsforlag.

Lassen, A. M., & Kjærgaard, T. (2022). Teknologiforståelser i professionerne. Learning Tech – Tidsskrift for Læremidler. *Didaktik og Teknologi*, (11), 15–43.

Lave, J., & Wenger, E. (1991). *Situated Learning: Legitimate Peripheral Participation*. Cambridge University Press. DOI: 10.1017/CBO9780511815355

Levande, J. S. (2003). A Curricular and Instructional Challenge: Teaching and Learning for Technological Literacy/Capability. *The Journal of Technology Studies*, *29*(2), 88–97. DOI: 10.21061/jots.v29i2.a.6

Locsin, R. C. (2017). The co-existence of technology and caring in the theory of technological competency as caring in nursing. *The Journal of Medical Investigation*, 64(1.2), 160-164.

Moudatsou, M., Stavropoulou, A., Philalithis, A., & Koukouli, S. (2020, January). The role of empathy in health and social care professionals. []. MDPI.]. *Health Care*, *8*(1), 26. PMID: 32019104

Nonaka, I., & Konno, N. (1998). The concept of 'Ba': Building a foundation for knowledge creation. *California Management Review*, *40*(3), 40–54. DOI: 10.2307/41165942

Robbins, D., & Dunn, P. (2019). Digital health literacy in a person-centric world. *International Journal of Cardiology*, *290*, 154–155. DOI: 10.1016/j.ijcard.2019.05.033 PMID: 31130277

Rolfe, G., & Freshwater, D. (2020). *Critical Reflection in Practice: Generating Knowledge for Care*. Blooms-bury Publishing.

Rožanec, J. M., Novalija, I., Zajec, P., Kenda, K., Tavakoli Ghinani, H., Suh, S., Veliou, E., Papamartzivanos, D., Giannetsos, T., Menesidou, S. A., Alonso, R., Cauli, N., Meloni, A., Recupero, D. R., Kyriazis, D., Sofianidis, G., Theodoropoulos, S., Fortuna, B., Mladenić, D., & Soldatos, J. (2023). Human-centric artificial intelligence architecture for industry 5.0 applications. *International Journal of Production Research*, *61*(20), 6847–6872. DOI: 10.1080/00207543.2022.2138611

Schön, D. (1983). *The Reflective Practitioner: How Professionals Think in Action*. Basic Books.

Schön, D. (1987). *Educating the Reflective Practitioner: toward a New Design for Teaching and Learning in the Professions*. Jossey-Bass.

Schön, D. A. (1992). The theory of inquiry: Dewey's legacy to education. *Curriculum Inquiry*, *22*(2), 119–139. DOI: 10.1080/03626784.1992.11076093

Shachak, A., Monkman, H., Lesselroth, B., Lee, W. W., & Alkureishi, M. L. A. (2024). Technological literacy as a framework for health professions education in the digital era. In *Digital Health and Informatics Innovations for Sustainable Health Care Systems* (pp. 1500–1504). IOS Press. DOI: 10.3233/SHTI240699

Tan, O. S. (2009). *Problem-Based Learning and Creativity*. Cengage: Learning Asia Pte Ltd: Singapore.

Tierney, A. A., Mosqueda, M., Cesena, G., Frehn, J. L., Payan, D. D., & Rodriguez, H. P. (2024). Telemedicine implementation for safety net populations: A systematic review. *Telemedicine Journal and e-Health*, *30*(3), 622–641. DOI: 10.1089/tmj.2023.0260 PMID: 37707997

Trocin, C., Mikalef, P., Papamitsiou, Z., & Conboy, K. (2023). Responsible AI for digital health: A synthesis and a research agenda. *Information Systems Frontiers*, *25*(6), 2139–2157. DOI: 10.1007/s10796-021-10146-4

Wahlgren, B., Høyrup, S., Pedersen, K., & Rattleff, P. (2002). *Refleksion og Læring: Kompetenceudvikling i Arbejdslivet*. Samfundslitteratur.

Wenger, E. (1998). *Communities of practice: Learning, Meaning, and Identity*. Cambridge University Press. DOI: 10.1017/CBO9780511803932

Young, A. T., Cole, J. R., & Denton, D. (2002). Improving technological literacy. *Issues in Science and Technology*, *18*(4), 73–79.

Zhou, C. (2012). Learning engineering knowledge and creativity by solving projects. *International Journal of Engineering Pedagogy*, *2*(1), 26–31. DOI: 10.3991/ijep.v2i1.1873

Zhou, C., & Lassen, A. M. (2024). Improving Technology Literacy among Health Professional Students. In *Proceedings of Nordic Education Research Association Conference 2024*. Malmö University.

Zhou, C., Michael Rosenberg Petri, S., & Bhattacharyya, S. (2025). AI Literacy and Professional Development in STEM Education. In Papadakis, S. (Ed.), *AI Roles and Responsibilities in Education*. Springer.

Chapter 3
Opportunities and Challenges of AI-Driven Transformation in Medical Education

Flaka Hoti
https://orcid.org/0000-0002-4780-5776
University of Gjakova "Fehmi Agani", Kosovo

Kamel Mouloudj
https://orcid.org/0000-0001-7617-8313
University of Medea, Algeria

Doruntina Kabashi
https://orcid.org/0009-0008-2696-8390
Main Family Medicine Center in Peja, Kosovo

Hasime Arif Bacaj Terziqi
University of Gjakova "Fehmi Agani", Kosovo

Antigona Ukëhaxhaj
University of Gjakova "Fehmi Agani", Kosovo & National Institute of Public Health, Kosovo

ABSTRACT

The integration of artificial intelligence (AI) and digital technologies is reshaping the landscape of medical education. This chapter explores how AI enhances clinical reasoning, personalizes learning pathways, and supports the digital transformation of teaching and assessment. Drawing on a narrative review of recent literature, the

DOI: 10.4018/979-8-3373-1519-5.ch003

chapter identifies both the opportunities and challenges associated with implementing AI in medical curricula. Particular attention is given to institutional resistance, ethical and data privacy concerns, infrastructural constraints, and the lack of faculty training. Recommendations are offered for educators, institutions, policymakers, and technology developers to facilitate responsible and effective adoption. By addressing these barriers and fostering collaboration across sectors, AI can serve as a powerful catalyst for innovation in medical education. The chapter concludes by emphasizing the need for ongoing investment, ethical oversight, and educator empowerment to ensure that AI contributes meaningfully to the development of future healthcare.

INTRODUCTION

In this rapidly advancing technological age, generative artificial intelligence (AI) has emerged as a transformative force, reshaping the landscape of education (Bahroun et al., 2023; Köse, 2023; Masters, 2019). Medical education, in particular, is undergoing a profound transformation driven by technological advancements and the integration of AI into healthcare and learning environments (Bouabdellah, 2023; Franco D'Souza et al., 2024; Levingston et al., 2024). This evolution is challenging traditional models of medical education—often characterized by passive learning and rigid curricula—and promoting more dynamic, learner-centered, and technology-enhanced approaches.

As healthcare systems evolve and patient care becomes more complex, the demand for competent, adaptable, and technologically literate healthcare professionals has never been greater. Recent developments in cognitive and learning sciences offer valuable insights, helping medical educators adopt more effective teaching strategies and improve the assessment process (Patel et al., 2009). According to Civaner et al. (2022), the majority of medical students viewed artificial intelligence as a supportive tool that could improve physicians' access to information (85.8%), enhance patient access to healthcare (76.7%), and decrease errors (70.5%). In this shifting landscape, the convergence of AI and digital tools holds the promise of revolutionizing not only what is taught but also how it is taught (Garcia et al., 2024). As a result, health professions education has already benefited from AI advancements and is poised to reap even greater rewards in the future (Grunhut et al., 2022; Köse, 2023; Masters, 2023).

AI is not a single, all-encompassing technology but rather comprises several subdomains, such as machine learning and deep learning, which can independently or collaboratively contribute intelligence to applications (Bajwa et al., 2021). AI has the potential to enhance clinical reasoning by offering clinical case simulations and can also support conversational learning, helping students develop responses to open-ended questions and improve their communication skills (Bouabdellah, 2023; Levingston et al., 2024). Additionally, AI can retrieve relevant details from patient histories, automatically generate medical summaries and treatment suggestions, and continuously update medical records in real time (Huo et al., 2025). AI-powered tools like chatbots can also deliver personalized learning experiences by adjusting to individual student knowledge levels (Levingston et al., 2024).

Conversely, Several ethical issues arise, such as the risk to data protection, the evolving dynamics of the patient-doctor relationship in healthcare, the creation of potential social disparities, and the advancement of AI robots that could eventually take over various professional roles, leading to higher unemployment rates (Bozorgi, 2023; Civaner et al., 2022). Therefore, while AI has the potential to significantly transform both medical education and healthcare (Franco D'Souza et al., 2024), it is essential for AI integration to be approached responsibly. Garcia et al. (2024) stress that effective AI integration into medical education is crucial for preparing healthcare professionals to meet the challenges of contemporary medicine. Moreover, it is necessary to ensure that AI does not become the primary driver of learning decisions. Coates (2025) argues for a cautious approach, ensuring that AI serves as a tool for learning rather than dictating the learning process.

Generative AI technologies are being adopted more widely across various sectors, sparking both significant interest and concern about their potential use in medical education (Preiksaitis & Rose, 2023). Preiksaitis and Rose (2023) identified several potential uses of generative AI in medical education, including facilitating self-directed learning, creating simulation scenarios, and offering writing support. As educators and institutions consider the potential of AI, it is crucial to have a thorough understanding of its implications and the potential concerns related to its responsible use (Grunhut et al., 2022; Franco D'Souza et al., 2024). In this context, Mouloudj et al. (2025a) note that the adoption of AI in educational settings can be enhanced by intuitive AI tools, clear advantages, positive perceptions, and institutional or peer support. However, Garcia et al. (2024) point out that despite the growing use of AI in healthcare, there remains a significant gap in research focused on its effective integration into medical education. Although the use of AI in learning, teaching, and assessment is expanding, further research is still required to fully understand its impact and potential (Chan & Zary, 2019).

Based on the above, the primary aim of this chapter is to explore the transformative impact of AI and digital technologies on medical education. Specifically, it seeks to answer key questions: How is AI reshaping clinical reasoning and decision-making skills among medical students? In what ways are digital technologies redefining the delivery of medical content and enhancing the student learning experience? What barriers hinder the effective implementation of AI in medical training? And what strategic recommendations can guide stakeholders in embracing these changes effectively? By addressing these questions, this chapter contributes to the growing body of research that advocates for rethinking medical education in the context of a technology-driven future (Tolsgaard et al., 2023).

This chapter is grounded in a narrative review methodology, allowing for a comprehensive, interpretive synthesis of the existing literature (Mouloudj et al., 2024). The analysis draws upon the latest peer-reviewed research, academic journal articles, relevant conference proceedings, and chapters from indexed scholarly books. By integrating diverse sources, the chapter aims to provide a holistic understanding of how technology and AI are shaping medical training in contemporary contexts.

Levingston et al. (2024) argue that while AI has made significant strides, its adoption in medical education remains relatively limited. In this context, medical education must move beyond mere digitization to achieve true innovation. Therefore, this chapter calls for a strategic and holistic approach to ensure that future medical professionals are not only clinically competent but also digitally fluent and ethically grounded in an AI-enabled healthcare system. Ultimately, the chapter emphasizes that while technology and AI offer substantial opportunities to improve medical education, their success depends on thoughtful implementation, evidence-based pedagogical strategies, and a willingness among institutions to embrace change.

To achieve these objectives, the chapter is organized into five key sections. The first section, *AI: Enhancing clinical reasoning and personalization*, discusses how AI technologies are supporting diagnostic reasoning, simulating clinical scenarios, and offering personalized learning paths. The second section, *the digital transformation of medical education*, examines broader digital innovations such as e-learning platforms, virtual simulations, and digital assessments, emphasizing their pedagogical implications. The third section, *Barriers to implementing AI in medical education*, addresses the institutional, ethical, and technical challenges that hinder AI adoption. The final section, *Recommendations*, outlines actionable steps for educators, policymakers, and institutions to foster innovation and overcome existing limitations.

AI: ENHANCING CLINICAL REASONING AND PERSONALIZATION

AI refers to the capacity of computing systems to perform tasks typically associated with human intellect, such as learning, reasoning, problem-solving, perception, and decision-making (Martínez Asanza et al., 2024). According to Garcia et al. (2024), AI involves the creation of algorithms that enable machines to perform functions traditionally dependent on human intelligence. It is a branch of computer science focused on developing tools and software that allow machines to sense their environment and use intelligence and learning to respond in ways that increase the likelihood of achieving predefined objectives (Russell & Norvig, 2021).

In healthcare, AI is increasingly employed to improve various aspects of clinical practice. It is used in radiology to enhance diagnostic accuracy, facilitate faster diagnoses, support cancer screening, assist in clinical trials and robotic surgery, and generate predictions from "electronic health records" (EHRs) (Levingston et al., 2024). As AI technology continues to develop, it offers significant potential for transforming healthcare (Alowais et al., 2023; Martínez Asanza, 2025a). AI technologies have a wide range of applications in healthcare, including improving patient engagement and adherence to treatment plans, enhancing medical imaging and diagnostic services, combating pandemics, providing virtual patient care, and reducing administrative burdens on healthcare professionals (Al Kuwaiti et al., 2023; Levingston et al., 2024).

Moreover, AI is driving innovation in drug and vaccine development, monitoring patient compliance with rehabilitation exercises, and performing gait analyses for technology-assisted rehabilitation (Alowais et al., 2023). AI has also shown promise in improving clinical laboratory testing, enhancing illness detection accuracy, and increasing efficiency and cost-effectiveness. Additionally, AI can help monitor population health, optimize pharmaceutical choices, and provide precise, real-time information to guide healthcare decisions (Alowais et al., 2023; Martínez Asanza, 2025b; Mouloudj et al., 2025b).

The global healthcare delivery has been changed by the entry of an AI that automates routine procedures and helps relieve clinicians from excessive paperwork (Martínez Asanza, 2025a). Medical scribes are technologies that enable automatic recording of appointment notes and storing them in a patient's medical file, thus granting extra time for the physicians to interact directly with the patient. Papery form filling is simplified with the assistance of AI drafting letters to patients, summarizing medical history, and helping choose the most appropriate therapies. In addition, it helps specialists create the workflow for reading medical images by detecting the abnormality and optimizing their workflow (Martínez Asanza, 2024). By performing the abovementioned functions, AI reduces mental fatigue and increases the possibility of professional burnout. Another role of AI is for ensuring high-quality and safe care (Franco D'Souza et al., 2024). It can sift through data to identify at-risk patients for issues like sepsis or opioid dependency in order to trigger early intervention. AI algorithms help map out the terrains where medication errors occurred along with decision support for clinical choices that analyze like cases. AI equips practitioners to instantly access information pertaining to complex diagnoses and aid in the realization of personalized treatment plans for every patient. In cases of rare diseases, AI is able to assist in deciphering the possible diagnoses and treatments of record, thus fast-tracking patient care and improving overall patient outcomes (Bouarar et al., 2024; Ellis, 2024).

The integration of AI into healthcare systems has significantly enhanced patient care, reduced medical errors, and streamlined treatment planning (Levingston et al., 2024). AI holds immense promise and is expected to play a pivotal role in healthcare decision-making in the future. When implemented effectively, AI can alleviate the burden on healthcare professionals by reducing errors, increasing accuracy, and enhancing the quality of care. Additionally, it empowers patients by giving them more control over their health decisions, helps prevent unnecessary hospitalizations, and contributes to the expansion of medical knowledge. AI can also support the development of improved clinical guidelines, ultimately advancing the field of healthcare (Bajwa et al., 2021; Huo et al., 2025).

THE DIGITAL TRANSFORMATION OF MEDICAL EDUCATION

Just as AI has significantly impacted healthcare, it has also brought about profound changes in medical education (Bahroun et al., 2023). One of AI's key advantages is its efficiency: it can process and analyze vast datasets far more quickly than humans, operating continuously without the limitations of fatigue. This ensures not only high accuracy but also rapid performance (Levingston et al., 2024). In the realm of healthcare education, AI is particularly valuable. It supports personalized learning, simulates clinical scenarios for training purposes, and updates educational content to reflect the latest research and clinical practices (Tozsin et al., 2024). Medical education is a lifelong learning process that spans undergraduate, graduate, specialty training, and beyond. AI can enhance this process for doctors, nurses, and other healthcare professionals by streamlining complex tasks and improving overall efficiency (Tolsgaard et al., 2023).

The ongoing revolution in education, driven by rapid technological advancements, signifies not just incremental changes but a fundamental shift in how teaching and learning are approached (Bahroun et al., 2023; Masters, 2019). Educators who embrace AI and concepts like precision education can become pioneers in the field. They will play a crucial role in determining when AI and personalized learning approaches are most beneficial and when traditional methods might still offer greater reliability (Coates, 2025).

As technology rapidly transforms both healthcare and medical education, it necessitates a reevaluation of conventional teaching methods. This is essential in the context of continuous advancements in medical knowledge, diagnostic tools, and treatment strategies (Martínez Asanza et al., 2024). AI can be applied across several key areas of medical education, including learning, assessment, and curriculum development. It can manage complex tasks, enhance classification accuracy, and reduce the time required to analyze curricula. Moreover, AI can illustrate how various parameters within a curriculum interact. For example, AI can assess the effectiveness of a curriculum and gauge medical students' overall satisfaction with their educational experience. Additionally, AI facilitates personalized, adaptive learning, enabling students to pinpoint knowledge gaps and address them (Garg, 2020).

Tokuç and Varol (2023) examine AI's role in medical education, discussing the advantages and challenges of using digital learning tools. They emphasize the importance of preserving the human element in doctor-patient relationships, even as technological advancements shape the educational landscape.

Garg (2020) conducted a study demonstrating how AI can tailor medical education to individual students by processing large amounts of data and utilizing adaptive intelligence. This customization not only helps in improving knowledge retention but also aids in the comprehension of complex medical concepts (Martínez Asanza et al., 2024). Furthermore, AI-driven platforms enhance students' understanding of diagnoses and treatment plans, leading to improved clinical decision-making skills.

Medical education is undergoing a transformation driven by technology, customization, and collaboration. Dr. David H. Roberts of Harvard Medical School underscores that, in order to equip students for a dynamic profession, educators must anticipate change. Dr. Sarah K. Wood highlights that communication and problem-solving skills are nurtured through diverse perspectives and collaborative learning. Platforms offering "precision education" and other flexible, data-driven methods provide students with individualized instruction. While AI and other advanced technologies offer benefits such as virtual tutoring and automated learning, Roberts stresses that AI should complement human instruction rather than replace it. Institutions like Harvard Medical School and the Harvard Macy Institute are investing in professional development and innovation to ensure that students are prepared for the evolving demands of healthcare. Through promoting adaptability, personalized learning, and AI integration, medical education is increasingly aligned with the future needs of healthcare (Ellis, 2024).

Technology plays a crucial role in modernizing medical education, providing flexibility and a more tailored learning experience. With AI as a virtual tutor or learning assistant, medical students can receive immediate feedback, access supplemental materials, and evaluate their readiness through quizzes (Levingston et al., 2024). AI also enables the automated evaluation of written responses and offers reliable feedback on interpreting medical images (Tolsgaard et al., 2023). While the long-term effects of such technologies on performance remain uncertain, Moran et al. (2018) argue that tools like e-learning, simulations, and virtual reality are effective in enhancing medical students' knowledge and skills. Social media, audience response systems, and multimedia content have also shown promise in increasing student engagement, although concerns about professional boundaries and social isolation have been raised. The authors emphasize that while technology presents vast opportunities for educational innovation, it is crucial to strike a balance between digital resources and the human elements of medical education. To fully optimize the benefits, educators should develop strategies that not only integrate technology effectively but also foster students' interpersonal skills.

The advantages, difficulties, and tactics of integrating AI technologies in the classroom are examined by Owoc et al. (2021). The study emphasizes how technological developments and the ever-changing nature of learning environments have led to the growing significance of AI in education. The authors list the benefits of AI, including how it might improve student learning and help teachers with instructional duties. But there is also discussion of difficulties like opposition to change and the requirement for sufficient resources. To facilitate the acceptance and efficient use of AI technology in educational settings, a five-stage implementation strategy is put forth, along with tactics customized for various higher education institutions.

Technology has revolutionized knowledge acquisition and management in healthcare professional education, improving pedagogical techniques' efficacy and accessibility (Bouarar et al., 2024; Martínez Asanza et al., 2024). According to Frenk et al. (2010), the advent of knowledge management systems has lessened the need for memorization, although artificial intelligence and digital technologies are still essential to learning. Additionally, since the COVID-19 outbreak, pedagogical innovations like integrated learning and flipped classrooms have proliferated, allowing for remote instruction via telemedicine and simulations. Nevertheless, issues like unequal access to technology and screen weariness persist in spite of these developments. In order to prepare healthcare workers for a constantly changing environment, it will be crucial to further integrate artificial intelligence and improve technological competencies.

A systematic study by McGee et al. (2024) looked at how digital technologies affected medical students' clinical skills education, particularly during the COVID-19 pandemic. When compared to conventional in-person instruction, the review discovered that digital learning techniques yielded results that were either equal to or better. Additionally, research found that digital tools were cost-effective and had a favorable impact on student satisfaction and assessment scores. However, the most thorough learning experience was achieved by combining conventional and digital approaches. The long-term efficacy of blended and digital learning in the development of clinical skills should be the main focus of future studies.

According to Chowdhury et al. (2024), MedTech has advanced impressively from multimedia resources to the pervasive usage of internet platforms and virtual reality simulations. With the development of AI, AR, and customized learning resources, they anticipate even more promise. In order to properly train healthcare workers for the demands of current medical practice, the authors stress the necessity for a balanced strategy that combines conventional bedside instruction with contemporary techniques.

Altintas and Sahiner (2024) draw attention to how new medical gadgets and technology are revolutionizing medical education. They highlight how AI, mobile devices, and simulations may enhance learning results by facilitating safe practice, ongoing resource access, and individualized instruction. The authors emphasize the necessity for educational practices to adjust to these improvements and urge more study to examine the long-term advantages of these changes.

Also, Jha (2022) asserts that in order to attain the best learning results, the use of contemporary technology into medical education needs to be carefully coordinated with conventional teaching techniques. Digital tools improve accessibility, self-directed learning, and student engagement, but how well they work relies on how well teachers and students use them. Even though technology has many benefits, such as virtual simulations and personalized learning, it cannot completely replace practical clinical training. Therefore, to maximize educational efficacy in medical training, a balanced strategy that incorporates both classic and current teaching methodologies is necessary.

The integration of AI in medical education and healthcare is reviewed by Sun et al. (2024), who concentrate on its use in clinical training and continuing education, specifically in radiology, surgery, and cardiology. Although AI increases efficiency and accuracy, the authors emphasize that policymakers, medical professionals, and educators must work together to address ethical issues and develop regulatory standards. They also discovered that the majority of medical students are in favor of the inclusion of AI-related courses, despite the fact that the quality of research in this area is still low.

The three-step digitization strategy gives teachers an easy way to turn traditional lectures into interesting digital information, increasing concentration, decreasing distractions, and boosting students' well-being, according to a research by Gellischet al. (2024), although the findings in microscopic anatomy are encouraging, the authors point out that more study is necessary to assess its cross-disciplinary applicability and encourage the use of integrated learning.

Mistry et al. (2023) draw attention to the increasing significance of virtual reality (VR) in medical education, pointing out how it has developed from simple screen-based techniques to engaging, interactive simulations. Through the use of VR, students may participate in realistic situations that enhance clinical competency, critical thinking, and decision-making while lowering patient risk and increasing operational efficiency. Immersion VR training improves student performance, according to the review, which makes it a useful tool for upcoming medical curricula, particularly in terms of fostering clinical skills and guaranteeing patient safety.

In their study, Gómez-González et al. (2020) classify the present and near-term uses of AI in healthcare according to their technological, social, and ethical ramifications. The study examines a range of AI technologies, such as surgical robotics, augmented reality, genetic testing tools, software, and personal monitoring gadgets. The writers discuss the idea of "extended personalized medicine" and look at how artificial intelligence is upending conventional therapy. They also draw attention to how, in a society with digital connectivity, the roles of physicians and patients are evolving. Additionally, the paper examines possible hazards, like the separation of medicine into "fake-based," "patient-generated," and "scientifically tailored" methods, and calls for more public discussion and investigation of these findings.

As AI becomes more integrated into clinical workflows, Ma et al. (2024) examine the significance of fostering AI competencies in medical education. They found 18 papers that offer guiding frameworks and 11 that detail practical training on AI in medicine in their scoping review of 1,699 publications. According to the review, current rules for teaching AI place more emphasis on ethics and AI evaluation than on more technical subjects like coding and data science. Lack of precise definitions of AI literacy, a lack of evidence of its clinical utility, and a teacher scarcity are among the difficulties. To help medical students navigate the pre-clinical, clinical, and clinical research phases of AI education, the authors provide a thorough framework for AI literacy that is divided into four dimensions: foundational, practical, experimental, and ethical.

The growing use of AI technology in oncology, particularly in medical imaging for cancer detection, is examined by Coccia (2019). The work demonstrates how deep learning methods may be used to analyze medical images and detect breast and lung cancer, assisting pathologists in identifying metastases, gene alterations, and cancer subtypes. According to the study, the demand for more precise diagnosis and efficient treatment applications is what is driving the growing use of AI in cancer imaging, especially in high-mortality malignancies like breast and lung cancer. Although more research is required before this "mortality-driven" trend can be widely adopted to enhance diagnostic procedures, it has the potential to revolutionize cancer diagnoses.

Regarding students' perception a bouts AI and technology in medical education, research shows that they have a positive perception. For example, a study by Li and Qin (2023) showed that 54.3% of 1,243 undergraduate and graduate students from 13 universities and 33 hospitals who participated in the study acknowledged having used medical AI before. According to their research, medical postgraduate students were more knowledgeable about the use of medical AI than undergraduate students. Performance anticipation, habit, hedonic incentive, and trust were all positively correlated with the intention to utilize medical AI.

Another study discovered this issue. The results showed that medical students had an overall positive attitude towards AI (80.3%), with most of them viewing it as a credible (58.4%) and effective (60.8%) learning tool in medical education. Students concurred that AI learning gave them the most recent medical facts (63.1%) and maximized their study time (60.3%). Notably, 66.8% of students said AI provided them with more accurate answers to their medical questions, and 65.7% of students said AI was more effective in helping them understand medical ideas than more conventional resources like books and lectures. The study found that 59% of medical students believe that existing tools are becoming more and more antiquated, underscoring the significance of incorporating AI into medical education and developing specialized AI tools for medical education (80%) (Sami et al., 2025).

Furthermore, Busch et al. (2024) conducted a survey involving 4,313 medical students, 205 dental students, and 78 veterinary students from 192 educational institutions spanning 48 countries. The findings revealed that while students generally held favorable attitudes toward the integration of AI in healthcare and expressed interest in receiving more education on the topic, they also acknowledged having minimal knowledge of AI. Many reported a shortage of AI-related courses in their curricula and felt ill-equipped to apply AI technologies in their future professional practice. Moreover, Mouloudj et al. (2025a) found that students' intentions to adopt AI for language learning are significantly and positively impacted by perceived ease of use, perceived usefulness, supportive attitudes toward AI, and the level of perceived support.

Rapidly becoming obsolete are the traditional learning materials, emphasizing the tangible and immediate necessity for incorporating AI in modernizing medical education. Advances in technology have caused a newer development in the field of medicine, proving insufficient for future healthcare professionals to be trained based only on traditional textbooks and resources. Integration of AI in medical education helps create dynamic personalized interactive learning experiences tailored to individual student needs and clinical scenarios. It's also the requirement for building domain-specific AI tools, not just cutting edge in technology but appropriate to the ethical, applicative, and pedagogical requirements in medical training. They might be used for support in diagnostic reasoning, clinical decision-making, procedural simulations-they promise to bring the quality and effectiveness of medical education forward.

BARRIERS TO IMPLEMENTING AI IN MEDICAL EDUCATION

Despite the growing potential of AI to enhance medical education, several significant barriers continue to impede its widespread integration. Currently, medical schools have not fully incorporated AI into their curricula, primarily due to challenges such as a lack of faculty expertise, limited evidence supporting students' increasing interest in AI, and the absence of formal guidance from accreditation bodies like the Liaison Committee on Medical Education (Grunhut et al., 2022). As noted by Civaner et al. (2022), there are concerns that the use of AI in medicine could devalue the medical profession, undermine trust, and negatively impact the patient-physician relationship. The existing literature highlights a variety of challenges, including issues related to academic integrity, the accuracy of data, and the potential negative effects on the quality of learning (Preiksaitis & Rose, 2023). Additionally, there are significant ethical concerns, such as threats to data security, shifts in the dynamics of the patient-physician relationship, the emergence of social inequalities, and the growing presence of AI robots that could replace many professional roles, leading to increased unemployment rates (Hoffman et al., 2025; Civaner et al., 2022). These challenges are multifaceted and span institutional, ethical, technical, and human-resource dimensions. This section will examine four key obstacles to the integration of AI in medical education: institutional resistance, ethical concerns and data privacy issues, infrastructure limitations, and the lack of faculty training.

Institutional Resistance

The integration of generative AI into medical education holds significant promise, yet it is accompanied by notable challenges—foremost among them is institutional resistance to change (Preiksaitis & Rose, 2023). Medical education has long relied on traditional pedagogical methods, including lectures, textbooks, and standardized assessments. The emergence of AI, a relatively unfamiliar and sometimes misunderstood technology, is often viewed not as a complement to these practices but as a disruption.

One of the key sources of resistance stems from concerns among faculty. Educators may fear that AI could eventually replace their teaching roles or erode the value of human interaction within the learning process. Compounding this issue is institutional leadership's hesitation to invest in AI technologies, particularly in the absence of clear evidence demonstrating pedagogical efficacy or return on investment. This reluctance is especially pronounced in resource-limited settings, where educators often lack both the motivation and institutional backing necessary to adopt emerging technologies in their teaching environments.

A study by Hoffman et al. (2025) revealed that across multiple focus groups, participants identified a critical barrier: the lack of communication and strategic guidance from leadership. Managers, senior colleagues, and clinical governance bodies were often silent on the topic of AI, signaling a broader disengagement from institutional leadership in driving digital innovation.

This leadership gap is particularly detrimental in developing regions, where resource constraints further hinder the adoption of AI. Institutions in these areas continue to lag behind, exacerbating the divide between medical graduates in developing versus developed countries. Without sufficient exposure to AI-driven tools, students in under-resourced settings risk being underprepared for a healthcare landscape that increasingly relies on AI for clinical decision-making and diagnostics (Civaner, 2022; Naseer et al., 2025).

Both faculty and students have stressed the vital role of institutional support in navigating this transformation; such support must go beyond providing access to technology—it requires fostering a culture that embraces innovation, encourages interdisciplinary collaboration, and promotes adaptability (Naseer et al., 2025). Institutions must also address regulatory barriers that contribute to institutional inertia, including unresolved questions around liability, governance, and policy development (Hoffman et al., 2025). These regulatory uncertainties can create a climate of caution and delay among decision-makers, further slowing the integration of AI into educational practices.

Overcoming institutional resistance demands a cultural shift led by visionary leadership. Institutions must cultivate a mindset that views AI as a powerful tool for enhancing—rather than replacing—human educators. Engaging stakeholders early in the process, encouraging open dialogue, and showcasing successful pilot programs are all effective strategies for easing resistance and building momentum for sustainable change. With intentional leadership and inclusive planning, institutions can begin to bridge the gap between innovation and implementation.

Ethical Concerns and Data Privacy

Ethics plays a fundamental role in shaping decision-making and behavior, especially in the context of education and healthcare (Vu Lan Oanh et al., 2024). Although the integration of AI into medical education offers numerous benefits—such as personalized learning, advanced data analysis, and enhanced diagnostics—it also raises a host of ethical concerns that present significant barriers to full adoption (Bozorgi, 2023; Franco D'Souza et al., 2024).

One of the most pressing issues is the potential threat to academic integrity. As AI technologies become more advanced and accessible, concerns are growing over their misuse. Generative AI, for instance, may be used to artificially boost assessment performance, generate content falsely presented as student-authored, or bypass essential learning processes meant to foster critical thinking and skill development (Preiksaitis & Rose, 2023). These possibilities challenge the foundational principles of fairness and authenticity in education.

Ethical concerns extend far beyond academic dishonesty. Health professions educators and administrators face complex questions regarding data gathering, privacy, consent, anonymity, data ownership, security, bias, transparency, responsibility, autonomy, and beneficence (Masters, 2023). AI systems often rely on large datasets, which may include sensitive information about patients, students, and educators. Improper handling of this data—whether through design flaws or intentional breaches—can lead to severe consequences, including violations of privacy and loss of trust (Chan & Zary, 2019).

Indeed, Civaner et al. (2022) found that while 44.7% of participants believed they could maintain professional confidentiality while using AI applications, a significant minority (16.1%) expressed concern that AI could lead to confidentiality breaches. Similarly, nearly 94% of respondents in the same study emphasized the importance of receiving dedicated training to address ethical challenges associated with AI. These findings underscore the urgent need for targeted educational efforts to equip future healthcare professionals with the ethical literacy required to navigate AI's complexities.

As the digital landscape continues to evolve, the ethical dimensions of AI usage must be anticipated and addressed with vigilance (Bozorgi, 2023; Vu Lan Oanh et al., 2024; Masters, 2023). Ethical considerations are particularly relevant in regions where regulatory structures may be underdeveloped or inconsistently enforced. Grunhut et al. (2022) highlight that most current physicians lack adequate knowledge of the ethical frameworks necessary to responsibly incorporate AI in line with modern care standards. As AI becomes more embedded in clinical and educational settings, ensuring that healthcare professionals understand and uphold ethical standards becomes critical.

AI systems also present additional risks, including algorithmic bias, lack of transparency, and over-reliance on machine-generated decisions—all of which can diminish human judgment and reinforce existing inequalities (Nagi et al., 2023; Naseer et al., 2025). These issues are especially concerning in medical education, where the accuracy and fairness of AI-driven assessments and recommendations can significantly impact a student's learning path and future clinical competence.

To address these challenges, institutions must develop localized policies that reflect their unique cultural, ethical, and legal contexts. These policies should safeguard academic integrity, protect data privacy, and promote inclusivity (Awadallah Alkouk & Khlaif, 2024). Ensuring compliance with data protection laws—such as the General Data Protection Regulation (GDPR) in Europe or the Health Insurance

Portability and Accountability Act (HIPAA) in the U.S.—is essential. Moreover, ethical review boards should be actively involved in the deployment of AI systems that interact with personal or sensitive data within educational environments.

Franco D'Souza et al. (2024) propose twelve key recommendations for addressing ethical issues in AI integration. These include promoting transparency, mitigating bias, validating educational content, securing data privacy, obtaining informed consent, fostering collaboration, training faculty, empowering learners, conducting regular audits, ensuring accountability, adhering to ethical guidelines, and establishing dedicated ethics committees to oversee implementation processes. As leaders in healthcare, physicians have a critical role to play in promoting transparency and accountability in the use of AI technologies. Rampton et al. (2020) emphasize that physicians must engage patients in discussions about AI, recognize their varied responses to digital tools, and advocate for a culture that clearly discloses the commercial and institutional interests behind AI systems. Educators, likewise, must be prepared to anticipate and manage the ethical dilemmas that arise in AI-enhanced learning environments (Franco D'Souza et al., 2024). This includes championing the principles of ethical AI—transparency, fairness, accountability, and data protection—from the design phase through deployment and evaluation (Vu Lan Oanh et al., 2024; Coates, 2025).

In conclusion, the ethical integration of AI in medical education cannot be an afterthought—it must be foundational. Institutions must prioritize ethical design and implementation, align AI tools with professional values, and provide robust training and policy frameworks. Doing so will not only ensure the responsible use of AI but also foster trust, equity, and long-term success in transforming medical education for the future.

Infrastructure Limitations

The successful integration of AI into medical education requires robust digital infrastructure, including high-speed internet, advanced computing systems, secure data storage, and reliable software platforms. However, many educational institutions, particularly in low- and middle-income countries, face significant challenges in providing such infrastructure. The lack of financial and technical resources in these settings hinders not only the initial deployment of AI systems but also the ongoing maintenance, updates, and scalability of these technologies.

In resource-limited environments, these infrastructural deficiencies create substantial barriers to the adoption of AI in medical education. Naseer et al. (2025) highlight that students in Pakistan identified several barriers to AI integration, including technological constraints, financial limitations, and restricted access to AI tools. These challenges reflect broader socio-economic factors that hinder learners in developing regions from benefiting fully from AI-enhanced educational tools. The high cost of acquiring advanced AI technologies, coupled with minimal institutional support, further exacerbates the problem. This underscores the urgent need for educational institutions to make investments in both physical and digital infrastructure to create a level playing field for all students, regardless of their socio-economic background.

The challenge of integrating AI into educational contexts is not only a matter of financial resources. Chan and Zary (2019) identify two primary challenges when incorporating AI into medical education: first, the difficulty in evaluating the effectiveness of AI in enhancing educational outcomes, and second, the technical difficulties encountered during the development and adaptation of AI technologies to meet the needs of diverse learners. Both of these challenges require substantial infrastructure to address, particularly in institutions where resources are limited.

Students, recognizing these challenges, have voiced a demand for free institutional access to subscription-based AI tools; Naseer et al. (2025) note that such a demand presents an opportunity for academic institutions to play a pivotal role in addressing resource disparities. By providing equitable access to cutting-edge AI tools, institutions can help democratize the use of AI in education, ensuring that all students, regardless of their economic background, have the opportunity to benefit from personalized, data-driven learning experiences. Without foundational infrastructure—such as cloud-based computing services or high-capacity servers—AI-powered platforms cannot function effectively in real-world academic settings, leaving many students excluded from the advantages AI can offer. Moreover, the digital divide presents a growing concern in medical education, potentially exacerbating existing educational inequalities. Institutions that can afford to invest in AI technologies will gain a competitive advantage, while those unable to do so will fall further behind. This disparity risks widening the gap between students educated in well-resourced environments and those in underfunded institutions. Thus, investment in infrastructure—both digital and physical—is not only crucial for the effective deployment of AI in medical education, but also for ensuring that all students have equitable access to these transformative technologies.

To mitigate this issue, educational leaders must prioritize infrastructure development as part of a broader strategy to incorporate AI into medical curricula. Only with comprehensive support structures in place can AI truly enhance medical education in a way that is inclusive and beneficial to all students.

Lack of Faculty Training

To effectively integrate AI into medical education, educators must have at least a basic understanding of AI's role in teaching and learning, as well as its potential impact on medical education (Masters, 2019). The development of AI systems tailored for educational purposes requires specialized expertise in both the subject area and the technology itself to ensure that these tools are embedded with relevant curriculum content and aligned with the specific educational context (Chan & Zary, 2019). However, AI tools are only as effective as the educators who use them. Many medical educators currently lack the necessary training to incorporate AI meaningfully into their teaching practices. This includes not only technical skills, such as using AI-powered simulations or learning analytics, but also a conceptual understanding of AI's capabilities and limitations (Hoffman et al., 2025). At present, AI has yet to become a standard part of medical curricula, potentially leaving future healthcare professionals underprepared for an increasingly AI-driven work environment (Levingston et al., 2024). A study by [Author et al., 2023] revealed that many medical educators expressed uncertainty about how to interpret AI-generated data or apply it effectively in pedagogical contexts. Furthermore, according to Grunhut et al. (2022), modern physicians are often inadequately trained to routinely integrate AI-generated recommendations into clinical decision-making processes.

The lack of faculty training extends beyond clinical applications to patient-facing scenarios. Civaner et al. (2022) found that only 6% of participants felt confident in their ability to explain the features and risks associated with AI to patients. Additionally, 96.2% of participants expressed the need for further knowledge and skills related to AI applications, and 95.8% sought training in AI tools to reduce medical errors. This highlights a significant gap in medical education that needs to be addressed to ensure that healthcare providers can safely and effectively utilize AI technologies. Moreover, the rapid development of AI technologies in healthcare, along with their integration into clinical practice and increasing use by patients, underscores the need to train medical professionals in managing experimental methods that are not yet widely accepted as part of conventional medical knowledge (Rampton et al., 2020).

A key concern for educators and healthcare providers is the issue of data accuracy. AI systems are known to "hallucinate" or generate false information, which raises critical issues regarding their reliability in clinical decision-making and educational contexts (Preiksaitis & Rose, 2023). As such, professional development for educators is crucial. Institutions must provide ongoing training programs to help faculty build confidence in using AI, stay informed about technological advancements, and adapt their teaching strategies accordingly (Awadallah Alkouk & Khlaif, 2024). In addition, interdisciplinary collaboration between educators, data scientists, and instructional designers can create a more integrated and supportive environment for the adoption of AI tools. Chan and Zary (2019) emphasize that experts in both medicine and education will need to work closely with data scientists to design AI tools that are not only technically accurate but also impactful in the context of medical education. Rampton et al. (2020) further suggest that physicians and educators will benefit from enhancing their digital literacy and engaging in ongoing education about AI, mathematical modeling, decision theory, and related fields. This is closely tied to recognizing biases in data and understanding how these biases can undermine claims that AI models offer objective, neutral outcomes.

In conclusion, the integration of AI into medical education is not simply about introducing new tools; it involves navigating complex institutional cultures, ethical frameworks, technical infrastructure, and the competencies of educators. Without addressing these foundational barriers, the full potential of AI-enhanced learning cannot be realized. A coordinated approach involving policy reforms, faculty development, infrastructure investment, and ethical oversight will be essential to ensure AI serves as a catalyst for innovation rather than a source of disruption or division.

RECOMMENDATIONS

To fully harness the potential of AI in medical education, a coordinated effort from all stakeholders—academic institutions, faculty, policymakers, technology developers, and accreditation bodies—is essential. First and foremost, medical schools and universities must cultivate an institutional culture that is receptive to innovation. AI should be integrated into the curriculum as a continuous component within existing disciplines (Grunhut et al., 2022). This requires strategic planning, clear leadership commitment, and the alignment of AI with long-term educational goals. Institutions must invest in the necessary digital infrastructure, including secure data systems, simulation labs, and cloud-based learning platforms that support AI technologies. Moreover, curricula must be updated to incorporate AI literacy, data ethics, and interdisciplinary competencies to ensure that students are well-prepared for AI-enhanced clinical environments. Several authors emphasize the importance of establishing well-defined policies regarding the appropriate use of generative AI in medical education (Preiksaitis & Rose, 2023). In this regard, Civaner et al. (2022) highlight the need to revise the medical curriculum to meet the demands of an AI-driven healthcare system.

Second, equally crucial is the development of faculty competencies to effectively integrate AI into teaching and assessment. Educators must be equipped with both the technical skills and conceptual understanding of AI's capabilities and limitations (Hoffman et al., 2025). This requires continuous professional development programs, mentorship from tech-savvy colleagues, and opportunities for educators to experiment with AI tools in low-risk settings. To ensure that future physicians are proficient in utilizing AI applications while maintaining professional values and rights, medical curricula should be updated accordingly (Civaner et al., 2022). Additionally, teacher training programs should focus on fostering critical thinking, creativity, and adaptability—essential skills for navigating the evolving landscape of AI-driven education (Awadallah Alkouk & Khlaif, 2024). Institutions should incentivize faculty participation in training programs through workload adjustments, recognition, and funding support for research on AI-enhanced pedagogy. Collaborative efforts between educators and developers will also help create more user-friendly tools that align with teaching needs and pedagogical objectives.

Third, policymakers and accreditation bodies have a pivotal role in fostering an environment conducive to AI integration. They must establish regulatory frameworks that promote innovation while ensuring ethical and equitable use of AI in education. These frameworks should address critical issues such as data governance, student privacy, and digital inclusion. Accreditation standards should evolve to recognize and reward institutions that responsibly incorporate AI into their programs. Funding agencies can further support these efforts by prioritizing grants and scholarships that encourage the use of technology in teaching and AI-related educational research.

Finally, Technology developers and EdTech companies must collaborate closely with medical educators to create AI tools that are pedagogically sound, ethically robust, and technically reliable. Co-design approaches involving educators, students, and IT specialists can ensure that AI tools are intuitive, relevant, and adaptable to diverse learning environments. Developers should also prioritize transparency by clearly disclosing the data sources used to train AI systems, allowing users to understand and challenge the outputs generated. This collaborative approach will help establish AI as a trusted and effective tool in the advancement of medical education.

CONCLUSION

The integration of technology and AI into medical education represents a transformative shift in how future healthcare professionals are trained. From adaptive learning platforms and intelligent tutoring systems to virtual simulations and diagnostic AI tools, these innovations provide unprecedented opportunities to enhance clinical reasoning, personalize learning experiences, and bridge the gap between theory and real-world practice. As explored throughout this chapter, AI has the potential to revolutionize not only the content and delivery of medical education but also the very pedagogical frameworks that underpin it.

However, this transformation is not without significant challenges. Persistent barriers—such as institutional resistance, ethical dilemmas, data privacy concerns, infrastructure limitations, and insufficient faculty training—continue to hinder the seamless and equitable adoption of AI in educational settings. These obstacles risk deepening disparities between institutions and regions, particularly in resource-constrained environments. Addressing them requires a unified commitment to fostering institutional readiness, developing ethical and regulatory frameworks, investing in digital infrastructure, and building educator capacity. Moreover, as Preiksaitis and Rose (2023) observe, while the literature reflects both enthusiasm and caution about AI's role in medical education, the broader perspectives of educators remain largely underexplored.

Moving forward, a strategic and collaborative approach is essential. Academic institutions must lead with vision and targeted investment. Faculty should be supported through continuous professional development and access to AI-driven teaching tools. Policymakers must create regulatory environments that encourage innovation while safeguarding ethical and equitable use. Meanwhile, technology developers must work closely with educators and students to design tools that are pedagogically sound, ethically grounded, and practically usable.

Ultimately, AI and digital technologies are not mere add-ons—they are actively reshaping the foundation of medical education. If harnessed responsibly and inclusively, these tools can help create more adaptive, effective, and equitable learning environments. To fully realize this potential, ongoing research, interdisciplinary collaboration, and reflective practice are essential. Together, these efforts can ensure that technology enhances—not disrupts—the core mission of medical education: to cultivate skilled, ethical, and compassionate healthcare professionals prepared for the demands of an evolving healthcare landscape.

ACKNOWLEDGMENT

This research received no specific grant from any funding agency in the public, commercial, or not-for-profit sectors.

REFERENCES

Al Kuwaiti, A., Nazer, K., Al-Reedy, A., Al-Shehri, S., Al-Muhanna, A., Subbarayalu, A. V., Al Muhanna, D., & Al-Muhanna, F. A. (2023). A Review of the Role of Artificial Intelligence in Healthcare. *Journal of Personalized Medicine*, *13*(6), 951. DOI: 10.3390/jpm13060951 PMID: 37373940

Alowais, S. A., Alghamdi, S. S., Alsuhebany, N., Alqahtani, T., Alshaya, A. I., Almohareb, S. N., Aldairem, A., Alrashed, M., Bin Saleh, K., Badreldin, H. A., Al Yami, M. S., Al Harbi, S., & Albekairy, A. M. (2023). Revolutionizing healthcare: The role of artificial intelligence in clinical practice. *BMC Medical Education*, *23*(1), 689. DOI: 10.1186/s12909-023-04698-z PMID: 37740191

Altintas, L., & Sahiner, M. (2024). Transforming medical education: The impact of innovations in technology and medical devices. *Expert Review of Medical Devices*, *21*(9), 797–809. DOI: 10.1080/17434440.2024.2400153 PMID: 39235206

Awadallah Alkouk, W., & Khlaif, Z. N. (2024). AI-resistant assessments in higher education: Practical insights from faculty training workshops. *Frontiers in Education*, *9*, 1499495. DOI: 10.3389/feduc.2024.1499495

Bahroun, Z., Anane, C., Ahmed, V., & Zacca, A. (2023). Transforming education: A comprehensive review of generative artificial intelligence in educational settings through bibliometric and content analysis. *Sustainability (Basel)*, *15*(17), 12983. DOI: 10.3390/su151712983

Bajwa, J., Munir, U., Nori, A., & Williams, B. (2021). Artificial intelligence in healthcare: Transforming the practice of medicine. *Future Healthcare Journal*, *8*(2), e188–e194. DOI: 10.7861/fhj.2021-0095 PMID: 34286183

Bouabdellah, M. (2023). Digital Innovation in Healthcare. In Bouarar, A., Mouloudj, K., & Martínez Asanza, D. (Eds.), *Integrating Digital Health Strategies for Effective Administration* (pp. 1–19). IGI Global., DOI: 10.4018/978-1-6684-8337-4.ch001

Bouarar, A. C., Asanza, D. M., Mouloudj, S., Bouarar, A., Mouloudj, K., & Bozorgi, M. (2024). Elderly's Intention to Use Teledentistry Services: Antecedents and Challenges. In Martínez Asanza, D. (Ed.), *Geriatric Dentistry in the Age of Digital Technology* (pp. 101–116). IGI Global., DOI: 10.4018/979-8-3693-0260-6.ch004

Busch, F., Hoffmann, L., Truhn, D., Ortiz-Prado, E., Makowski, M. R., Bressem, K. K., Adams, L. C., Abdala, N., Navarro, Á. A., Aerts, H. J. W. L., Águas, C., Aineseder, M., Alomar, M., Angkurawaranon, S., Angus, Z. G., Asouchidou, E., Bakhshi, S., Bamidis, P. D., Barbosa, P. N. V. P., & Zhang, L. (2024). Global cross-sectional student survey on AI in medical, dental, and veterinary education and practice at 192 faculties. *BMC Medical Education*, *24*(1), 1066. DOI: 10.1186/s12909-024-06035-4 PMID: 39342231

Chan, K. S., & Zary, N. (2019). Applications and challenges of implementing artificial intelligence in medical education: Integrative review. *JMIR Medical Education*, *5*(1), e13930. https://preprints.jmir.org/preprint/13930. DOI: 10.2196/13930 PMID: 31199295

Chowdhury, P. N., Vaish, A., Puri, B., & Vaishya, R. (2024). Medical education technology: Past, present and future. *Apollo Medicine*, *21*(4), 374–380. DOI: 10.1177/09760016241256202

Civaner, M. M., Uncu, Y., Bulut, F., Chalil, E. G., & Tatli, A. (2022). Artificial intelligence in medical education: A cross-sectional needs assessment. *BMC Medical Education*, *22*(1), 772. DOI: 10.1186/s12909-022-03852-3 PMID: 36352431

Coates, W. C. (2025). Precision education–a call to action to transform medical education. *International Journal of Emergency Medicine*, *18*(1), 21. DOI: 10.1186/s12245-025-00819-1 PMID: 39924527

Coccia, M. (2019). Artifical intelligence technology in cancer imaging: Clinical challenges for detection of lung and breast cancer. *Journal of Social and Administrative Sciences*, *6*(2), 82–98. DOI: 10.1453/jsas.v6i2.1888

Ellis, L. D. (August 30, 2024). Exploring current trends in medical education. Harvard Medical School. https://postgraduateeducation.hms.harvard.edu/trends-medicine/benefits-latest-ai-technologies-patients-clinicians

Franco D'Souza, R., Mathew, M., Mishra, V., & Surapaneni, K. M. (2024). Twelve tips for addressing ethical concerns in the implementation of artificial intelligence in medical education. *Medical Education Online*, *29*(1), 2330250. DOI: 10.1080/10872981.2024.2330250 PMID: 38566608

Frenk, J., Chen, L. C., Chandran, L., Groff, E. O. H., King, R., Meleis, A., & Fineberg, H. V. (2022). Challenges and opportunities for educating health professionals after the COVID-19 pandemic. *Lancet*, *400*(10362), 1539–1556. DOI: 10.1016/S0140-6736(22)02092-X PMID: 36522209

Garcia, M. B., Arif, Y. M., Khlaif, Z. N., Zhu, M., de Almeida, R. P., de Almeida, R. S., & Masters, K. (2024). Effective Integration of Artificial Intelligence in Medical Education: Practical Tips and Actionable Insights. In Garcia, M., & de Almeida, R. (Eds.), *Transformative Approaches to Patient Literacy and Healthcare Innovation* (pp. 1–19). IGI Global., DOI: 10.4018/979-8-3693-3661-8.ch001

Garg, T. (2020). Artificial intelligence in medical education. *The American Journal of Medicine*, *133*(2), e68. DOI: 10.1016/j.amjmed.2019.08.017 PMID: 31954481

Gellisch, M., Morosan-Puopolo, G., Brand-Saberi, B., & Schäfer, T. (2024). Adapting to new challenges in medical education: A three-step digitization approach for blended learning. *BMC Medical Education*, *24*(1), 1–15. DOI: 10.1186/s12909-024-05503-1 PMID: 38807088

Gómez-González, E., Gomez, E., Márquez-Rivas, J., Guerrero-Claro, M., Fernández-Lizaranzu, I., Relimpio-López, M. I., & Capitán-Morales, L. (2020). Artificial intelligence in medicine and healthcare: A review and classification of current and near-future applications and their ethical and social. *Impact.* Advance online publication. arXiv2001.09778. DOI: 10.48550/arXiv.2001.09778

Grunhut, J., Marques, O., & Wyatt, A. T. (2022). Needs, challenges, and applications of artificial intelligence in medical education curriculum. *JMIR Medical Education*, *8*(2), e35587. DOI: 10.2196/35587 PMID: 35671077

Hoffman, J., Wenke, R., Angus, R. L., Shinners, L., Richards, B., & Hattingh, L. (2025). Overcoming barriers and enabling artificial intelligence adoption in allied health clinical practice: A qualitative study. *Digital Health*, *11*, 20552076241311144. DOI: 10.1177/20552076241311144 PMID: 39906878

Huo, W., Li, Q., Liang, B., Wang, Y., & Li, X. (2025). When healthcare professionals use AI: Exploring work well-being through psychological needs satisfaction and job complexity. *Behavioral Sciences (Basel, Switzerland)*, *15*(1), 88. DOI: 10.3390/bs15010088 PMID: 39851892

Jha, S. (2022). Role of technology in medical education: SWOC analysis. *SBV Journal of Basic. Clinical and Applied Health Science*, *5*(1), 19–21. DOI: 10.5005/jp-journals-10082-03131

Köse, A. (2023). Artificial Intelligence in Health and Applications. In Bouarar, A., Mouloudj, K., & Martínez Asanza, D. (Eds.), *Integrating Digital Health Strategies for Effective Administration* (pp. 20–31). IGI Global., DOI: 10.4018/978-1-6684-8337-4.ch002

Levingston, H., Anderson, M. C., & Roni, M. A. (2024). From theory to practice: Artificial intelligence (AI) literacy course for first-year medical students. *Cureus*, *16*(10), e70706. DOI: 10.7759/cureus.70706 PMID: 39493023

Li, Q., & Qin, Y. (2023). AI in medical education: Medical student perception, curriculum recommendations and design suggestions. *BMC Medical Education*, *23*(1), 1–18. DOI: 10.1186/s12909-023-04700-8 PMID: 37946176

Ma, Y., Song, Y., Balch, J. A., Ren, Y., Vellanki, D., Hu, Z., Shickel, B. (2024). Promoting AI competencies for medical students: a scoping review on frameworks, programs, and tools. *arXiv preprint*:2407.18939. https://doi.org/10.48550/arXiv.2407.18939

Martínez Asanza, D. (Ed.). (2024). *Geriatric Dentistry in the Age of Digital Technology*. IGI Global., DOI: 10.4018/979-8-3693-0260-6

Martínez Asanza, D. (2025a). Emerging Trends and Future Perspectives in Digital Dentistry for Rural Areas: An Update. In Martínez Asanza, D. (Ed.), *Transforming Dental Health in Rural Communities: Digital Dentistry* (pp. 1–20). IGI Global., DOI: 10.4018/979-8-3693-7165-7.ch001

Martínez Asanza, D. (Ed.). (2025b). *Transforming Dental Health in Rural Communities: Digital Dentistry*. IGI Global., DOI: 10.4018/979-8-3693-7165-7

Martínez Asanza, D., Rojas Herrera, I. A., Njoku, A. U., Reyes Puig, A. C., Mouloudj, F., Capote, I. G., & Maupome, G. (2024). Study Plans and Programs Supporting Geriatric Dentistry Teaching in Cuba: An Update. In Martínez Asanza, D. (Ed.), *Geriatric Dentistry in the Age of Digital Technology* (pp. 174–191). IGI Global., DOI: 10.4018/979-8-3693-0260-6.ch007

Masters, K. (2019). Artificial intelligence in medical education. *Medical Teacher*, *41*(9), 976–980. DOI: 10.1080/0142159X.2019.1595557 PMID: 31007106

Masters, K. (2023). Ethical use of artificial intelligence in health professions education: AMEE Guide No. 158. *Medical Teacher*, *45*(6), 574–584. DOI: 10.1080/0142159X.2023.2186203 PMID: 36912253

McGee, R. G., Wark, S., Mwangi, F., Drovandi, A., Alele, F., & Malau-Aduli, B. S.ACHIEVE Collaboration. (2024). Digital learning of clinical skills and its impact on medical students' academic performance: A systematic review. *BMC Medical Education, 24*(1), 1477. DOI: 10.1186/s12909-024-06471-2 PMID: 39696150

Mistry, D., Brock, C. A., & Lindsey, T. (2023). The present and future of virtual reality in medical education: A narrative review. *Cureus, 15*(12), e51124. DOI: 10.7759/cureus.51124 PMID: 38274907

Moran, J., Briscoe, G., & Peglow, S. (2018). Current technology in advancing medical education: Perspectives for learning and providing care. *Academic psychiatry: the journal of the American Association of Directors of Psychiatric Residency Training and the Association for Academic Psychiatry, 42*(6), 796–799. https://doi.org/DOI: 10.1007/s40596-018-0946-y

Mouloudj, F., Aljaeed, S. A., & Asanza, D. M. (2025a). Understanding Students' Intentions to Use AI for English Language Learning. In Ali, M., Anwar, M., Fazal, S., & Ayyaz, S. (Eds.), *AI Applications for English Language Learning* (pp. 157–178). IGI Global., DOI: 10.4018/979-8-3693-9077-1.ch007

Mouloudj, K., Bouarar, A. C., Martínez Asanza, D. A., & Dimitrova, M. (2025b). Understanding Customers' Intentions to use Digital Dental Health Services: An Expanded Technology Acceptance Model. In Martínez Asanza, D. (Ed.), *Transforming Dental Health in Rural Communities: Digital Dentistry* (pp. 173–194). IGI Global., DOI: 10.4018/979-8-3693-7165-7.ch007

Mouloudj, K., Vu Lan Oanh, L., Bouarar, A., Bouarar, A. C., Asanza, D. M., & Srivastava, M. (2024). Adopting Artificial Intelligence in Healthcare: A Narrative Review. In Teixeira, S., & Remondes, J. (Eds.), *The use of Artificial Intelligence in Digital Marketing: Competitive Strategies and Tactics* (pp. 1–20). IGI Global., DOI: 10.4018/978-1-6684-9324-3.ch001

Nagi, F., Salih, R., Alzubaidi, M., Shah, H., Alam, T., Shah, Z., & Househ, M. (2023). Applications of artificial intelligence (AI) in medical education: A scoping review. *Studies in Health Technology and Informatics, 305*, 648–651. DOI: 10.3233/SHTI230581 PMID: 37387115

Naseer, M. A., Saeed, S., Afzal, A., Ali, S., & Malik, M. G. R. (2025). Navigating the integration of artificial intelligence in the medical education curriculum: A mixed-methods study exploring the perspectives of medical students and faculty in Pakistan. *BMC Medical Education, 25*(1), 273. DOI: 10.1186/s12909-024-06552-2 PMID: 39979912

Owoc, M. L., Sawicka, A., & Weichbroth, P. (2021). Artificial intelligence technologies in education: Benefits, challenges and strategies of implementation. In *IFIP advances in information and communication technology*. Springer International Publishing.

Patel, V. L., Yoskowitz, N. A., & Arocha, J. F. (2009). Towards effective evaluation and reform in medical education: A cognitive and learning sciences perspective. *Advances in Health Sciences Education : Theory and Practice*, *14*(5), 791–812. DOI: 10.1007/s10459-007-9091-1 PMID: 18214707

Preiksaitis, C., & Rose, C. (2023). Opportunities, challenges, and future directions of generative artificial intelligence in medical education: Scoping review. *JMIR Medical Education*, *9*, e48785. DOI: 10.2196/48785 PMID: 37862079

Rampton, V., Mittelman, M., & Goldhahn, J. (2020). Implications of artificial intelligence for medical education. *The Lancet. Digital Health*, *2*(3), e111–e112. DOI: 10.1016/S2589-7500(20)30023-6 PMID: 33328081

Russell, S. J., & Norvig, P. (2021). *Artificial Intelligence: A Modern Approach* (4th ed.). Pearson.

Sami, A., Tanveer, F., Sajwani, K., Kiran, N., Javed, M. A., Ozsahin, D. U., Muhammad, K., & Waheed, Y. (2025). Medical students' attitudes toward AI in education: Perception, effectiveness, and its credibility. *BMC Medical Education*, *25*(1), 1–12. DOI: 10.1186/s12909-025-06704-y PMID: 39833834

Sun, L., Yin, C., Xu, Q., & Zhao, W. (2023). Artificial intelligence for healthcare and medical education: A systematic review. *American Journal of Translational Research*, *15*(7), 4820–4828. PMID: 37560249

Tokuç, B., & Varol, G. (2023). Medical Education in the Era of Advancing Technology. *Balkan Medical Journal*, *40*(6), 395–399. DOI: 10.4274/balkanmedj.galenos.2023.2023-7-79 PMID: 37706676

Tolsgaard, M. G., Pusic, M. V., Sebok-Syer, S. S., Gin, B., Svendsen, M. B., Syer, M. D., Brydges, R., Cuddy, M. M., & Boscardin, C. K. (2023). The fundamentals of Artificial Intelligence in medical education research: AMEE Guide No. 156. *Medical Teacher*, *45*(6), 565–573. DOI: 10.1080/0142159X.2023.2180340 PMID: 36862064

Tozsin, A., Ucmak, H., Soyturk, S., Aydin, A., Gozen, A. S., Fahim, M. A., Güven, S., & Ahmed, K. (2024). The role of artificial intelligence in medical education: A systematic review. *Surgical Innovation*, *31*(4), 415–423. DOI: 10.1177/15533506241248239 PMID: 38632898

Vu Lan Oanh, L., Tettamanzi, P., Tien Minh, D., Comoli, M., Mouloudj, K., Murgolo, M., & Dang Thu Hien, M. (2024). How ethical behavior is considered in different contexts: A bibliometric analysis of global research trends. *Administrative Sciences*, *14*(9), 200. DOI: 10.3390/admsci14090200

KEY TERMS AND DEFINITIONS

Artificial Intelligence (AI): A branch of computer science focused on creating systems capable of performing tasks that normally require human intelligence, such as decision-making, problem-solving, and learning.

Data Privacy: The protection of personal or sensitive information from unauthorized access, use, or disclosure, especially in the context of digital learning tools and educational data.

Digital Transformation: The integration of digital technologies into all areas of education, fundamentally changing how teaching, learning, and assessment are designed and delivered.

EdTech (Education Technology): The use of digital tools and technologies to support, enhance, and optimize teaching and learning processes across various educational settings.

Ethical Concerns: Moral questions or dilemmas that arise from the use of AI and technology, such as fairness, bias, transparency, and responsibility in decision-making processes.

Faculty Development: Institutional efforts to enhance the teaching, technical, and professional skills of educators, particularly in adapting to innovations like AI in the classroom.

Infrastructure Limitations: The lack of essential digital resources, such as high-speed internet, computing devices, or secure data storage systems that hinders the adoption of new technologies.

Personalized Learning: An educational approach that tailors learning experiences, content, and pacing to the individual needs, preferences, and progress of each student, often supported by AI tools.

Chapter 4
AI for Personalized Learning in Medical Education

Hayatullah Niazai
Ahmad Shah Abdali Medical College, Afghanistan

Wali Khan Monib
https://orcid.org/0000-0002-9575-9305
Shaikh Zayed University, Afghanistan

ABSTRACT

Personalized learning involves tailoring learning experiences to individual learners' needs, preferences, and progress. However, ensuring personalized learning remains a challenging task. Artificial intelligence (AI) usage can be an opportunity to enhance personalized learning. This chapter explores AI role in enhancing personalized learning in medical education. The chapter covers content development, AI-assisted tutoring, adaptive case-based learning, automated assessments, immediate feedback, and clinical decision-making in personalized medical education. It further discusses AI in conducting literature reviews and knowledge synthesis in medical education. Moreover, it provides insights into AI risks and ethical considerations in medical education, including potential bias, data privacy, accuracy and reliability challenges, and over-reliance on this technology. It emphasizes the need to promote AI literacy among medical learners, offering insights into effective AI-assisted personalized learning in medical education.

DOI: 10.4018/979-8-3373-1519-5.ch004

1. INTRODUCTION

The world is advancing rapidly, and there is a vast transformation in various aspects of our lives where we need new skills, competencies, and ways of learning (Abubakari et al., 2024; Monib, 2023). The transformation has been deep in the education landscape, particularly in medical education, driven by the technological wave (Salloum et al., 2024). There is mounting pressure to adjust continually to technological and educational changes (Çakmakkaya et al., 2025). Didactic methods commonly do not meet the needs for interactive and personalized learning that a medical education program calls for (Salloum et al., 2024), in keeping with sustaining engagement or helping students develop skills in critical thinking (Ali et al., 2025). It tends to be fairly good in finding solutions to only part of it, dealing with just the ever-growing body of knowledge and ever-shifting science, more and more complex concepts to teach and learn (Aslam & Nisar, 2023), and a diverse range of learning needs among learners. To some degree, the answer to those challenges has been personalized learning, which offers some solutions by creating learning experiences built around individual competencies, learning styles, and progress. But is it still applicable at scale due to resource constraints and curriculum complexities? In this context, perhaps AI would offer a more fitting concept for personalizing medical learning. In its basic form, it may enhance learning through content adaptability, instant diagnostics, and virtual simulations calibrated to every learner's learning requirements. This can support diagnostic reasoning, procedural training, and clinical decision support, extracting learning patterns to prescribe personal guidance to fill critical gaps in static education models. This chapter aims to conduct a comprehensive review of AI for personalized learning in medical education. The chapter is organized into sections, as depicted in Figure 1. Section 2 explores literature, including (1) personalized learning and (2) an overview of AI. Section 3 encompasses the method. Section 4 is about the results and discussion, including (1) AI usage, (2) AI risks, (3) AI literacy, and (4) case studies. Section 5 presents the conclusion. Section 6 highlights the limitations, and Section 7 provides directions for future research.

Figure 1. Structure of the Chapter (Authors' Creation Using Napkin.ai)

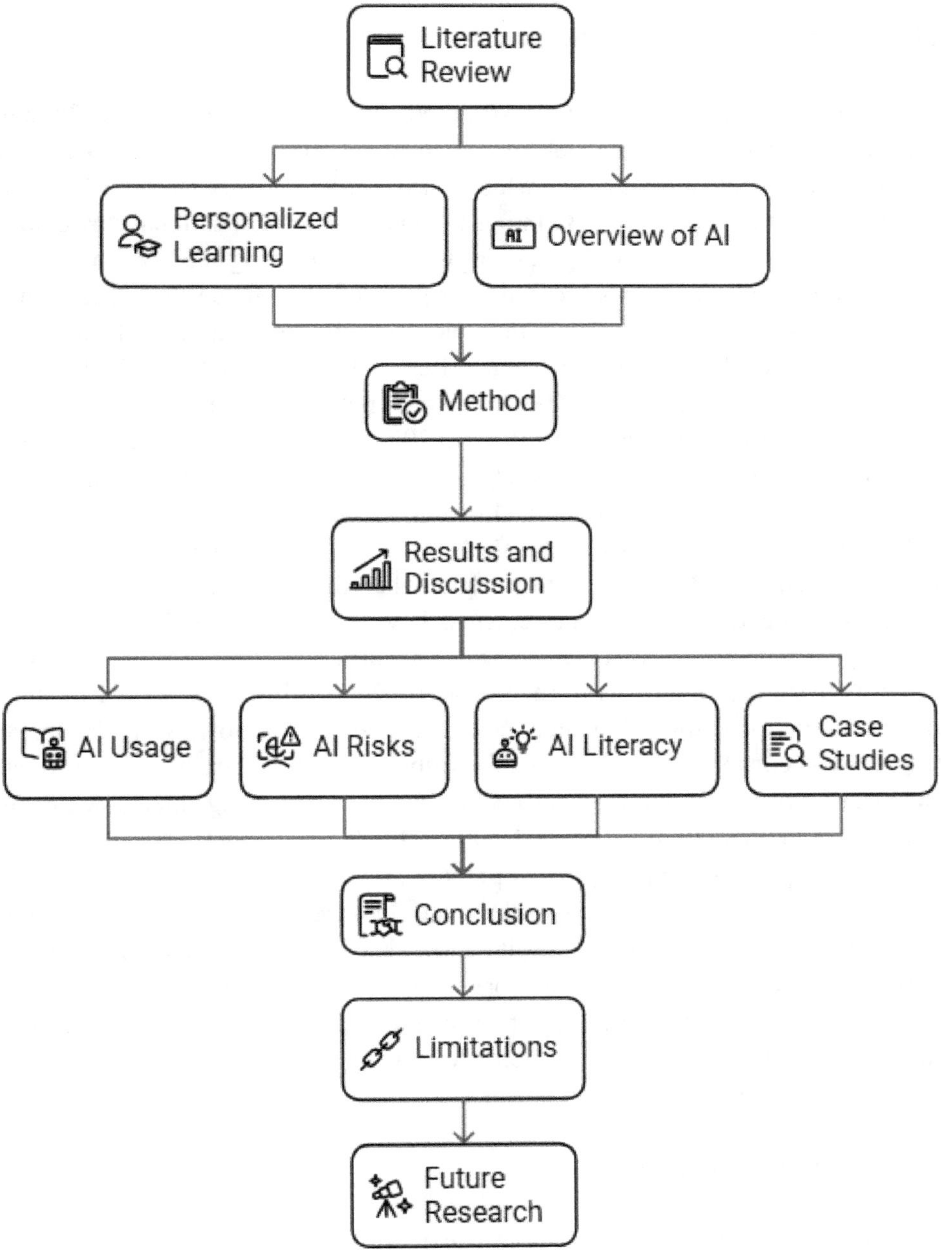

2. LITERATURE REVIEW

2.1. Personalized Learning

Educational needs are growing as fast as medical science moves forward (Rhoney et al., 2021). The success of the most modern medical services is directly connected to well-trained healthcare providers, which places medical education at the forefront of higher education disciplines. By imposing one standardized national curriculum for all learners without considering adapting to different learning needs and styles, the traditional medical education system hinders the success of modernized healthcare services. The same national curriculum cannot be applied to the quality of education practice across levels (Karataş et al., 2024). Research has proven that a rigid curriculum may not engage learners well because it does not consider learners' differential learning capabilities (Martin-Alguacil et al., 2024). Indeed, learners differ in their capability to acquire and retain knowledge, way of learning, objectives, motivation, and effort—all of which can affect the learning process.

A learning experience based on the skill and pace of each learner can be achieved through personalized learning. For example, when the educational process is designed according to individual requirements, they can better gain and apply medical knowledge in practice. Research has shown that learner-centered learning enhances the ability of students to retain information and develop skills, such as critical thinking and problem-solving, in medical education; new and innovative pedagogical technology is converging toward feasible, fully personalized learning for medical students. Recent evidence tells us well about personalized learning, thus showing this convergence trend and preparing medical learners for varied patient-care settings. However, to optimize the pedagogical process through the personalization path, a deep knowledge of each learner's background, knowledge, engagement, learning style, and preference is needed. Thus, it is very challenging to personalize learning according to the needs of individual learners. On the other hand, the development of AI, especially GenAI, speeds up the process of eliminating this problem. For example, ChatGPT, as a GenAI tool, can offer content retrieved in several languages and customized for diverse learning needs.

2.2. An Overview of AI

Artificial intelligence (AI) can be understood simply by imitating human intelligence processes with machines, especially computer systems (Mitra & Chitra, 2024). In contrast to the natural intelligence displayed by humans and animals, AI is demonstrated by machines whose known intellectual features include learning (the acquisition of information and rules for using the information), reasoning (the use of rules to attain definite conclusions), and creativity (such as playing chess). AI includes executing tasks by computer systems that would typically require human intelligence, such as developing tasks that require human intelligence, using algorithms and neural networks with machine learning and deep learning. There are three categories of AI: narrow, general, and super (Thayyib et al., 2023). Narrow consists of those systems developed to operate very efficiently within a specific domain, such as robotics, machine learning, natural language processing, and computer vision (Rashid & Kausik, 2024). This is the only type of AI used today; the others are hypothetical. General AI is a theoretical concept about machinery that will perform human functions autonomously at par with human cognitive capabilities, while Super AI is another theoretical concept above human intelligence. No actual systems now fit into the categories of general AI or super AI (IBM Data and AI Team, 2023). It is further maintained that all existing systems, including language models, image recognition, and self-driving cars, qualify as narrow AI.

Based on functionality, they categorized AI into theory of mind AI, self-aware AI, reactive AI, and limited memory AI. Theory of Mind AI is a class of AI under General AI. Although this type of AI is unattained, it will understand thoughts and emotions and be able to simulate human-like relationships. This AI could infer human motives, personalizing interactions based on emotional needs. It would also contextualize artwork and essays, unlike current GenAI tools. Self-aware AI, another theoretical class, would possess super AI capabilities, understanding its traits and human emotions, with emotions and beliefs of its own. Reactive AI and limited memory AI fall under narrow AI. Reactive AI involves systems that react based on presently available data with no memory, exemplified by IBM Deep Blue. Limited Memory AI can keep and remember past events and outcomes. It uses past and current data to determine the best action to achieve a goal. However, this type of AI only retains past data for a limited time and cannot store information for long-term use. Examples include virtual assistants like Siri and Alexa, using natural language processing combined with Limited Memory AI; self-driving cars, which understand their environment in real-time to make informed decisions on speed and direction; and GenAI tools like ChatGPT and Bard, which predict content. GenAI represents a subset within a broader classification of AI that can create unique and original content, such as text, images, sounds, or other forms of media (Monib, Qazi, Apong, et al., 2024). It does so by learning from existing data and generating new examples resembling the learned patterns. Suppose a GenAI model is trained on different paintings; it can create entirely new artwork, generating novel output rather than merely replicas. Conversely, non-GenAI systems typically analyze, classify, or manipulate data without creating novel content. The AI model trained to detect fake artwork is non-generative; instead, it analyses authenticity.

3. METHOD

This chapter employs a comprehensive literature review of AI in personalized learning in medical education (Monib, Qazi, Apong, et al., 2024). The literature search covered multiple databases, e.g., Scopus, ScienceDirect, PubMed, Springer, Taylor & Francis, and Google Scholar. The search was performed on the publications' titles, abstracts, and keywords sections. Various relevant keywords were searched, such as AI, GenAI, AI tools, or ChatGPT, and personalized learning, and medical education. Other keywords included content development, tutoring, case-based learning, automated assessments, immediate feedback, clinical decision-making, risks, ethical considerations, or AI literacy.

The chapter focused on peer-reviewed publications published in English, including the keywords, and relevant to the topic. A specific, strict date range was not employed to provide greater flexibility in capturing relevant publications (Monib, Qazi, Apong, et al., 2024). Publications were excluded if they did not focus on personalized learning in medical education, lacked substantial discussion on AI applications, were published in languages other than English, or were non-peer-reviewed publications. An expert in the field validated the result of the analysis (Grant & Booth, 2009).

4. RESULT AND DISCUSSION

This section discusses AI in personalized medical education, focusing on its usage, associated risks, literacy requirements, and practical case studies (see Figure 2). These highlight AI transformative potential in medical education while addressing its challenges. AI literacy is crucial in ensuring the responsible and effective use of AI-driven technologies. Following this discussion, case studies are presented to further illustrate these concepts in real-world applications.

Figure 2. AI in Personalized Learning Usage, AI Risks, AI Literacy, and Case Studies (Authors' Creation Using Napkin.ai)

4.1. AI Usage

Personalized education considers a learner's knowledge level, preferences, and learning pace to provide customized educational experiences. Why not use AI in learning? AI is already there and cannot be neglected. There is a paradigm shift from traditional to AI-assisted learning (Monib et al., 2025), particularly in personalized learning (Monib, Qazi, Silva, et al., 2024). If someone is avoiding cutting-edge technologies such as AI, they might be replaced by those who are using them, as they are more efficient. The key themes where AI might benefit from personalized medical learning are presented in Figure 3.

Figure 3. AI Usage in Personalized Learning (Authors' Creation Using Napkin.ai)

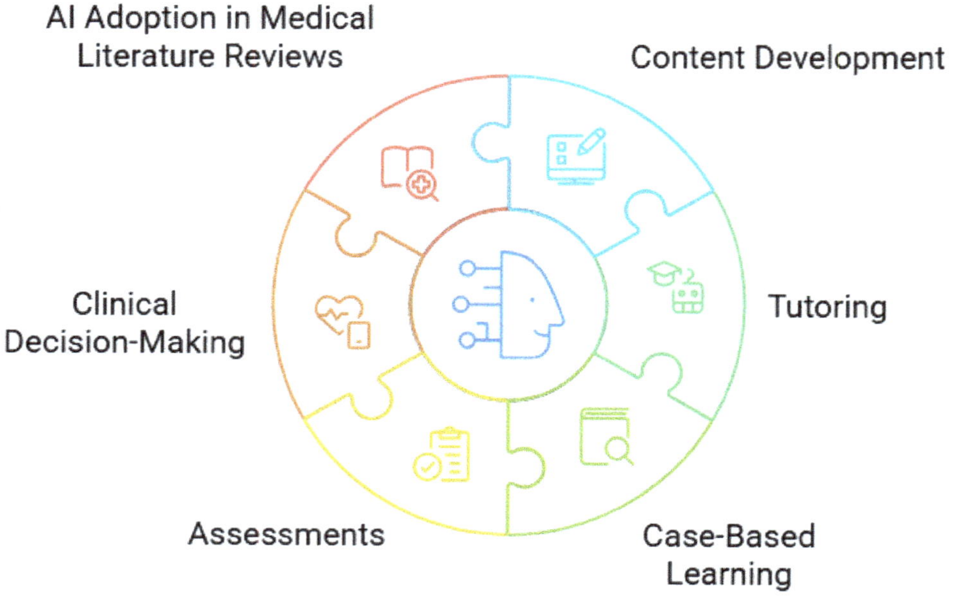

4.1.1. Content Development

To produce custom educational resources tailored to specific medical learners' needs, AI can customize learning materials. For example, GenAI could optimize instructional material design (Ranuharja et al., 2025). It would generate personalized summaries, flashcards, practice questions, and quizzes based on the interests and existing knowledge of the learners. In that way, study materials can be created to focus on areas where the learner needs help, whether compliance with a treatment guideline or accurate knowledge of a medical specialty. If a learner struggles, say, for example, with pathophysiology, the GenAI would develop specific study aids directed at directly addressing the most difficult concepts experienced by the learner during their studies. A study found that integrating GenAI in, e.g., occupational therapy curriculum could improve intervention planning and enhance the clinical readiness of learners (Ranuharja et al., 2025). On the other hand, GenAI flashcards might revisit the content topics the learner had a difficult time with in the past—this will encourage targeted, active revisit practice.

4.1.2. Tutoring

AI can be used to support intelligent tutoring systems (ITS) that can offer one-to-one tutoring similar to that of a human tutor (Kamalov et al., 2023). The incorporation of advanced AI in modern ITS enables advanced learner-centered learning capable of flexibly applied effects in diverse educational settings. Such systems feature active integration of human-centered models intended to enrich learning for learners in every aspect. By using sophisticated machine learning algorithms, ITS can adjust instruction in response to learners' highly diverse learning needs based on their unique interactions and differentiation of learning preferences. Natural Language Processing (NLP) allows them to properly interpret learner input and generate highly timely and relevant responses. For example, Affective Intelligent Tutoring Systems (ATSs) would adjust content based on real-time assessment of learners' emotions and engagement, which can significantly uplift overall learner engagement and learning outcomes (Fernández-Herrero, 2024). In applied situations, AI tutors have been found to deliver practical guidance and feedback suitable in the context and in the language preferred by the learner so that everything is accessible and well-comprehended. An example is a need for a potentially complex, e.g., neurology explanation, based on learner-specific performance metrics resulting from multiple forms of evaluations, tests, homework, or quiz assignments, as mentioned by Karpouzis et al. (2024). AI tutors provide multiple optional interpretations for complex sentences or concepts encountered in medical content. The systems can offer in-depth alternative definitions of new terms or abstract scientific language with contextual details and clarity that enhance learning to a large extent, helping learners comprehend difficult research findings and experimental results more easily. This plays a key role in building a more potent and effective environment conducive to significant intellectual growth and enduring success among diverse learners, making a real difference in their medical education.

4.1.3. Case-Based Learning

Using real medical examples in case-based learning is what instructors do with learners to integrate and solve problems under their guidance (Mejeh & Rehm, 2024). Personalization of real-world cases adjusts to a learner, thereby increasing the ability to solve problems. Technologies that allow adaptive learning can adjust learning based on individual learner needs. They help in gap identification, content recommendation, and the assessment of progress (Mejeh & Rehm, 2024). AI adaptive CBL, at the core, is considered a breakthrough pedagogical innovation that welcomes AI in building highly individualized clinical cases designed for learners. Consider, for example, a learner working through a case on cardiovascular disease.

In this case, AI monitors the learner's diagnostic choices, responses, and reasoning processes throughout the learning episode. It could be used to adjust the case if the learner is unable to come to the proper diagnosis. It could give more tips and additional clues. This personalization is essential because it allows for the reinforcement of understanding without going overwhelmed. In the same way, AI would increase the case complexity for students who have shown a higher level of competency. This might mean offering more vague symptoms or possible diagnoses with cases that would need a deeper level of critical thinking and analysis. The educational experience is thus customized to optimize learning results by staying clear of the problems of very complicated cases that create frustration and overly simple cases that create boredom.

4.1.4. Assessments

AI might play an ever more significant role in the automatic assessments of medical education by enabling immediate assessment of learners' work. AI can help significantly transform the assessment process by ensuring quick delivery of results to learners so they can understand their weaknesses and work on them to improve (Mejeh & Rehm, 2024). These innovations help improve current practices and fundamentally change the paradigm of how assessment should be performed. It can be used equally by both teachers and learners. Learners can use it for self-assessment in self-directed learning. Teachers can use it to prepare assessments (Khlaif et al., 2024) and automate the grading of the assessments (Arslan et al., 2024), including both formative and summative assessments (Khlaif et al., 2024), which may encompass multiple-choice questions, detailed essays, and even spoken responses. AI can be used to identify weaknesses and provide real-time, personalized formative assessment tailored to the unique needs of each learner. It pinpoints what areas of learning need concentration and improvement as informed by formative assessment. Conventional grading takes considerable time to assess and sometimes lacks consistency in grading work (Misut & Misutova, 2017). AI-driven tools can carry out an almost immediate analysis of a broad spectrum of submissions by learners and return individualized recommendations in perpetuity for enhancement. Rapid feedback can drive learners to engage more with the materials and reduce teachers' workload (Khlaif et al., 2024). AI could also be used to improve the homogeneity of the grading process in assignment evaluation. Human graders often become susceptible to unconscious biases and inconsistencies, especially within subjective evaluations like essay writing, where there are vast differences in personal interpretation. AI filters out these biases and disparities by its standardized criteria for evaluation. Studies found that AI evaluations are considered more objective, fair (Turner et al., 2024), consistent, and highly efficient (Himi et al., 2024). This can be within large classrooms and even online, where manual evaluation methods can be excessively cumbersome for the teacher. Besides, AI might be handy in finding common trends within the group's performance; such trends are essential for proper gap detection and furthering the area. The introduction of AI technology in the assessment of the learning process in medical education is a move toward the realization of an educational terrain that is learner-centered, efficient, and equitable for all learners (Turner et al., 2024). AI-generated questions have been successfully integrated into medical education, providing formative assessments that align with learning outcomes and curriculum guidelines (Ahmed et al., 2025; Sridharan & Sequeira, 2024). This integration supports continuous learning and helps prepare students for clinical practice. It redefines and enhances the landscape of educational assessment, forever, a provision aimed at making learning within its structures suitable for all learners. However, it is yet a critical function to be executed cautiously under human control to be valid, reliable, and fair to all (Arslan et al., 2024). The discussion on AI feedback in personalized medical learning is of particular importance. This is because the Feedback is immediate, consistent, and without bias (Francis et al., 2025). AI tools can provide immediate language refinement and creative writing enhancement, which benefits medical students and professionals (Pakdel et al., 2025). For instance, it can flag recurring issues and make meaningful recommendations for improvement. Immediate feedback to learners is instrumental in academic settings, especially when medical instructors are limited. However, occasional suggestion inaccuracies have been noted, indicating the need for human oversight (Nasra et al., 2025; Pakdel et al., 2025).

4.1.5. Decision-making

AI can help support decisions by analysing patient symptoms, medical history, and test results to suggest potential diagnoses and treatment options. For example, decision-making under uncertainty, multidisciplinary consults, drug information retrieval, identifying labelling errors, and prescription interpretation (Shin et al., 2024). Its use in billing, diagnosis, treatment, and research could make healthcare delivery more efficient, equitable, and effective (Reddy, 2024). GenAI can help produce new insights and content, and non-GenAI can help analyze existing medical datasets to improve patient care continuously. These two approaches also interact by identifying and eliminating redundancy to make better decisions in the healthcare industry (Hasan et al., 2025). For example, suppose a patient complains of chest pain. In that case, AI might be used to analyze their ECG, evaluate previous medical history, and risk factors to gauge the likelihood of myocardial infarction. The findings of Muzammil et al. (2024) confirm that AI-supported ECG analysis, particularly based on deep-learning CNN (convolutional neural network), provides high sensitivity and specificity for the early and precise diagnosis of cardiovascular abnormalities. Research indicates that supervised GenAI improves end-users' decision-making accuracy and trust in the emergency healthcare environment's real-time analyses at the expense of response time (Ebnali Harari et al., 2025). The support and accuracy level might vary depending on the type of AI tool and version. For example, a study by Currie et al. (2023) indicated that ChatGPT-3.5 provided friendly information to the patient; however, it was incomplete and outdated for clinical use. However, GPT-4 improved appropriateness, accuracy, and currency, although some omissions remained. Nevertheless, it should perform in an assistive capacity only, assigning the final decision at all times to the medical users since there are errors and biases in such tools. AI may come up with wrong diagnoses, misinformation, or even ethical issues that may compromise patient safety. Therefore, medical learners should remain the final decision-makers using AI as an adjunct to expert and judgmental humans, not as a replacement for them.

4.1.6. The Adoption of AI in Medical Literature Reviews

AI is redefining the work of conducting reviews of medical literature. AI tools facilitate rapid draft generation, literature summarization, and/or consistency in medical documentation (Kumar et al., 2025; Thaichana et al., 2025). A study by Van Veen et al. (2024) provides evidence of LLMs outperforming medical experts in clinical text summarization across multiple tasks. This activity previously would take time to extract relevant insights for building meaningful conclusions. However, modern AI-based tools enable researchers to automate this arduous process, which helps significantly reduce the workload and time required (Zhang et al., 2022). AI is able to handle huge datasets, aggregating information from many different sources. It can assist in drafting and maintaining consistency in medical documentation (Thaichana et al., 2025). In a literature search, Scopus AI can quickly summarize insights from vast data. Similarly, AI tools like ChatGPT can be used to extract specific key ideas and themes. Automation would tremendously quicken the review process; however, the requirement for human intervention to verify AI-generated outputs, as well as its compliance with high scientific standards, remains extremely important. GenAI tools like ChatGPT can help generate specific hypotheses (Sengar et al., 2024). However, limited studies were found on AI in medical literature reviews, which warrants further investigation.

4.2. AI Risks

Massive investments in AI technologies and research have been driving its widespread advent in every sector of human life. AI impacts varied dimensions of medical education and healthcare and calls for the development of guidelines that do not yet exist and need a high level of expertise (Franco D'Souza et al., 2024). There are a number of concerns with AI. Some of the common are presented in Figure 4 and discussed below.

Figure 4. AI Risks (Authors' Creating Using Napkin.ai)

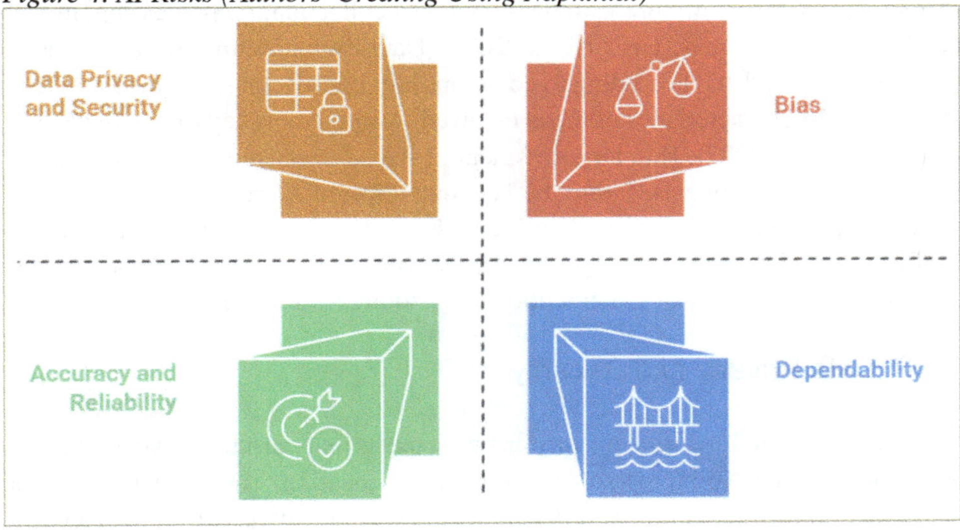

4.2.1. Bias

Bias is a complex issue that can permeate AI models in many forms (Templin et al., 2024). AI models are trained on large datasets that may contain historical biases, such as the under-representation of certain demographic groups (Aquino et al., 2023; Luu, 2025; Sun & Harris, 2024). This bias results from inadequate representation of select demographic groups within the clinical datasets (Mihan et al., 2024). In turn, it often results in a situation where there is a misdiagnosis for groups of patients, most commonly gender and ethnic minorities (Mihan et al., 2024; Norori et al., 2021). Historically, clinical studies and trials have predominantly focused on healthy, young, or middle-aged males, particularly white males, as the "standard," while females were excluded or seen as complicating results due to fluctuating hormone levels and reproductive factors (National Academies of Sciences et al., 2022). Therefore, AI, trained based on male data, may imperfectly recognize these symptoms in females; hence, it generates mistakes in detection. Research shows that gender disparities in the data used to train AI algorithms for diagnosing heart diseases reduced the accuracy of the algorithms for female patients relative to male patients (Larrazabal et al., 2020). Similarly, the correctness of AI technology in identifying skin disease impairments is limited for darker skin because they are mainly based on light-skinned data. This may be less effective for a case like melanoma detection for individuals with dark skin because it was relatively less trained against different shades of dark pigmentation (Patel et al., 2023). Bias can be inadvertently introduced during various stages of AI development, including data collection, preprocessing, model training, and deployment (Griffin et al., 2024). Datasets for training AI models need to be regularly updated according to contemporary improvements in medicine and changes in the characteristics of those involved. Awareness is key to not worsening with AI (Moore, 2022). Human assessment of the AI-created outputs is critical to finding and correcting biased outputs. The joint effort of AI developers, healthcare professionals, and educators must work together to create a more just and inclusive medical education system through the empowerment of AI to enhance rather than obstruct the preparation of the practitioners of future healthcare.

4.2.2. Data Privacy and Security

Data privacy and security are very critical aspects that must be considered while trying to integrate AI into personalized medical education. There is large amount of sensitive information involved in health care (Lilhore et al., 2024) with a number of very strict laws regulating privacy regarding data like the Health Insurance Portability and Accountability Act (HIPAA) (McGraw & Mandl, 2021). Since AI operates using a large volume of data for training, ensuring correct data handling and protection against unauthorized access becomes a significant priority. Unauthorized access and misuse of patient data can lead to privacy infringements and data breaches (Lilhore et al., 2024; Teo et al., 2024), particularly having access to large datasets of patient medical records. Such records are not adequately secured; patient identifiable information breaches could occur. For example, within a patient history and diagnostic data medical simulation, any system vulnerabilities would allow access to patient-sensitive information (Teo et al., 2024). Complete anonymization is challenging, and there can be a risk of re-identification, especially with unique medical histories or conditions (Ru et al., 2025; Wang et al., 2024). Ensuring the security of AI systems is crucial to maintaining trust and reliability (Mohsin Khan et al., 2025).

4.2.3. Accuracy and Reliability

The accuracy and reliability of AI in medical education is a serious concern and, therefore, has to be addressed very cautiously since it relies heavily on the quality and representativeness of the data they are trained on. Poor data quality can lead to inaccurate predictions and decisions, which is particularly dangerous in medical contexts (McMahon, 2024). Research indicates that GenAI is used for disease detection and diagnosis and in various medical fields related to screening, like radiology, cardiology, gastrointestinal medicine, and diabetes (Yim et al., 2024). For example, research into the response of GenAI to Familial Mediterranean Fever (FMF) noticed inaccuracy and unreliability (La Bella et al., 2024). Moreover, AI models may not always account for the complexity of human physiology. It, for instance, falls short of characterizing patient-related idiosyncrasies and nuances accurately (Atkinson et al., 2024). This, in turn, would lead the learners to misread the symptoms or make incorrect treatment decisions (Gu et al., 2025). For instance, AI models trained on limited or non-diverse datasets may not generalize well to the broader population, including women with atypical CVD presentations (Cai et al., 2024). Such models are defined as "black boxes" (Lovat, 2024), and they do not all the time reveal their decision-making processes. This presents a significant issue within medical education due to the need for learners to understand why a clinical decision was made so they can develop their critical thinking skills.

The GenAI ability to deal with edge cases and complex medical cases (Kernberg et al., 2024) is another source of concern with regard to accuracy and reliability. Models that are trained on large datasets may perform well on common conditions, but results would vary for rare diseases/and or unusual presentations of common conditions. For example, in the diagnosis of common conditions such as acne, eczema, psoriasis, and rosacea, AI could perform to expectation limits yet be inept at recognizing complex diseases and nuances (Venkatesh et al., 2024). This would, therefore, leave learners with actual knowledge shortcomings that would be worrisome if reflected in real-world healthcare conditions. Human oversight, transparency, and monitoring ensure AI maintains quality in medical education without compromising the ability of the learner to develop critical thinking and diagnostic skills for effective patient care.

4.2.4. Dependability

Over-reliance on AI in general and personalized medical education in specific can result in several potential risks that might undermine the development of critical thinking skills. Though these AI tools might bring about better educational experiences by providing information quickly and efficiently, over-dependence on them can bring about adverse effects such as decreased problem-solving skills (Liberatore et al., 2025). This is a significant concern that learners may become overly reliant on GenAI (Fawaz et al., 2025) and AI content in medical cases, diagnostic simulations, and treatment recommendations. The over-dependency can reduce learners' engagement in active learning, such as problem-solving, self-confidence, critical thinking, creative thinking, and collaboration skills (Wijaya et al., 2024). It may undermine clinical skills and judgement. For example, learners may rely on AI for diagnostics and treatment planning rather than developing their own clinical judgment (Wu et al., 2024). Similarly, a healthcare trainee who uses AI to propose treatment options for a complicated case without first fully assessing all critical factors related to the individual patient may risk patient safety. While these systems are trained on vast datasets, they can make mistakes, provide inaccurate information, outdated content (Giannakopoulos et al., 2023), or biased recommendations (Uribe et al., 2025). Misinformation or misleading information can creep into their practice if learners rely on these means without cross-referencing information from trustworthy medical sources.

Moreover, the use of AI in medical education may pose a threat in terms of healthcare empathy. Medical practice involves understanding the human side of patient care, as well as the emotions, wishes, and personal experiences. Patient care must be delivered with more than data and compassion. Therefore, AI should be used as a pedagogic aid rather than a replacement. It may be used as an assisting tool for information, simulating cases, and encouraging clinical decisions, provided there is monitoring, peer collaboration, and real contact with patients.

4.3. Literacy

AI literacy refers to the capability to comprehend, apply, and critically evaluate AI systems and results that AI comes up with (Lintner, 2024). It involves understanding and the ability to use and evaluate its content effectively and use such knowledge responsibly in medical practices (Simms, 2025). One of the key aspects of AI literacy is awareness and knowledge of AI tools like ChatGPT (Wang et al., 2023). If students lack the knowledge, they may put trust in the output by AI, which can trigger inaccurate knowledge acquisition, misdiagnosis, or irrelevant choice of therapy. In addition to awareness, the learners need to know its effective use in the impartation of medical education. It is broadly used in clinical documentation, taking a history, diagnosing, and building empathetic interactions (Blease & Rodman, 2024).

They must have the ability to evaluate AI, another pillar of literacy (Wang et al., 2023). In turn, the learners should be able to distinguish between different GenAI tools, those built according to health-privacy standards, and those more commercial (Blease & Rodman, 2024). They should be able to critique their content accuracy, reliability, and relevance as they can be hazardous by producing inaccuracies, inconsistencies, hallucinations, and bias in clinical decision-making (Blease & Rodman, 2024). For example, outdated guidelines or failure to include new therapies would not meet the present criteria. Learners should recognize the discrepancies and think about the information based on reliable medical literature or perhaps discuss with an experienced health provider. Medical learners must consider the content, such as recommendations, by referring to region-specific guidelines, such as those provided by the local health ministry or the World Health Organisation.

Moreover, AI literacy involves understanding its ethical implications in medical education and practice (Blease & Rodman, 2024; Simms, 2025; Wang et al., 2023). Medical learners must be aware of ethical issues, particularly data privacy and security, when interacting with GenAI tools (Simms, 2025), bias, and transparency (Robinson et al., 2025). It needs to be used responsibly (Simms, 2025) and consider patient safety implications (Huo et al., 2025). Most of these systems are used with access to highly sensitive data related to health. The data must be handled in compliance with data privacy regulations, which makes this task of utmost importance. Having recognized these ethical dilemmas, GenAI learners will be able to embrace responsible use and support fairer healthcare policies (Simms, 2025). Above all, learners need to understand that AI is not a substitute for their expertise but only increases it.

Technical practicums of AI literacy in medical education could be during conferences, workshops, seminars, and mentorship. Ensuring that AI is used responsibly and ethically is essential for fostering critical thinking and maintaining the humanistic core of medical practice (Reuben et al., 2024; Wu et al., 2024).

4.4. Case Studies

The following case studies are evidence of AI applications within medical education. AI provides great promises and opportunities, but is equally fraught with challenges regarding accuracy, reliability, and ethical considerations in medical applications.

Sauder et al. (2024) applied GenAI, specifically ChatGPT, in a case-based, active learning, pre-clerkship curriculum within medical education. The paper concentrated on how well ChatGPT could develop educational materials, pose medical assessment questions, and be involved in clinical reasoning. Although ChatGPT managed well with questions related to the epidemiology, diagnosis, and treatment of cases, it sometimes failed to keep pace with more complex medical questions and sometimes responded with errors or incomplete information. This finding raises red flags on the dependability of such a solution for learners in medicine. It thus highlights the necessity for an instructor to guide learners in the correct application.

The study authenticates the hope and the limitations involved in integrating GenAI into curricula for medical research.

The study by Wu et al. (2020) discussed the application of AI-facilitated PBL in ophthalmology and evaluated its impact on student performance. In this study, thirty-eight second-year medical students were randomly assigned to two groups: one using the AI-tutoring PBL module, Group A, and the other receiving traditional lectures, Group B. The results show statistically significant improvements in test scores for both groups. However, Group A shows a larger gain in diagnostic skills. On the whole, the students in the AI-tutoring group had high satisfaction, and the module turned out to be very effective in promoting critical and creative thinking. The study implies that AI-enhanced learning may improve the comprehension of medical signs by the learners, of course, with human instructors.

Su et al. (2024) instituted MEKAS, a system designed to effect adaptive learning of core clinical medical knowledge (CCMK) in otolaryngology. MEKAS, a system that enables the merging of AI-driven knowledge aggregation, is provided for personalized assessments of medical trainees. In one month, a much higher improvement in their CCMK scores was delivered by the experimental group, using the MEKAS system, compared to the control group. High satisfaction was reported by its users both with the adaptive capabilities of the system and with the quality of its interface. The application of AI to self-directed learning appears feasible, while the extendibility of the MEKAS system to other medical professions is likely.

ChatGPT, a large language model, had its capabilities evaluated by the researchers for educational use in community pharmacies and clinics in Shin et al. (2024). ChatGPT was tested on tasks such as checking drug information, spotting labeling errors, and making clinical decisions. The tool returned good results in that it provided correct information about drugs and was able to perceive and report issues with medications in clinical scenarios. ChatGPT found empirical testing challenging within more complex, multicategorical environments. While thus limited, the study still ensured that LLMs, such as ChatGPT, found enormous potential within pharmacy education, with further validation and improvements yet required within such tools to ensure their accuracy and reliability.

Van Veen et al. (2024) focused on applications of LLMs for clinical text summarization in radiology report summaries, progress notes, and doctor-patient dialogues. It demonstrated that well-adapted LLMs will sometimes provide summaries as accurate as those of the human expert generation. The study also highlighted concerns about the risks of LLM-induced fiction or information incompleteness that may generate medical errors. Despite some risks, the research implies that LLMs can attenuate overhead documentation for clinicians and preserve increased time for more direct patient care, although applied with much scrutiny for general practice. The last touchpoint must be directed to the ethical implications of AI's application to education in health professions. As AI incorporation in the medical education domain augments, educators must ensure that the tools are used ethically and responsibly.

Habs et al. (2025) evaluated ChatGPT 4.0's effectiveness in proofreading neurology reports, comparing it to a human expert. The AI detected up to 75% of errors and was significantly faster, with accuracy depending on the prompt. The study highlights ChatGPT's potential to improve medical documentation efficiency and suggests that careful prompt design is essential for optimal use in clinical and educational contexts.

Stogiannos et al. (2025) explored ethical challenges associated with AI deployment in medical imaging, identifying data protection, governance, accountability, and staff deskilling concerns. The study called for stronger legislation, updated education, and ongoing monitoring to ensure ethical and responsible AI use in healthcare.

DeCook et al. (2024) compared ChatGPT's content generation with orthopaedic fellows' performance in producing educational material on total joint arthroplasty. ChatGPT outperformed the fellows in speed and quality, although human experts excelled in integrating references and key points. The study underscores the potential of AI as a supplementary tool in medical training.

Lastly, Gravina et al. (2024) assessed ChatGPT 3.5 and Perplexity AI's performance on gastroenterology questions from the 2023 Italian national residency exam. ChatGPT 3.5 achieved 94.11% accuracy, outperforming Perplexity AI, but the study highlighted the need for caution and clear guidelines when integrating AI tools into medical education.

5. CONCLUSION

AI has a great potential to reshape personalized learning in medical education using content that suits the individual, tutoring and assessment delivered to the individual, clinical decision support targeted at the individual, and reviewing the medical literature. All these must be well managed during integration to mitigate the ethical issues involved: bias, data privacy, and over-reliance. Building AI literacy among medical learners is essential to guide responsible and appropriate application in practice. Just as there is an imperative drive toward evidence, implementation, and evaluation through research as the field moves forward, so too is the need for action research to realize the wealth of potential that AI holds in medical education. Future research can investigate personalization through AI in terms of its impact on medical learning outcomes, and longitudinal studies could explore how the use of AI impacts clinical competency in the long term and its relationship with the standards of accreditation that allow sustained and productive use of AI technology in medical education.

6. LIMITATIONS

This review has several limitations that need to be considered. First, the review did not follow a systematic approach to the literature review. Second, the review focused on publications from specific databases, which may have excluded other relevant publications. Third, AI models, applications, and methodologies in medical education are continuously advancing, which leads to potential gaps in the current chapter coverage of the latest innovations. Fourth, the chapter did not focus on specific AI tools, which may influence the interpretation of the findings, as specific AI tools may be better, for example, in accuracy level, while others may not.

7. FUTURE RESEARCH

Suggestions for future improvements include alternative approaches to address the identified limitations, such as systematic literature reviews, scoping reviews, and bibliometric analysis. In the future, researchers should also consider expanding the scope of the databases and conducting a robustness check of the included publications. Further empirical research is required to evaluate AI tools usage in personalized learning, such as instructional content development, individual tutoring, case-based learning, assessment, clinical decision-making, and conducting the literature review. Additionally, more research is needed to evaluate the AI risks in personalized medical education and provide policies and guidelines. Future research should also focus on developing specialized AI tools for the medical field with supervised large and diverse data sets to improve the accuracy and reliability of the outputs. Finally, reviews in the future should concentrate on specific AI tools and possibly their comparison in medical education.

REFERENCES

Abubakari, M. S., Shafik, W., & Hidayatullah, A. F. (2024). Evaluating the potential of artificial intelligence in Islamic religious education: A SWOT analysis overview. In *AI-Enhanced Teaching Methods* (pp. 216–239). IGI Global., DOI: 10.4018/979-8-3693-2728-9.ch010

Ahmed, A., Kerr, E., & O'Malley, A. (2025). Quality assurance and validity of AI-generated single best answer questions [Article]. *BMC Medical Education*, *25*(1), 300. Advance online publication. DOI: 10.1186/s12909-025-06881-w PMID: 40001164

Ali, R., Afzal, A., Shakil, S., Sultan, A., Babar, S., Rehman, J., Malik, M. G. R., Qadir, M. S., Khan, S., & Saeed, S. (2025). Transforming Education: Case-Based Integrated Learning Development and Implementation – A Mixed Methods Study at a Private Medical College [Article]. *Journal of Advances in Medical Education & Professionalism*, *13*(1), 49–58. DOI: 10.30476/jamp.2024.104285.2048 PMID: 39906080

Aquino, Y. S. J., Carter, S. M., Houssami, N., Braunack-Mayer, A., Win, K. T., Degeling, C., Wang, L., & Rogers, W. A. (2023). Practical, epistemic and normative implications of algorithmic bias in healthcare artificial intelligence: A qualitative study of multidisciplinary expert perspectives [Article]. *Journal of Medical Ethics*, jme-2022-108850. Advance online publication. DOI: 10.1136/jme-2022-108850 PMID: 36823101

Arslan, B., Lehman, B., Tenison, C., Sparks, J. R., López, A. A., Gu, L., & Zapata-Rivera, D. (2024). 2024-October-07). Opportunities and challenges of using generative AI to personalize educational assessment [Perspective]. *Frontiers in Artificial Intelligence*, *7*, 1460651. Advance online publication. DOI: 10.3389/frai.2024.1460651 PMID: 39434872

Aslam, M. S., & Nisar, S. (2023). *Artificial intelligence applications using ChatGPT in education: Case studies and practices* [Book]. IGI Global., DOI: 10.4018/978-1-6684-9300-7

Atkinson, C. J., Seth, I., Xie, Y., Ross, R. J., Hunter-Smith, D. J., Rozen, W. M., & Cuomo, R. (2024). Artificial Intelligence Language Model Performance for Rapid Intraoperative Queries in Plastic Surgery: ChatGPT and the Deep Inferior Epigastric Perforator Flap [Article]. *Journal of Clinical Medicine*, *13*(3), 900. Advance online publication. DOI: 10.3390/jcm13030900 PMID: 38337594

Blease, C., & Rodman, A. (2024). 2024/12/09). Generative Artificial Intelligence in Mental Healthcare: An Ethical Evaluation. *Current Treatment Options in Psychiatry, 12*(1), 5. DOI: 10.1007/s40501-024-00340-x

Cai, Y. Q., Gong, D. X., Tang, L. Y., Cai, Y., Li, H. J., Jing, T. C., Gong, M., Hu, W., Zhang, Z. W., Zhang, X., & Zhang, G. W. (2024). Pitfalls in Developing Machine Learning Models for Predicting Cardiovascular Diseases: Challenge and Solutions [Article]. *Journal of Medical Internet Research*, *26*, e47645. Advance online publication. DOI: 10.2196/47645 PMID: 38869157

Çakmakkaya, Ö. S., Jaremko, K. M., Kitapçıoğlu, D., & Wolpaw, J. (2025). Orthopedic Anesthesia Training: A Narrative Review on Program Development [Article]. *Current Anesthesiology Reports*, *15*(1), 4. Advance online publication. DOI: 10.1007/s40140-024-00669-2

Currie, G., Robbie, S., & Tually, P. (2023). ChatGPT and Patient Information in Nuclear Medicine: GPT-3.5 Versus GPT-4 [Article]. *Journal of Nuclear Medicine Technology*, *51*(4), 307–313. DOI: 10.2967/jnmt.123.266151 PMID: 37699647

DeCook, R., Muffly, B. T., Mahmood, S., Holland, C. T., Ayeni, A. M., Ast, M. P., Bolognese, M. P., Guild, G. N.III, Sheth, N. P., Pean, C. A., & Premkumar, A. (2024). 2024/06/01/). AI-Generated Graduate Medical Education Content for Total Joint Arthroplasty: Comparing ChatGPT Against Orthopaedic Fellows. *Arthroplasty Today*, *27*, 101412. https://doi.org/https://doi.org/10.1016/j.artd.2024.101412. DOI: 10.1016/j.artd.2024.101412 PMID: 38912098

Ebnali Harari, R., Altaweel, A., Ahram, T., Keehner, M., & Shokoohi, H. (2025). A randomized controlled trial on evaluating clinician-supervised generative AI for decision support [Article]. *International Journal of Medical Informatics*, *195*, 105701. Advance online publication. DOI: 10.1016/j.ijmedinf.2024.105701 PMID: 39631268

Fawaz, M., El-Malti, W., Alreshidi, S. M., & Kavuran, E. (2025). Exploring Health Sciences Students' Perspectives on Using Generative Artificial Intelligence in Higher Education: A Qualitative Study [Article]. *Nursing & Health Sciences*, *27*(1), e70030. Advance online publication. DOI: 10.1111/nhs.70030 PMID: 39797529

Fernández-Herrero, J. (2024). Evaluating Recent Advances in Affective Intelligent Tutoring Systems: A Scoping Review of Educational Impacts and Future Prospects [Review]. *Education Sciences*, *14*(8), 839. Advance online publication. DOI: 10.3390/educsci14080839

Francis, N. J., Jones, S., & Smith, D. P. (2025). 2025-January-09). Generative AI in Higher Education: Balancing Innovation and Integrity [Review]. *British Journal of Biomedical Science*, *81*, 14048. Advance online publication. DOI: 10.3389/bjbs.2024.14048 PMID: 39850144

Franco D'Souza, R., Mathew, M., Mishra, V., & Surapaneni, K. M. (2024, December 31). Twelve tips for addressing ethical concerns in the implementation of artificial intelligence in medical education. *Medical Education Online*, *29*(1), 2330250. DOI: 10.1080/10872981.2024.2330250 PMID: 38566608

Giannakopoulos, K., Kavadella, A., Salim, A. A., Stamatopoulos, V., & Kaklamanos, E. G. (2023). Evaluation of the Performance of Generative AI Large Language Models ChatGPT, Google Bard, and Microsoft Bing Chat in Supporting Evidence-Based Dentistry: Comparative Mixed Methods Study [Article]. *Journal of Medical Internet Research*, *25*(1), e51580. Advance online publication. DOI: 10.2196/51580 PMID: 38009003

Grant, M. J., & Booth, A. (2009, June). A typology of reviews: An analysis of 14 review types and associated methodologies. *Health Information and Libraries Journal*, *26*(2), 91–108. DOI: 10.1111/j.1471-1842.2009.00848.x PMID: 19490148

Gravina, A. G., Pellegrino, R., Palladino, G., Imperio, G., Ventura, A., & Federico, A. (2024). 2024/08/01/). Charting new AI education in gastroenterology: Cross-sectional evaluation of ChatGPT and perplexity AI in medical residency exam. *Digestive and Liver Disease*, *56*(8), 1304–1311. https://doi.org/https://doi.org/10.1016/j.dld.2024.02.019. DOI: 10.1016/j.dld.2024.02.019 PMID: 38503659

Griffin, A. C., Wang, K. H., Leung, T. I., & Facelli, J. C. (2024). Recommendations to promote fairness and inclusion in biomedical AI research and clinical use [Article]. *Journal of Biomedical Informatics*, *157*, 104693. Advance online publication. DOI: 10.1016/j.jbi.2024.104693 PMID: 39019301

Gu, T., Pan, W., Yu, J., Ji, G., Meng, X., Wang, Y., & Li, M. (2025). Mitigating bias in AI mortality predictions for minority populations: A transfer learning approach [Article]. *BMC Medical Informatics and Decision Making*, *25*(1), 30. Advance online publication. DOI: 10.1186/s12911-025-02862-7 PMID: 39825353

Habs, M., Knecht, S., & Schmidt-Wilcke, T. (2025, 2025/03/18/). Using artificial intelligence (AI) for form and content checks of medical reports: Proofreading by ChatGPT4.0 in a neurology department. *Zeitschrift für Evidenz, Fortbildung und Qualität im Gesundheitswesen*. https://doi.org/https://doi.org/10.1016/j.zefq.2025.02.007

Hasan, S. S., Woo, J. J., Cote, M. P., & Ramkumar, P. N. (2025). Generative Versus Nongenerative Artificial Intelligence [Article]. *Arthroscopy*, *41*(3), 545–546. DOI: 10.1016/j.arthro.2024.12.001 PMID: 39929595

Himi, S. T., Monalisa, N. T., Sultana, S., Afrin, A., & Hasib, K. M. (2024, 25-26 Sept. 2024). Automated Exam Script Checking using Zero-Shot LLM and Adaptive Generative AI. *2024 IEEE International Conference on Computing, Applications and Systems (COMPAS)*, 1-6. https://doi.org/DOI: 10.1109/COMPAS60761.2024.10795949

Huo, B., Boyle, A., Marfo, N., Tangamornsuksan, W., Steen, J. P., McKechnie, T., Lee, Y., Mayol, J., Antoniou, S. A., Thirunavukarasu, A. J., Sanger, S., Ramji, K., & Guyatt, G. (2025). Large Language Models for Chatbot Health Advice Studies: A Systematic Review. *JAMA Network Open*, *8*(2), e2457879–e2457879. DOI: 10.1001/jamanetworkopen.2024.57879 PMID: 39903463

IBM Data and AI Team. (2023). *Understanding the different types of artificial intelligence*. IBM. https://www.ibm.com/think/topics/artificial-intelligence-types

Kamalov, F., Santandreu Calonge, D., & Gurrib, I. (2023). New Era of Artificial Intelligence in Education: Towards a Sustainable Multifaceted Revolution. *Sustainability (Basel)*, *15*(16), 12451. Advance online publication. DOI: 10.3390/su151612451

Karataş, F., Eriçok, B., & Tanrikulu, L. (2024). Reshaping curriculum adaptation in the age of artificial intelligence: Mapping teachers' AI-driven curriculum adaptation patterns [Article]. *British Educational Research Journal*. Advance online publication. DOI: 10.1002/berj.4068

Karpouzis, K., Pantazatos, D., Taouki, J., & Meli, K. (2024, 8-11 May 2024). Tailoring Education with GenAI: A New Horizon in Lesson Planning. *2024 IEEE Global Engineering Education Conference (EDUCON)*, 1-10. https://doi.org/DOI: 10.1109/EDUCON60312.2024.10578690

Kernberg, A., Gold, J. A., & Mohan, V. (2024). Using ChatGPT-4 to Create Structured Medical Notes From Audio Recordings of Physician-Patient Encounters: Comparative Study [Article]. *Journal of Medical Internet Research*, *26*(1), e54419. Advance online publication. DOI: 10.2196/54419 PMID: 38648636

Khlaif, Z. N., Ayyoub, A., Hamamra, B., Bensalem, E., Mitwally, M. A. A., Ayyoub, A., Hattab, M. K., & Shadid, F. (2024). University Teachers' Views on the Adoption and Integration of Generative AI Tools for Student Assessment in Higher Education [Article]. *Education Sciences*, *14*(10), 1090. Advance online publication. DOI: 10.3390/educsci14101090

Kumar, I., Yadav, N., & Verma, A. (2025). Navigating Artificial Intelligence in Scientific Manuscript Writing: Tips and Traps [Review]. *The Indian Journal of Radiology & Imaging*, *35*(1), S178–S186. DOI: 10.1055/s-0044-1800801 PMID: 39802715

La Bella, S., Attanasi, M., Porreca, A., Di Ludovico, A., Maggio, M. C., Gallizzi, R., La Torre, F., Rigante, D., Soscia, F., Ardenti Morini, F., Insalaco, A., Natale, M. F., Chiarelli, F., Simonini, G., De Benedetti, F., Gattorno, M., & Breda, L. (2024). Reliability of a generative artificial intelligence tool for pediatric familial Mediterranean fever: Insights from a multicentre expert survey [Article]. *Pediatric Rheumatology Online Journal*, *22*(1), 78. Advance online publication. DOI: 10.1186/s12969-024-01011-0 PMID: 39180115

Larrazabal, A. J., Nieto, N., Peterson, V., Milone, D. H., & Ferrante, E. (2020, June 9). Gender imbalance in medical imaging datasets produces biased classifiers for computer-aided diagnosis. *Proceedings of the National Academy of Sciences of the United States of America*, *117*(23), 12592–12594. DOI: 10.1073/pnas.1919012117 PMID: 32457147

Liberatore, G., Kim, A., Brenner, J., & Milanaik, R. (2025). Artificial intelligence impacts in education and pediatric mental health [Review]. *Current Opinion in Pediatrics*, Article . https://doi.org/DOI: 10.1097/MOP.0000000000001453

Lilhore, U. K., Simaiya, S., Poongodi, M., & Dutt, V. (2024). *Federated learning and privacy-preserving in healthcare AI* [Book]. IGI Global. https://doi.org/DOI: 10.4018/979-8-3693-1874-4

Lintner, T. (2024, 2024/08/06). A systematic review of AI literacy scales. *npj Science of Learning*, *9*(1), 50. https://doi.org/DOI: 10.1038/s41539-024-00264-4

Lovat, L. B. (2024). Artificial intelligence in gastroenterology: Where are we and where are we going? [Article]. *Gastrointestinal Nursing*, *22*(Sup3), S6–S13. DOI: 10.12968/gasn.2024.22.Sup3.S6

Luu, H. S. (2025). Laboratory Data as a Potential Source of Bias in Healthcare Artificial Intelligence and Machine Learning Models [Review]. *Annals of Laboratory Medicine*, *45*(1), 12–21. DOI: 10.3343/alm.2024.0323 PMID: 39444135

Martin-Alguacil, N., Avedillo, L., Mota-Blanco, R., & Gallego-Agundez, M. (2024). Student-Centered Learning: Some Issues and Recommendations for Its Implementation in a Traditional Curriculum Setting in Health Sciences. *Education Sciences*, *14*(11), 1179. https://www.mdpi.com/2227-7102/14/11/1179. DOI: 10.3390/educsci14111179

McGraw, D., & Mandl, K. D. (2021). 2021/01/04). Privacy protections to encourage use of health-relevant digital data in a learning health system. *npj. Digital Medicine*, *4*(1), 2. DOI: 10.1038/s41746-020-00362-8 PMID: 33398052

McMahon, G. T. (2024). The Risks and Challenges of Artificial Intelligence in Endocrinology [Article]. *The Journal of Clinical Endocrinology and Metabolism*, *109*(6), e1468–e1471. DOI: 10.1210/clinem/dgae017 PMID: 38471009

Mejeh, M., & Rehm, M. (2024). 2024/06/01). Taking adaptive learning in educational settings to the next level: Leveraging natural language processing for improved personalization. *Educational Technology Research and Development*, *72*(3), 1597–1621. DOI: 10.1007/s11423-024-10345-1

Mihan, A., Pandey, A., & Van Spall, H. G. (2024). Mitigating the risk of artificial intelligence bias in cardiovascular care [Review]. *The Lancet. Digital Health*, *6*(10), e749–e754. DOI: 10.1016/S2589-7500(24)00155-9 PMID: 39214762

Mitra, N. K., & Chitra, E. (2024). Glimpses of the Use of Generative AI and ChatGPT in Medical Education [Review]. *Education in Medicine Journal*, *16*(2), 155–164. DOI: 10.21315/eimj2024.16.2.11

Mohsin Khan, M., Shah, N., Shaikh, N., Thabet, A., alrabayah, T., & Belkhair, S. (2025). Towards secure and trusted AI in healthcare: A systematic review of emerging innovations and ethical challenges [Review]. *International Journal of Medical Informatics*, *195*, 105780. Advance online publication. DOI: 10.1016/j.ijmedinf.2024.105780 PMID: 39753062

Monib, W. K. (2023). Implementation of 21st Century Skills in EFL Classroom: Perceptions of Lecturers and Students. [IJonSES]. *International Journal on Social & Education Sciences*, *5*(3), 536–559. https://doi.org/https://doi.org/10.46328/ijonses.544. DOI: 10.46328/ijonses.544

Monib, W. K., Qazi, A., Apong, R. A., Azizan, M. T., De Silva, L., & Yassin, H. (2024). Generative AI and future education: A review, theoretical validation, and authors' perspective on challenges and solutions. *PeerJ. Computer Science*, *10*, e2105. DOI: 10.7717/peerj-cs.2105 PMID: 39650462

Monib, W. K., Qazi, A., De Silva, L., & Mahmud, M. M. (2024). Exploring Learners' Experiences with ChatGPT in Personalized Learning. *2024 6th International Workshop on Artificial Intelligence and Education (WAIE)*, 66-70. https://doi.org/ DOI: 10.1109/WAIE63876.2024.00019

Monib, W. K., Qazi, A., & Mahmud, M. M. (2025). 2025/01/01). Exploring learners' experiences and perceptions of ChatGPT as a learning tool in higher education. *Education and Information Technologies*, *30*(1), 917–939. DOI: 10.1007/s10639-024-13065-4

Moore, C. M. (2022). 2022/01/01/). The challenges of health inequities and AI. *Intelligence-Based Medicine*, *6*, 100067. https://doi.org/https://doi.org/10.1016/j.ibmed.2022.100067. DOI: 10.1016/j.ibmed.2022.100067

Muzammil, M. A., Javid, S., Afridi, A. K., Siddineni, R., Shahabi, M., Haseeb, M., Fariha, F. N. U., Kumar, S., Zaveri, S., & Nashwan, A. J. (2024). 2024/03/01/). Artificial intelligence-enhanced electrocardiography for accurate diagnosis and management of cardiovascular diseases. *Journal of Electrocardiology*, *83*, 30–40. https://doi.org/https://doi.org/10.1016/j.jelectrocard.2024.01.006. DOI: 10.1016/j.jelectrocard.2024.01.006 PMID: 38301492

Nasra, M., Jaffri, R., Pavlin-Premrl, D., Kok, H. K., Khabaza, A., Barras, C., Slater, L. A., Yazdabadi, A., Moore, J., Russell, J., Smith, P., Chandra, R. V., Brooks, M., Jhamb, A., Chong, W., Maingard, J., & Asadi, H. (2025). Can artificial intelligence improve patient educational material readability? A systematic review and narrative synthesis [Review]. *Internal Medicine Journal*, *55*(1), 20–34. DOI: 10.1111/imj.16607 PMID: 39720869

Norori, N., Hu, Q., Aellen, F. M., Faraci, F. D., & Tzovara, A. (2021). Addressing bias in big data and AI for health care: A call for open science. *Patterns (New York, N.Y.)*, *2*(10), 100347. Advance online publication. DOI: 10.1016/j.patter.2021.100347 PMID: 34693373

Pakdel, F., Khojasteh, L., Kafipour, R., & Shahsavar, Z. (2025). Navigating AI writing tools in medical education: A SWOT analysis of L2 academic writing perspectives [Article]. *Language Teaching Research*, 13621688251322953. Advance online publication. DOI: 10.1177/13621688251322953

Patel, R. H., Foltz, E. A., Witkowski, A., & Ludzik, J. (2023, September 23). Analysis of Artificial Intelligence-Based Approaches Applied to Non-Invasive Imaging for Early Detection of Melanoma: A Systematic Review. *Cancers (Basel)*, *15*(19), 4694. Advance online publication. DOI: 10.3390/cancers15194694 PMID: 37835388

Ranuharja, F., Rizal, F., Langeveldt, D., Ejjami, R., Torres-Toukoumidis, A., & Jalinus, N. (2025). Relevance and Impact of Generative AI in Vocational Instructional Material Design: A Systematic Literature Review [Review]. *Salud, Ciencia y Tecnología*, *5*, 1336. Advance online publication. DOI: 10.56294/saludcyt20251336

Rashid, A. B., & Kausik, M. D. A. K. (2024, 2024/12/01/). AI revolutionizing industries worldwide: A comprehensive overview of its diverse applications. *Hybrid Advances, 7*, 100277. https://doi.org/https://doi.org/10.1016/j.hybadv.2024.100277

Reddy, S. (2024). Generative AI in healthcare: An implementation science informed translational path on application, integration and governance [Article]. *Implementation Science : IS*, *19*(1), 27. Advance online publication. DOI: 10.1186/s13012-024-01357-9 PMID: 38491544

Reuben, J. S., Meiri, H., & Arien-Zakay, H. (2024). AI's pivotal impact on redefining stakeholder roles and their interactions in medical education and health care [Article]. *Frontiers in Digital Health*, *6*, 1458811. Advance online publication. DOI: 10.3389/fdgth.2024.1458811 PMID: 39564581

Rhoney, D. H., Singleton, S., Nelson, N. R., Anderson, S. M., & Hubal, R. (2021). Forces driving change in pharmacy education: Opportunities to take academic, social, technological, economic, and political into the future [Article]. *Journal of the American College of Clinical Pharmacy: JAACP*, *4*(5), 639–651. DOI: 10.1002/jac5.1407

Robinson, J. R., Stey, A., Schneider, D. F., Kothari, A. N., Lindeman, B., Kaafarani, H. M., & Haines, K. L. (2025, 2025/02/10/). Generative Artificial Intelligence in Academic Surgery: Ethical Implications and Transformative Potential. *Journal of Surgical Research*. https://doi.org/https://doi.org/10.1016/j.jss.2024.12.059

Ru, Z. J., Panchal, O., Chen, C. T., Jonnagaddala, J., Dai, H. J., & Hsueh, S. C. (2025). Utilizing Large Language Models for Privacy Protection and Advancing Medical Digitization [Conference paper]. *Communications in Computer and Information Science*, *2148*, 177–188. DOI: 10.1007/978-981-97-7966-6_13

Salloum, A., Alfaisal, R., & Salloum, S. A. (2024). Revolutionizing Medical Education: Empowering Learning with ChatGPT. In *Studies in Big Data* (Vol. 144, pp. 79-90). Springer Science and Business Media Deutschland GmbH. https://doi.org/ DOI: 10.1007/978-3-031-52280-2_6

Sauder, M., Tritsch, T., Rajput, V., Schwartz, G., & Shoja, M. M. (2024, January). Exploring Generative Artificial Intelligence-Assisted Medical Education: Assessing Case-Based Learning for Medical Students. *Cureus*, *16*(1), e51961. DOI: 10.7759/cureus.51961 PMID: 38333501

Sengar, S. S., Hasan, A. B., Kumar, S., & Carroll, F. (2024). 2024/08/14). Generative artificial intelligence: A systematic review and applications. *Multimedia Tools and Applications*. Advance online publication. DOI: 10.1007/s11042-024-20016-1

Shin, E., Hartman, M., & Ramanathan, M. (2024). Performance of the ChatGPT large language model for decision support in community pharmacy [Article]. *British Journal of Clinical Pharmacology*, *90*(12), 3320–3333. DOI: 10.1111/bcp.16215 PMID: 39191671

Simms, R. C. (2025). 2025/03/01/). Generative artificial intelligence (AI) literacy in nursing education: A crucial call to action. *Nurse Education Today*, *146*, 106544. https://doi.org/https://doi.org/10.1016/j.nedt.2024.106544. DOI: 10.1016/j.nedt.2024.106544 PMID: 39708405

Sridharan, K., & Sequeira, R. P. (2024). Artificial intelligence and medical education: Application in classroom instruction and student assessment using a pharmacology & therapeutics case study [Article]. *BMC Medical Education*, *24*(1), 431. Advance online publication. DOI: 10.1186/s12909-024-05365-7 PMID: 38649959

Stogiannos, N., Georgiadou, E., Rarri, N., & Malamateniou, C. (2025). 2025/01/01/). Ethical AI: A qualitative study exploring ethical challenges and solutions on the use of AI in medical imaging. *European Journal of Radiology Artificial Intelligence*, *1*, 100006. https://doi.org/https://doi.org/10.1016/j.ejrai.2025.100006. DOI: 10.1016/j.ejrai.2025.100006

Su, J.-M., Hsu, S.-Y., Fang, T.-Y., & Wang, P.-C. (2024). 2024/08/01/). Developing and validating a knowledge-based AI assessment system for learning clinical core medical knowledge in otolaryngology. *Computers in Biology and Medicine*, *178*, 108765. https://doi.org/https://doi.org/10.1016/j.compbiomed.2024.108765. DOI: 10.1016/j.compbiomed.2024.108765 PMID: 38897143

Sun, C., & Harris, S. L. (2024). Reducing bias in healthcare artificial intelligence: A white paper [Article]. *Health Informatics Journal*, *30*(4), 14604582241291410. Advance online publication. DOI: 10.1177/14604582241291410 PMID: 39541598

Templin, T., Perez, M. W., Sylvia, S., Leek, J., & Sinnott-Armstrong, N. (2024, May). Addressing 6 challenges in generative AI for digital health: A scoping review. *PLOS Digital Health*, *3*(5), e0000503. DOI: 10.1371/journal.pdig.0000503 PMID: 38781686

Teo, Z. L., Quek, C. W. N., Wong, J. L. Y., & Ting, D. S. W. (2024). 2024/07/01/). Cybersecurity in the generative artificial intelligence era. *Asia-Pacific Journal of Ophthalmology*, *13*(4), 100091. https://doi.org/https://doi.org/10.1016/j.apjo.2024.100091. DOI: 10.1016/j.apjo.2024.100091 PMID: 39209217

Thaichana, P., Oo, M. Z., Thorup, G. L., Chansakaow, C., Arworn, S., & Rerkasem, K. (2025). Integrating Artificial Intelligence in Medical Writing: Balancing Technological Innovation and Human Expertise, with Practical Applications in Lower Extremity Wounds Care [Review]. *The International Journal of Lower Extremity Wounds*, 15347346241312814. Advance online publication. DOI: 10.1177/15347346241312814 PMID: 39801150

Thayyib, P. V., Mamilla, R., Khan, M., Fatima, H., Asim, M., Anwar, I., Shamsudheen, M. K., & Khan, M. A. (2023). State-of-the-Art of Artificial Intelligence and Big Data Analytics Reviews in Five Different Domains: A Bibliometric Summary. *Sustainability (Basel)*, *15*(5), 4026. https://www.mdpi.com/2071-1050/15/5/4026. DOI: 10.3390/su15054026

Turner, L., Hashimoto, D. A., Vasisht, S., & Schaye, V. (2024). Demystifying AI: Current State and Future Role in Medical Education Assessment [Article]. *Hepatology (Baltimore, Md.)*, *99*(4), S42–S47. DOI: 10.1097/ACM.0000000000005598 PMID: 38166201

Uribe, S. E., Maldupa, I., & Schwendicke, F. (2025). Integrating Generative AI in Dental Education: A Scoping Review of Current Practices and Recommendations [Article]. *European Journal of Dental Education*, *29*(2), 341–355. Advance online publication. DOI: 10.1111/eje.13074 PMID: 39891376

Van Veen, D., Van Uden, C., Blankemeier, L., Delbrouck, J.-B., Aali, A., Bluethgen, C., Pareek, A., Polacin, M., Reis, E. P., Seehofnerová, A., Rohatgi, N., Hosamani, P., Collins, W., Ahuja, N., Langlotz, C. P., Hom, J., Gatidis, S., Pauly, J., & Chaudhari, A. S. (2024). 2024/04/01). Adapted large language models can outperform medical experts in clinical text summarization. *Nature Medicine*, *30*(4), 1134–1142. DOI: 10.1038/s41591-024-02855-5 PMID: 38413730

Venkatesh, K. P., Raza, M. M., Nickel, G., Wang, S., & Kvedar, J. C. (2024). 2024/02/10). Deep learning models across the range of skin disease. *npj. Digital Medicine*, *7*(1), 32. DOI: 10.1038/s41746-024-01033-8 PMID: 38341516

Wang, B., Rau, P.-L. P., & Yuan, T. (2023). 2023/07/04). Measuring user competence in using artificial intelligence: Validity and reliability of artificial intelligence literacy scale. *Behaviour & Information Technology*, *42*(9), 1324–1337. DOI: 10.1080/0144929X.2022.2072768

Wang, Y., Liu, C., Zhou, K., Zhu, T., & Han, X. (2024). Towards regulatory generative AI in ophthalmology healthcare: A security and privacy perspective [Review]. *The British Journal of Ophthalmology*, *108*(10), 1349–1353. DOI: 10.1136/bjo-2024-325167 PMID: 38834290

Wijaya, T. T., Yu, Q., Cao, Y., He, Y., & Leung, F. K. S. (2024). Latent Profile Analysis of AI Literacy and Trust in Mathematics Teachers and Their Relations with AI Dependency and 21st-Century Skills [Article]. *Behavioral Sciences (Basel, Switzerland)*, *14*(11), 1008. Advance online publication. DOI: 10.3390/bs14111008 PMID: 39594308

Wu, D., Xiang, Y., Wu, X., Yu, T., Huang, X., Zou, Y., Liu, Z., & Lin, H. (2020, June). Artificial intelligence-tutoring problem-based learning in ophthalmology clerkship. *Annals of Translational Medicine*, *8*(11), 700. DOI: 10.21037/atm.2019.12.15 PMID: 32617320

Wu, Z., Liu, Z., & Zhang, Z. (2024). Research on the current situation and future governance of artificial intelligence in the field of medical education [Article]. *Chinese Medical Ethics*, *37*(9), 1093–1100. DOI: 10.12026/j.issn.1001-8565.2024.09.12

Yim, D., Khuntia, J., Parameswaran, V., & Meyers, A. (2024). Preliminary Evidence of the Use of Generative AI in Health Care Clinical Services: Systematic Narrative Review [Article]. *JMIR Medical Informatics*, *12*, e52073. Advance online publication. DOI: 10.2196/52073 PMID: 38506918

Zhang, Y., Liang, S., Feng, Y., Wang, Q., Sun, F., Chen, S., Yang, Y., He, X., Zhu, H., & Pan, H. (2022). Automation of literature screening using machine learning in medical evidence synthesis: A diagnostic test accuracy systematic review protocol [Review]. *Systematic Reviews*, *11*(1), 11. Advance online publication. DOI: 10.1186/s13643-021-01881-5 PMID: 35031074

Chapter 5
Teaching Medicine With Generative Artificial Intelligence (GenAI): A Review of Practices, Pitfalls, and Possibilities in Medical Education

Manuel B. Garcia
https://orcid.org/0000-0003-2615-422X
FEU Institute of Technology, Philippines

Raquel Simões de Almeida
https://orcid.org/0000-0003-4703-1712
Polytechnic of Porto, Portugal

Dharel P. Acut
https://orcid.org/0000-0002-9608-1292
Cebu Technological University, Philippines

Rui Pedro Pereira de Almeida
https://orcid.org/0000-0001-7524-9669
University of Algarve, Portugal

Precious S. Garcia
Jose Rizal University, Philippines

Eleonora Stefani
https://orcid.org/0009-0005-0540-157X
University of Padova, Italy

ABSTRACT

Once confined to science fiction and speculative futures, generative artificial intelligence (GenAI) has swiftly entered the lecture halls of modern medical education. Despite its expanding use, a synthesis of its implementation, limitations, and educational value remains underexplored. This review aims to critically examine current applications, identify pedagogical pitfalls, and delineate future trajectories for GenAI in medical training. Key innovations include AI-driven content generation tailored to curricular benchmarks, automated assessments with real-time diagnostic feedback, and immersive virtual patient simulations replicating complex pathophysiologies.

DOI: 10.4018/979-8-3373-1519-5.ch005

Additional advances span multilingual knowledge translation, anatomically precise surgical training environments, and adaptive learning systems powered by intelligent tutoring frameworks. As discussed herein, GenAI holds transformative potential for advancing clinical competence in an evolving medical landscape—provided its integration is evidence-based, ethically sound, and educationally coherent.

INTRODUCTION

The journey of becoming a physician is often compared to drinking from a firehose—a vivid metaphor that fails to mention that the hose also occasionally sprays Latin terminology, unexpected ethical dilemmas, and a growing existential crisis. This lighthearted analogy does not even capture the sheer volume of information medical students must absorb, as it only scratches the surface of what truly makes medical education both rigorous and essential. Beyond the endless stream of lectures, clinical rotations, and late-night study sessions fueled by caffeine and sheer determination, medical training is an intricate process that shapes the very mindset and resilience of future physicians. More importantly, medical education is not simply about knowledge transfer but about cultivating clinical reasoning, ethical judgment, and the ability to navigate the complexities of patient care (Kirch & Sadofsky, 2021; Ogden et al., 2023; Yazdani & Abardeh, 2019). The effectiveness of medical training depends not only on what is taught but also on how it is taught. Therefore, traditional methods such as didactic lectures and rote memorization, while still valuable, are increasingly being supplemented by more dynamic, student-centered pedagogies designed to enhance engagement and retention (Buja, 2019).

As the landscape of medical education evolves, instructional technologies have emerged as powerful tools to bridge the gap between traditional learning and modern medical practice (Chowdhury et al., 2024; Garcia, de Almeida, et al., 2025). For instance, a systematic review of immersive technology applications highlights empirical evidence demonstrating their effectiveness in improving practical and procedural skills among medical students and professionals (Tang et al., 2022). The review further emphasized that immersive technologies, including augmented reality (AR), virtual reality (VR), mixed reality (MR), and extended reality (XR), are widely implemented in surgery and anatomy training to overcome limitations in cadaver availability and the associated financial, ethical, and supervision challenges that are particularly significant in neuroanatomy. In another systematic review, McGee et al. (2024) underscored the use of digital tools in teaching clinical skills as a viable alternative to traditional face-to-face instruction. Their findings suggest that these technologies can enhance educational outcomes, improve student satisfaction, and potentially reduce costs. This shift reflects the broader digital transformation in medical education, where technology-driven approaches are reshaping how clinical training is delivered, assessed, and scaled to meet the evolving needs of healthcare professionals (Almeida, 2023). With these advancements, the question is no longer whether technology should be integrated into medical education but how can it be leveraged effectively to enhance learning without compromising the critical human elements of medicine.

LITERATURE REVIEW

The Role of Artificial Intelligence in Medical Education

Medical education has long embraced technological advancements to enhance learning, from early computer-assisted instruction to modern immersive simulations. However, no innovation has generated as much excitement and apprehension as Artificial Intelligence (AI). At its core, AI refers to computational systems capable of performing cognitive tasks typically associated with human intelligence, such as pattern recognition, reasoning, decision-making, and problem-solving. The conceptual foundations of AI can be traced back to Alan Turing, who proposed that machines could mimic human intelligence (Jackson et al., 2024). This vision has since evolved into sophisticated algorithms capable of analyzing vast datasets, adapting to learner needs, and transforming medical instruction (Acharya et al., 2023). Recent literature reviews highlight its expanding role across various stages of medical training, specialties, and instructional applications (Gordon et al., 2024). The integration of AI into medical training aligns with broader global initiatives, as organizations like the World Health Organization (WHO) recognize AI-driven technologies as critical components of modern healthcare systems (Zarei et al., 2024).

With medical students expressing a strong eagerness to acquire competencies in the use of AI in medicine (Krive et al., 2023), the need for structured guidance on its effective integration into medical education has become increasingly important. Garcia, Arif, et al. (2024) addressed this need by offering practical strategies and actionable insights for seamlessly incorporating AI into medical training. Key among their recommendations is cultivating a culture of innovation to better prepare future physicians to leverage AI-driven advancements in diagnostics, treatment planning, and medical research. This approach is particularly crucial as AI continues to evolve beyond automation, now enabling more sophisticated applications such as real-time decision support (Elhaddad & Hamam, 2024), predictive analytics (Dixon et al., 2024), and personalized learning (Feigerlova et al., 2025). Unless we expect physicians-in-training to learn from textbooks that still refer to AI as science fiction, these growing technical capabilities necessitate a parallel evolution in medical education to ensure thoughtful integration and evaluation. With each new technological advancement, the trajectory sets the stage for the next generation of AI-driven innovations that will further redefine the landscape of medical education.

Generative AI for Teaching and Learning in Medicine

The emergence of Generative AI (GenAI) marks a new era in medical education, where AI is no longer just an analytical tool but an active creator of educational content, clinical scenarios, and personalized learning pathways (Cervantes et al., 2024; Stretton et al., 2024). GenAI refers to AI systems that can autonomously produce text, images, code, simulations, and other forms of content by learning patterns from vast datasets. A key component of GenAI is large language models (LLMs), which are designed to process and generate human-like text. These models enable applications such as AI-powered tutoring, automated case studies, and interactive clinical reasoning exercises. Some examples include OpenAI's *ChatGPT*, Google's *Gemini*, Anthropic's *Claude*, and the newest addition, *DeepSeek*. Since the popularization of GenAI in late 2022, various studies have explored its role in medical education, assessing its impact across undergraduate (Hale et al., 2024) and postgraduate (Janumpally et al., 2024) training. While it is too early to draw definitive conclusions, early implementations of GenAI in medical and health education indicate significant promise in reshaping pedagogical methodologies (Thomae et al., 2024).

Researchers such as Saleem et al. (2024) described it as an innovative heutagogical tool that fosters self-directed learning in medical education. This concept is put into practice through AI-driven platforms that craft personalized study strategies, analyze student progress to refine resource recommendations, and offer on-demand feedback (Garcia, Rosak-Szyrocka, et al., 2025). In addition to personalized learning, Boscardin et al. (2024) underscored the ability of GenAI to simulate real-world clinical scenarios. This setup allows students to refine their diagnostic reasoning, decision-making, and communication skills, which are key competencies for effective healthcare practice. Han et al. (2024) also emphasized that GenAI can assist educators by automating content development, generating assessment questions, and enhancing curriculum planning. With these capabilities, GenAI allows educators to focus more on student engagement and higher-order instructional strategies rather than spending excessive time on administrative tasks. A growing body of literature (e.g., Aster et al., 2024) reinforces these insights by documenting the expanding role of GenAI in supporting both faculty and student learning.

The Promise and Pitfalls of LLMs and GenAI in Medical Training

While advancements in GenAI and LLMs offer exciting possibilities, their increasing use also raises important concerns regarding implementation, reliability, and ethical considerations. A scoping review by Preiksaitis and Rose (2023) identified key challenges, including academic integrity, data accuracy, and the risk of AI dependence undermining critical thinking and deeper learning. However, while these concerns are frequently discussed, they are often emphasized disproportionately compared to the actual benefits and successful implementations of these technologies in medical education – or vice versa. Many studies outline the risks, but fewer offer balanced discussions on the practical applications, instructional benefits, and adaptive strategies that educators are already employing to integrate AI effectively. This imbalance presents a critical research gap where discussions surrounding GenAI and LLMs often focus on their theoretical pitfalls while overlooking real-world implementations that demonstrate their potential (Acut et al., 2025). There is a need to stop treating AI in medical education as either a miraculous teaching assistant or an ominous threat to academic integrity. A more balanced and comprehensive discussion is warranted—one that does not just highlight what could go wrong but also explores what is already going right and how we can refine best practices moving forward.

MAIN FOCUS OF THE CHAPTER

This chapter takes a thoughtful dive into the practices, pitfalls, and possibilities of GenAI in medical education. It aims to examine how educators are currently integrating AI-powered tools into teaching while also analyzing the challenges that come with its adoption. By balancing success stories with cautionary tales, this chapter seeks to bridge the gap between theoretical excitement and real-world implementation. More importantly, this chapter looks ahead to the future possibilities of GenAI in medical training by exploring how it could evolve from an efficient assistant to an indispensable partner in education. These insights can provide future physicians, medical educators, healthcare policymakers, and academic institutions with a roadmap for making GenAI a trusted ally rather than a questionable experiment. Thus, the significance of this chapter is in its effort to steer away from extremes, neither glorifying GenAI as the ultimate teaching savior nor condemning it as a disruptive force destined to erase human wisdom. Instead, it takes a grounded, balanced approach to show how AI tools can enhance medical education while keeping ethics and critical thinking at the heart of learning. Table 1 summarizes key practices and pitfalls that serve as a basis for future possibilities in AI-driven medical education and training.

Table 1. Summary of Practices and Pitfalls of AI Integration in Medical Education

Application	Practice	Pitfall	References
Automated Content Generation	Automate lecture slides, quizzes, and notes for medical courses.	Risk of generating inaccurate or overly generic content.	(Cox et al., 2024; Dao et al., 2021; Giannakos et al., 2024; Liu, 2025)
AI-Generated Assessments and Feedback	Offer instant evaluation and promote iterative learning.	Assessments may be biased or fail to align with educational standards.	(Khojasteh et al., 2025; Nguyen, 2024; Xia et al., 2024)
Virtual Patient Simulations	Enhance hands-on training with lifelike patient interactions.	It may lack the complexity and unpredictability of real-world cases.	(Cook, 2024; Guraya, 2024; Potter & Jefferies, 2024; Vaughn et al., 2024)
Virtual Anatomy and Surgical Training	Offer immersive, hands-on learning in a controlled virtual environment.	Oversimplify anatomical complexity or fail to replicate tactile feedback.	(Dai & Ke, 2022; Elendu et al., 2024; Lin & Chen, 2024; Sun et al., 2024)
Language Translation and Simplification	Increase accessibility for non-native speakers and underprepared students.	Loss of intended meaning or accuracy in critical medical concepts.	(Genovese et al., 2024; Lin et al., 2023; Naveen & Trojovský, 2024)
Medical Research Assistance	Reduce the time and effort required for academic research.	Risks introducing inaccuracies, bias, or ethical concerns in research	(Dixon et al., 2024; Hossain et al., 2023; Serrano et al., 2024)
Adaptive Learning Systems	Improve individual learning outcomes by tailoring content.	Risks of over-reliance on AI, which may limit independent learning	(Capuano & Caballé, 2020; Kabudi et al., 2021; Martin et al., 2020)
Intelligent Tutoring System	Makes learning more accessible and offers on-demand assistance.	Undermine the vital role of human instructors and nuanced teaching.	(As'ad, 2024; Garcia & Garcia, 2023; Yang & Shulruf, 2019)

METHODS

The methods employed in this chapter combine an integrative literature review with reflective analysis grounded in scholarly expertise. Specifically, the authors adopted a hermeneutic approach, drawing upon their disciplinary knowledge in medical education and educational technology to critically synthesize existing research and contextualize emerging themes in generative AI applications. This dual-method strategy anchored in expert interpretation and systematic examination of contemporary literature enabled a comprehensive exploration of pedagogical practices, instructional affordances, and ethical considerations related to GenAI in medical training. By merging evidence-based insights with domain-informed perspectives, this methodology ensures both theoretical rigor and practical relevance in evaluating the transformative potential of AI-driven tools in medical education.

A targeted and purposive search was conducted across PubMed, Scopus, and IEEE to capture a broad yet focused range of perspectives. The search was conducted using Boolean combinations of "generative AI", and "medical education." The review was restricted to sources published from 2018 to 2025 as a reflection of the post-deep learning boom and emergence of transformer-based AI tools in education. Studies were included if they addressed (1) the pedagogical use of GenAI in clinical or pre-clinical medical education, (2) instructional design strategies involving AI-powered tools, and (3) ethical and sociotechnical implications of using GenAI in learning contexts. Studies were excluded if they focused solely on technical aspects of AI model architecture or performance, or if they lacked substantive engagement with instructional outcomes or pedagogical frameworks. To support methodological robustness, selected findings were compared against established instructional frameworks in medical education (e.g., Bloom's taxonomy, Miller's pyramid, and constructivist models) to assess coherence and pedagogical relevance. Rather than offering a statistical synthesis, this approach foregrounds interpretive integration and theoretical insight, which are essential in a domain where technological developments often outpace traditional evidence synthesis methodologies.

DISCUSSION

Automated Content Generation

GenAI is transforming content creation in medical education by streamlining the development of high-fidelity, evidence-based instructional materials aligned with competency-based curricula. Given the administrative burdens faced by educators, GenAI tools facilitate the rapid generation of diverse pedagogical resources (e.g., competency maps, case-based learning scenarios, and structured assessment instruments). This technology optimizes instructional design by automating the synthesis of peer-reviewed medical literature, generating adaptive quizzes, and structuring didactic content to enhance pedagogical efficacy. AI-driven content generation likewise enables the dynamic reconfiguration of learning materials. For example, AI-generated lecture slides can present key definitions, structured outlines, and explanatory visuals to improve student engagement (Giannakos et al., 2024), while adaptive quizzes adjust question difficulty based on student performance to support personalized learning (Mustafa et al., 2024). GenAI also facilitates just-in-time curriculum updates to ensure medical education remains aligned with evolving clinical guidelines and translational research advancements. Empirical evidence supports GenAI's efficacy, such as its integration into AI-assisted authorship of open educational resources in orthopedic training (Cox et al., 2024) and its role in automating multimedia content for MOOCs (Dao et al., 2021). Furthermore, AI-driven content adaptation enhances accessibility by incorporating inclusive design principles, accommodating neurodiverse learners, and supporting multimodal instructional strategies, as exemplified by initiatives at Open University UK. Overall, GenAI provides a scalable framework for medical education that optimizes instructional efficiency, personalization, and accessibility.

Despite its pedagogical advantages, the integration of GenAI into medical education presents epistemic and ethical challenges, particularly regarding content validity, inferential accuracy, and contextual appropriateness. AI-generated instructional materials may inadvertently propagate epistemic distortions or factual inconsistencies, which could compromise clinical decision-making in high-stakes domains (Nguyen, 2024). For example, AI-generated lecture content may oversimplify pathophysiological mechanisms, resulting in knowledge gaps that hinder diagnostic reasoning. Additionally, generative models often lack the domain-specific heuristics necessary to critically evaluate the nuances of complex medical phenomena, leading to the production of reductionist or mechanistic explanations (Narayanan et al., 2023). Algorithmic biases embedded within large language models pose another significant concern, as they can distort the representation of disease prevalence, therapeutic efficacy, or population-specific clinical guidelines, potentially exacerbating disparities in medical education and practice (Mustafa et al., 2024). Furthermore, over-reliance on AI-generated content may lead to cognitive disengagement among educators, diminishing opportunities for contextual scaffolding required for deep learning (Khojasteh et al., 2025). As such, its deployment in medical education necessitates robust human oversight, including expert curation, validation through peer review, and alignment with best practices in instructional design and evidence-based medicine (Giannakos et al., 2024).

AI-Generated Assessments and Feedback

The integration of AI in assessment design and feedback mechanisms has transformed medical education by enabling real-time evaluation, adaptive testing, and personalized competency-based learning trajectories. AI-driven assessment platforms generate diverse evaluative formats, including high-fidelity multiple-choice questions, case-based reasoning tasks, and interactive problem-based learning (PBL) scenarios. These systems leverage natural language processing (NLP) and machine learning (ML) algorithms to provide formative feedback, allowing learners to identify cognitive gaps and receive scaffolded remediation strategies tailored to their proficiency levels (Nissen et al., 2025). Additionally, adaptive AI-powered assessments utilize item response theory (IRT) and Bayesian modeling to dynamically calibrate question difficulty based on learner performance, optimizing challenge levels for knowledge retention and skill acquisition (Mustafa et al., 2024). GenAI further enhances the evaluation process by automating the grading of complex assignments, including structured clinical examinations and written reflections. LLMs perform linguistic and content analysis of written submissions, detecting coherence, diagnostic reasoning accuracy, and critical appraisal depth while generating individualized, criterion-referenced feedback. Furthermore, AI-driven integrity verification tools employing stylometry and semantic analysis detect potential academic misconduct and safeguard assessment validity. By automating these routine evaluative functions, AI liberates educators to focus on higher-order mentorship, clinical skill development, and professional identity formation (Liu, 2025). The immediacy and adaptability of AI-generated feedback promote self-regulated learning that strengthens students' diagnostic reasoning and metacognitive skills over time.

While AI-enhanced assessments offer efficiency, scalability, and personalized learning pathways, they also present epistemological and ethical challenges. A primary concern is the potential for algorithmic bias in AI-generated evaluations, particularly if training datasets lack representational diversity or embed latent inaccuracies (Xia et al., 2024). Such biases can produce skewed competency appraisals, disproportionately disadvantaging underrepresented student populations and undermining assessment fairness. Moreover, AI-generated test items and automated feedback may not always align with competency-based medical education (CBME) frameworks, potentially leading to assessments that lack the depth required for clinical reasoning, procedural fluency, and higher-order cognitive engagement (Bozkurt et al., 2024; Khojasteh et al., 2025). Over-reliance on AI-generated evaluations may also reduce students' engagement in critical thinking and self-directed inquiry, impeding their ability to navigate the complex, ambiguous nature of real-world medical practice (Nguyen, 2024). Additionally, while AI-generated feedback provides immediacy, it often lacks the contextual nuance and case-specific insights that human educators bring to clinical training. Authentic assessment, which emphasizes situated cognition and complex clinical scenario-based tasks, remains essential in fostering deep learning, professional competence, and the development of domain-specific expertise (Lobo et al., 2024). Consequently, while AI-driven assessments enhance efficiency and accessibility, their implementation must be subject to rigorous validation, continuous faculty oversight, and alignment with best practices in medical education to uphold assessment integrity, mitigate bias, and preserve the pedagogical rigor necessary for competent clinical training.

Virtual Patient Simulations

AI and ML are also transforming healthcare simulation by facilitating the development of highly interactive, data-driven virtual patient (VP) models with unprecedented realism. Recent advancements in LLMs demonstrate the feasibility of generating responsive VPs for competency-based medical training (Potter & Jefferies, 2024). These AI-enhanced simulations leverage NLP and reinforcement learning to enable adaptive patient interactions that augment the fidelity of clinical scenarios. AI-driven simulation platforms also allow learners to engage with lifelike virtual patients in structured, risk-free environments, fostering procedural mastery and clinical decision-making through iterative, experiential learning. These systems employ real-time physiological modeling to adjust patient responses dynamically based on user inputs, ensuring tailored feedback and scenario complexity modulation aligned with the learner's expertise level (Cook, 2024). Moreover, AI-powered VPs facilitate high-resolution anatomical visualization, enabling real-time exploration of three-dimensional anatomical structures. AR and VR applications further enrich this learning paradigm by integrating haptic feedback and immersive, interactive surgical simulations that replicate dynamic physiological and pathological states with high granularity (Guraya, 2024). This convergence of AI, VR, and AR in medical simulation optimizes skill acquisition, procedural competency development, and patient safety by allowing for repeated, deliberate practice in a controlled setting. A prime example is ALEX GenAI Lite (Figure 1), an advanced patient communication simulator that integrates GenAI-driven speech recognition and real-time physiological response modeling. ALEX supports multilingual clinical interviews, mimics vital physiological functions, and provides real-time auscultation feedback for cardiac and pulmonary assessments. The synergy of AI-driven naturalistic communication and physiological realism enhances the scope and effectiveness of simulation-based education.

Figure 1. Simulated Patient Encounter Using PCS Alex Virtual Simulator (PCS, 2025)

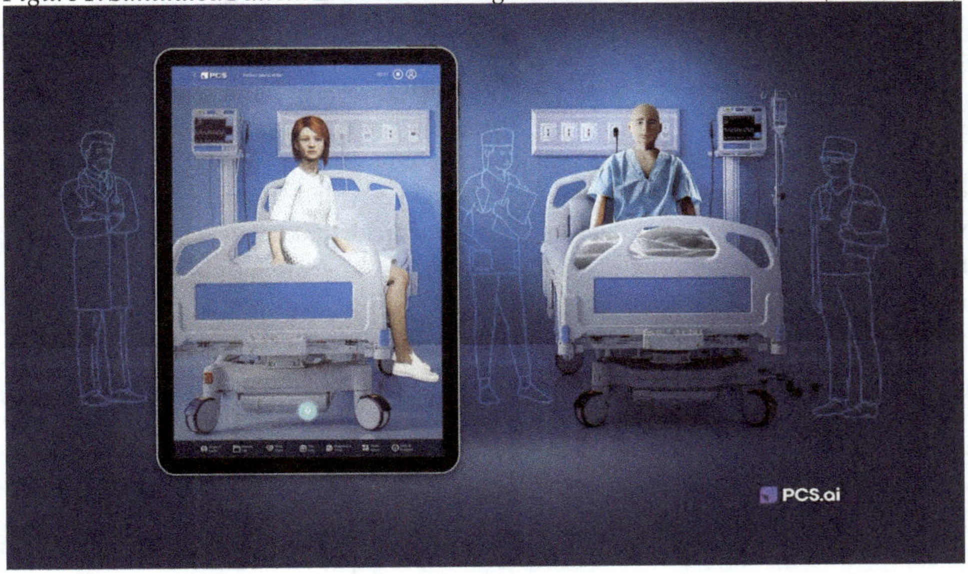

Despite its transformative potential, AI-powered virtual patient simulations present notable limitations. While GenAI platforms can streamline the design of intricate clinical case scenarios, expert oversight remains crucial to ensure content validity, contextual accuracy, and adherence to evidence-based medical education frameworks (Vaughn et al., 2024). One critical limitation is the potential oversimplification of anatomical and physiological variability, as AI-generated models may not fully replicate the complex heterogeneity of real-world patient presentations (Cook, 2024). Additionally, while AI-based simulations provide high cognitive fidelity, they often lack the tactile realism required for procedural skill development, posing challenges for mastering techniques (e.g., suturing, palpation, and fine motor surgical maneuvers). The absence of realistic haptic sensations may constrain the translation of virtual training into practical clinical proficiency (Guraya, 2024). Another key concern is the cost of deploying high-fidelity AI-driven simulations, particularly in resource-constrained settings where infrastructure and technical support may be limited. Furthermore, effective curriculum integration is essential to ensure that AI-based simulations function as a complementary, rather than substitutive, modality for experiential learning. Without structured faculty guidance and rigorous instructional scaffolding, learners may develop an over-reliance on virtual simulations, potentially affecting their clinical performance in real-world patient care settings. Consequently, while AI-driven medical simulations offer significant advancements in healthcare education, their implementation must be carefully designed to balance technological innovation with pedagogical integrity, ensuring alignment with competency-based medical training objectives.

Virtual Anatomy and Surgical Training

GenAI has also redefined virtual anatomy education and surgical training by delivering a precision-driven learning experience within a controlled digital environment. AI-powered simulations enable medical trainees to explore intricate anatomical structures through high-fidelity three-dimensional models (Elendu et al., 2024). Unlike static cadaveric dissections or two-dimensional textbook representations, AI-driven platforms generate volumetric reconstructions of human anatomy. This feature allows learners to manipulate, segment, and visualize physiological structures from multiple spatial perspectives with real-time biomechanical accuracy (Dai & Ke, 2022). These models integrate adaptive learning algorithms that tailor complexity levels based on learner progression, fostering an individualized, competency-based educational experience (Elendu et al., 2024; Lin & Chen, 2024). AI-driven surgical training environments also provide a risk-free, interactive setting where trainees refine procedural techniques and operative decision-making through virtual simulations. These platforms (Figure 2) realistically simulate surgical workflows with millimeter-level precision, allowing learners to practice incisions, suturing techniques, and instrument handling before transitioning to live clinical settings (Riddle et al., 2024). AI-based analytics further enhance surgical training by systematically assessing technical performance, identifying cognitive and motor skill deficiencies, and delivering targeted, data-driven feedback to optimize proficiency. Moreover, AI-enabled remote simulation platforms bridge the educational divide for students in resource-limited settings, providing scalable access to high-fidelity anatomical and procedural training that would otherwise require cadaveric laboratories or advanced surgical training centers (Sun et al., 2024; Zidoun & Mardi, 2024). As a cost-effective and scalable approach, AI-driven virtual anatomy and surgical simulations align with competency-based medical education paradigms, equipping learners with a robust foundation in anatomical and procedural knowledge before direct patient interaction.

Figure 2. Medical VR Solutions for Teaching Anatomy Without a Cadaver (MAI, 2025)

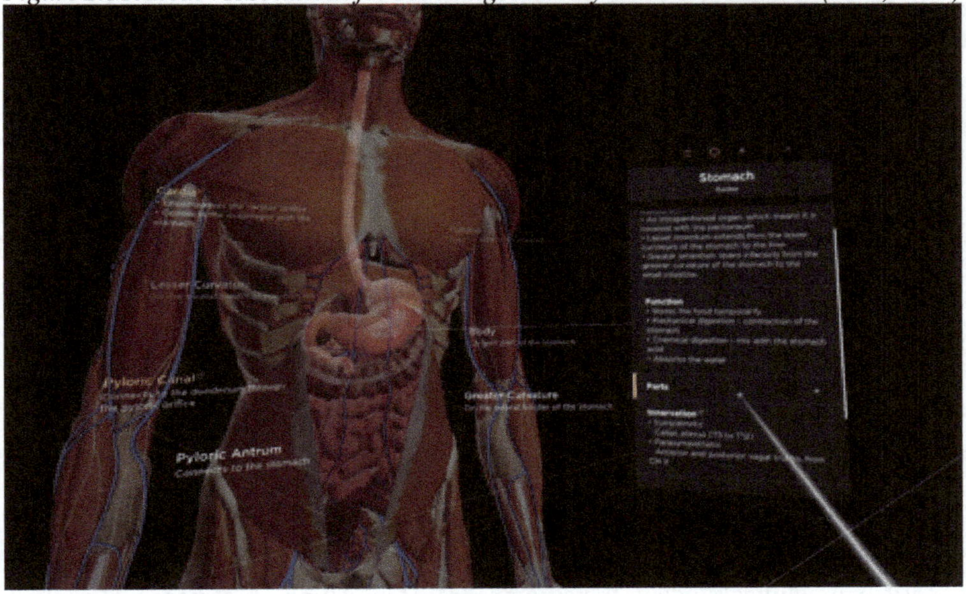

Although undoubtedly beneficial, this GenAI application also presents inherent limitations in its capacity to replicate the full spectrum of anatomical variability and haptic sensory feedback critical for surgical dexterity. Human anatomical variation, including differences in vascular configurations, pathological anomalies, and tissue elasticity, is often underrepresented in AI-generated models. While AI-driven simulations offer visually precise anatomical reconstructions, subtle morphological nuances essential for complex surgical decision-making may be absent (Zhai et al., 2024). A primary drawback of AI-based surgical training is the deficit in haptic feedback, which is a crucial factor in developing kinesthetic proficiency. Traditional surgical education relies on cadaveric dissection, animal models, or live patient training to cultivate an intuitive understanding of tissue resistance, elasticity, and force modulation (Pirri et al., 2021). While advancements in haptic gloves offer partial tactile replication, current VR and AR systems remain limited in mirroring the biomechanical complexity of human-tissue interaction. Following our previous remark, over-reliance on AI-driven simulations may create a disparity between theoretical competency and practical execution (Riddle et al., 2024). Infrastructure requirements pose another significant challenge, as AI-enhanced surgical training demands high-performance computing, sophisticated VR hardware, and continuous software updates. Ethical concerns also arise regarding the shift from traditional mentorship-based surgical apprenticeship models to AI-mediated training. This transition raises questions about the development of professional judgment, clinical intuition, and the humanistic aspects of medical practice (Satapathy et al., 2023). While AI-driven surgical education remains a radical advancement, its implementation must function as an adjunct to hands-on clinical exposure to ensure holistic skill acquisition.

Language Translation and Simplification

Another pivotal advancement in GenAI within medical education is its role in language translation and medical content simplification, which enhances accessibility for linguistically diverse learners and underprepared students. AI-driven translation systems facilitate domain-specific translations of medical textbooks, didactic materials, and peer-reviewed literature with semantic preservation (Genovese et al., 2024). These computational linguistics models mitigate lexical asymmetry between source and target languages, ensuring that non-native speakers gain unobstructed access to specialized medical knowledge. Additionally, AI-powered NLP pipelines execute lexical simplification and syntactic restructuring, which deconstructs complex biomedical nomenclature into more cognitively digestible formats—a critical benefit for preclinical students transitioning from foundational biosciences to applied clinical reasoning (Mir et al., 2023). Beyond static translation, adaptive AI-driven knowledge dissemination systems utilize reinforcement learning algorithms to calibrate content granularity based on real-time learner analytics. Dynamic knowledge graphs and intelligent tutoring systems (ITS) further enhance comprehension by contextually encoding medical ontologies, adjusting explanatory depth through personalized, multimodal instructional strategies, including interactive schematic overlays and three-dimensional anatomical annotations (Garcia & Garcia, 2023; Lin et al., 2023). These cognitive augmentation technologies enhance pedagogical inclusivity to ensure that heterogeneous learner cohorts engage with evidence-based medical curricula. Furthermore, AI-facilitated language interoperability extends its utility beyond didactic instruction, enabling cross-border knowledge transfer and multilingual clinical communication, particularly in transnational healthcare ecosystems (Barwise et al., 2024). By redefining linguistic accessibility in medical education, AI scaffolds the development of globally attuned healthcare professionals.

However, neural sequence modeling in AI-driven translation introduces epistemic vulnerabilities, particularly in semantic fidelity and terminological precision. A paramount concern is that probabilistic autoregressive models may generate lexical perturbations and polysemous ambiguities, leading to clinically consequential mistranslations (Naveen & Trojovský, 2024). Biomedical phraseology in domains such as pharmacokinetics, neuropathophysiology, and oncological pathology is semantically dense, where even marginal distortions in translingual encoding may compromise diagnostic accuracy. Additionally, LLMs, despite their contextual embedding optimizations, may produce algorithmically induced epistemic distortions, where explanatory reductionism leads to excessive abstraction of mechanistic pathophysiology (Khosravi et al., 2024). This didactic attenuation risks impairing medical reasoning schemas, disrupting diagnostic pattern recognition, and eroding clinical inferencing fidelity (Jin et al., 2024). A further structural limitation arises from AI-mediated lexical disambiguation failures, particularly in homonymous biomedical lexemes, where polysemic constructs (e.g., "lead" as a toxicant vs. an electrocardiographic waveform descriptor) may be contextually misattributed (Naveen & Trojovský, 2024). Moreover, algorithmic textual simplification lacks the heuristic adaptability of expert educators, who contextualize didactic materials based on learner epistemology and clinical reasoning progression. Without ontological validation and expert curation, AI-generated content risks propagating epistemic opacity, where learners unknowingly assimilate suboptimal or semantically compromised medical knowledge (Zhai et al., 2024). Hybridized AI-human instructional frameworks are imperative to mitigate these epistemological risks. Integrated validation pipelines, where automated translation outputs undergo expert peer review, ensure semantic coherence, domain specificity, and clinical applicability.

Medical Research Assistance

Medical and academic research methodologies are likewise being transformed through the integration of GenAI. NLP architectures, coupled with unsupervised and supervised ML algorithms, facilitate the rapid analysis of large-scale biomedical corpora, extracting clinically relevant insights and identifying emerging research trajectories (Hossain et al., 2023). These automated knowledge synthesis models surpass manual review methodologies, mitigating human-induced selection bias while optimizing semantic indexing and evidence mapping. Unlike traditional bibliometric approaches, which are resource-intensive and susceptible to inter-reviewer variability, LLM-powered meta-analytic pipelines accelerate literature synthesis with algorithmic precision and contextual coherence (Xiao et al., 2025). Beyond bibliographic aggregation, AI augments hypothesis generation and research design by using predictive modeling, identifying statistical correlations, and proposing novel exploratory variables for empirical investigation (Dixon et al., 2024). Impressively, advanced generative architectures simulate hypothetical clinical scenarios and allow researchers to model potential causative relationships and refine research inquiries based on historical epidemiological trends. Automated data synthesis engines also generate structured narrative abstracts, visualize multivariate datasets, and employ dimensionality reduction techniques to uncover latent data patterns. These capabilities redefine research productivity by enabling investigators to prioritize experimental validation and inferential rigor over preliminary data acquisition. The scalability of

AI in biomedical informatics fosters knowledge acceleration, driving high-impact scientific discoveries across translational medicine and clinical research paradigms (Serrano et al., 2024).

However, algorithmic-driven knowledge synthesis introduces epistemology, particularly regarding content validity, inferential generalizability, and methodological transparency. Alternatively, a critical limitation is that GenAI leverages pre-trained corpora, which may contain embedded inaccuracies, historical biases, or epistemic distortions (Hanna et al., 2025). In high-stakes biomedical research, AI hallucinations pose risks to evidence-based medicine and translational accuracy. Moreover, AI-generated hypotheses—although computationally derived—often lack epistemic depth and heuristic reasoning, potentially yielding superficial, mechanistic, or non-actionable research inquiries. Algorithmic bias in AI-driven metaresearch is another paramount concern, as LLMs inherent selection biases from skewed training datasets (Cross et al., 2024). For instance, biomedical models trained predominantly on Eurocentric clinical trials may generate non-generalizable findings. Over-reliance on automated synthesis models also risks circumventing essential peer-review mechanisms, which are foundational to scientific integrity and methodological reproducibility (Resnik & Hosseini, 2024). Further ethical concerns arise from AI-generated citation fabrications, where synthetically generated references can exacerbate concerns of research integrity violations and scientific fraudulence (Acut et al., 2024). AI-assisted research outputs must undergo rigorous cross-validation to ensure that algorithmic inferences align with empirically verified sources. Hybridized peer-review frameworks, wherein AI-augmented literature synthesis undergoes expert vetting, are essential to preserving scholarly rigor and epistemic accountability. Implementing AI governance policies, promoting algorithmic transparency, and enforcing ethical compliance guidelines will balance computational efficiency with academic credibility, safeguarding the integrity of AI-integrated medical research.

Adaptive Learning Systems

The integration of AI in Adaptive Learning Systems (ALS) has revolutionized medical education by enabling data-driven instructional modulation tailored to individual learner profiles (Capuano & Caballé, 2020). Unlike traditional pedagogical frameworks, which implement standardized curricular models, AI-enhanced ALS deploys ML algorithms to optimize knowledge retention, cognitive engagement, and metacognitive regulation (Alawneh et al., 2024). In medical education, AI-driven systems continuously analyze performance metrics, response latency, and interaction patterns to identify conceptual deficiencies and administer targeted remediation strategies (Kabudi et al., 2021). Adaptive learning platforms also leverage predictive analytics and neural network-based optimization to sequence instructional content. For instance, an ALS-integrated diagnostic reasoning module may intensify radiological image interpretation drills for students exhibiting suboptimal pattern recognition performance in electrocardiogram (ECG) waveform differentiation. Empirical research underscores the efficacy of AI-driven scaffolded instruction in not only amplifying academic performance but also enhancing conceptual transferability through interactive cognitive scaffolding and hierarchical content structuring (Lajoie & Gube, 2018). According to Martin et al. (2020), a comprehensive learning framework comprises three interdependent models: (1) *Learner Model*, which captures cognitive attributes, prior knowledge schemas, and individualized learning preferences; (2) *Content Model*, which delineates conceptual hierarchies and disciplinary complexity, structuring content to optimize domain coherence; and (3) *Instructional Model*, which modulates sequencing, pacing, and formative feedback loops to maximize learner efficacy. They argued that adaptive feedback mechanisms and AI-curated navigation pathways constitute some of the most efficacious AI methodologies for optimizing personalized learning trajectories. By integrating immediate diagnostic feedback, AI ensures that learners receive contextually relevant, precision-targeted instructional guidance while maintaining an optimal cognitive challenge threshold.

However, despite its pedagogical advancements, ALS introduces critical epistemological and cognitive risks, particularly in the attenuation of self-regulated learning capacities (Strielkowski et al., 2024). Clinical competency development necessitates metacognitive regulation, diagnostic reasoning, and heuristic decision-making, yet excessive dependence on AI-driven content modulation may diminish cognitive autonomy and analytical depth. Empirical studies highlight that when students passively engage with ALS technologies, they exhibit reduced engagement in self-directed inquiry (Lajoie & Gube, 2018). Another pressing concern is algorithmic bias in AI-mediated instructional decision-making, wherein non-representative training datasets can lead to disparities in content recommendations (Capuano & Caballé, 2020; Kabudi et al., 2021). AI-generated assessments may also lack the contextual granularity and ethical complexity that expert human educators provide, particularly in medical scenarios requiring clinical judgment and bioethical reasoning. While adaptive learning enhances personalized knowledge scaffolding, designing ALS to foster cognitive agency is imperative (Martin et al., 2020). The most pedagogically effective ALS implementations integrate AI-driven adaptivity with metacognitive enhancement techniques (e.g., student self-assessment frameworks, reflective learning analytics, and PBL methodologies) to ensure that learners retain agency over their cognitive trajectories. To mitigate these risks, hybrid instructional models once again offer the optimal equilibrium between automation and cognitive empowerment. Ensuring educational efficacy and preserving the epistemic integrity of medical training necessitates iterative curriculum recalibration and rigorous algorithmic monitoring.

Intelligent Tutoring Systems

A further significant development in medical education is the integration of ITS to create adaptive learning environments. ITS functions as cognitive scaffolding agents that emulate human tutoring methodologies by dynamically adjusting instruction and delivering context-sensitive feedback. These systems integrate domain-specific knowledge, learner modeling algorithms, and evidence-based pedagogical frameworks to facilitate competency-driven learning trajectories (Castro-Schez et al., 2021). ITS has demonstrated high efficacy in medical education by generating multimodal learning spaces that adapt to heterogeneous learner needs through adaptive content sequencing and intelligent feedback loops. AI-driven cognitive diagnostic models analyze user interactions, error patterns, and response latencies (Singh et al., 2022). In medical training, ITS applications span multiple disciplinary domains. For instance, Garcia and Garcia (2023) used ITS as an instructional technology for teaching and learning nutrition concepts (Figure 3). Similarly, Mirchi et al. (2020) used ITS in surgical education, where procedural simulations provide competency-based feedback. ITS embedded with NLP, such as the model by As'ad (2024), enhances conversational AI tutoring and allows learners to engage in context-aware discussions where AI tutors explain complex medical concepts in natural language. Like ALS, one of the most salient advantages of ITS is its ability to foster self-regulated learning. ITS have been empirically validated to enhance clinical knowledge acquisition and learner confidence beyond conventional didactic methodologies (Yang & Shulruf, 2019). By orchestrating structured problem-solving tasks, providing real-time diagnostic feedback, and reducing cognitive overload, ITS enhances conceptual engagement and cognitive scaffolding of learners.

Figure 3. Nutrition Intelligent Tutoring System for Primary Education (Garcia & Garcia, 2023)

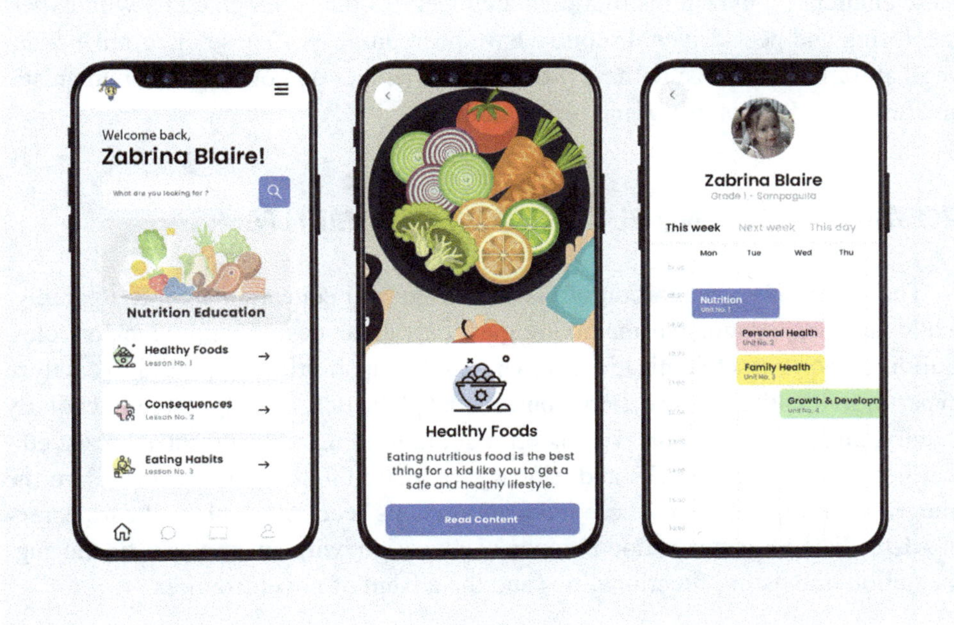

However, the integration of ITS in medical education introduces critical epistemological, pedagogical, and ethical challenges. One of the primary concerns is a potential attenuation of human educator engagement, which may impede the development of critical reasoning and clinical decision-making competencies. While ITS expedite formative feedback, they often lack the depth of heuristic reasoning and ethical contextualization that human educators provide, particularly in complex patient care scenarios where clinical decisions transcend algorithmic recommendations (Mousavinasab et al., 2018). ITS also faces integration challenges within competency-based medical curricula, as overreliance on automated tutoring environments may diminish learner autonomy and analytical dexterity, leading to passive information assimilation rather than active inquiry (Singh et al., 2022). Moreover, algorithmic biases in ITS pose a systemic risk to equitable medical education, as models trained on non-diverse clinical datasets may exacerbate knowledge disparities and skew competency assessments (As'ad, 2024). This issue is particularly critical in algorithmic competency evaluation, where training-set homogeneity may result in a disproportionate representation of certain clinical presentations, disadvantaging underrepresented medical conditions or minority populations. Overdependence on AI-mediated tutoring frameworks risks fostering algorithmic dependency, wherein learners prioritize computational guidance over independent critical inquiry and collaborative problem-solving (Gantalao et al., 2025; Singh et al., 2022). To mitigate these challenges, hybrid instructional architectures that synergize ITS with expert mentoring and peer-driven discourse have been proposed. These integrative pedagogical frameworks ensure that AI-driven efficiencies do not erode the humanistic and heuristic dimensions of medical training.

POSSIBILITIES AND FUTURE ADVANCEMENTS

The progressive integration of GenAI in medical education signals a paradigmatic shift in pedagogical methodologies, curricular design, and educator roles. Building upon extant applications, emergent AI capabilities are poised to catalyze hyper-individualized instruction, multimodal didactics, AI-augmented scholarly inquiry, and real-time clinical decision-making training. Concurrently, robust ethical governance frameworks and efficacy validation are imperative to ensure the integrity and inclusivity of these innovations. This section examines the trajectory of AI-mediated transformation in medical education, with an emphasis on the augmentation of existing functionalities and the advent of novel frontiers.

AI-Driven Personalization and Clinical Decision Support

AI in medical education is progressing toward anticipatory and dynamically responsive pedagogical architectures. Forthcoming ITS will integrate predictive modeling, leveraging deep learning and longitudinal learner analytics to preemptively identify cognitive lacunae and recalibrate instructional delivery in real time. This proactive optimization mitigates cognitive overload, reinforces knowledge retention, and cultivates advanced clinical reasoning competencies (Capuano & Caballé, 2020; Potter & Jefferies, 2024). Next-generation AI tutors will also supersede rule-based interactivity by incorporating situational awareness, case-based reasoning, and dialogic learning frameworks. These systems will iteratively refine their inferential capacity via federated ML paradigms, continuously assimilating de-identified, globally sourced learner interaction data to enhance pedagogical precision (Martin et al., 2020; Singh et al., 2022). Furthermore, multimodal AI frameworks will revolutionize virtual patient simulations, engendering fully adaptive, biofeedback-sensitive clinical environments. Through the integration of biometric telemetry, affective computing, and real-time performance metrics, AI systems will modulate clinical scenarios to align with learners' cognitive states, thus enhancing diagnostic fidelity and fostering metacognitive reflection. Such innovations will be particularly transformative in high-acuity domains such as surgical education, trauma response training, and telemedicine, where temporal precision and decision-making under duress are paramount.

Ethical and Regulatory Frameworks to Address Systemic Risks

The deployment of AI in medical pedagogy introduces substantive bioethical, legal, and regulatory challenges. Salient among these are concerns regarding algorithmic opacity, model bias, and the integrity of autonomous evaluative systems (Garcia, Garcia, et al., 2024; Strielkowski et al., 2024). Given that AI algorithms are inherently reflective of their training corpora, there exists a significant risk of perpetuating sociocultural and diagnostic inequities, particularly within underrepresented demographic cohorts (Kabudi et al., 2021). Meanwhile, the aggregation and processing of granular learner data (e.g., behavioral analytics, biometric feedback, and clinical reasoning trajectories) require stringent adherence to data protection mandates such as the GDPR, HIPAA, and analogous international statutes. AI-driven simulation platforms exacerbate vulnerability to cybersecurity threats, necessitating end-to-end encryption, differential privacy protocols, and institutional accountability mechanisms (Chen & Esmaeilzadeh, 2024). These issues necessitate preserving the primacy of human oversight through rigorous validation, ethical auditing, and governance mechanisms that uphold professional autonomy.

Human-AI Synergy in Enhancing Pedagogical Outcomes

The optimal integration of AI in medical education is predicated upon a collaborative paradigm wherein AI functions as an augmentative cognitive tool rather than a pedagogical surrogate. Interdisciplinary co-development involving clinical educators, computational scientists, and instructional designers is imperative to ensure that AI applications align with epistemological objectives and curricular standards (Schubert et al., 2025). Contemporary AI platforms already automate granular tasks such as rubric-aligned grading, curriculum mapping, and algorithmic content curation, liberating educators to concentrate on high-order cognitive scaffolding, ethical deliberation, and clinical contextualization (Narayanan et al., 2023). AI tutors of the next generation will employ semantic understanding, contextual inference, and case-based narrative analytics to facilitate personalized, longitudinal mentorship. Their continual refinement through federated learning ensures global scalability and cultural adaptability (Cox et al., 2024). Institutionalizing AI literacy within medical curricula is essential to cultivate informed practitioners capable of interrogating AI outputs, recognizing algorithmic fallibility, and engaging responsibly with emerging technologies. These programs must encompass epistemic training in

AI interpretability, model limitations, and sociotechnical ethics to foster judicious integration into clinical training (Genovese et al., 2024; Yazdani & Abardeh, 2019).

Equitable Deployment of GenAI in Global and Resource-Constrained Contexts

GenAI possesses the potential to democratize access to high-fidelity medical training in under-resourced and linguistically diverse settings. Multilingual AI language models can localize complex clinical knowledge, which enhances cognitive accessibility for non-English-speaking trainees and facilitating culturally congruent pedagogy (Genovese et al., 2024). Infrastructurally minimal yet pedagogically robust solutions (e.g., AI-enabled mobile platforms and low-bandwidth virtual simulations) offer scalable alternatives to traditional cadaveric or apprenticeship-based training. These technologies support competency-based skill acquisition in diagnostic and procedural domains, which directly address global disparities in clinical education (McGee et al., 2024; Potter & Jefferies, 2024). Moreover, AI-augmented tele-mentorship ecosystems and cloud-based collaborative platforms facilitate synchronous and asynchronous engagement between learners and global clinical experts. These systems enable case-based learning, peer interaction, and dynamically tailored feedback, which are all modulated via AI-driven learning analytics (Dixon et al., 2024). Equitable dissemination of such technologies necessitates infrastructural investment, policy support, and cross-border collaboration. Ensuring that AI-driven educational tools are accessible, linguistically adaptable, and pedagogically validated is critical to fostering globally inclusive, competency-driven medical training environments (Elendu et al., 2024).

CONCLUSION

Even in a learning environment as intense as medical school, where complexity is the norm and cognitive overload a constant companion, GenAI offers relief with purpose. Rather than adding pressure to the already overwhelming torrent of information, GenAI can serve as a well-calibrated valve that channels learning in ways that are more adaptive and responsive to individual needs. As this review has shown, its strengths lie not in replacing educators or simplifying medicine but in enhancing how knowledge is delivered, contextualized, and retained. At the same time, its integration is not without friction: questions of accuracy, bias, accountability, and pedagogical misalignment must temper uncritical enthusiasm. The way we train future physicians today profoundly influences how they will practice medicine, lead their communities, and drive innovation in the years ahead. As such, the thoughtful adoption of GenAI in medical education is not just a matter of instructional design but an investment in the future of healthcare itself.

REFERENCES

Acharya, V., Padhan, P., Bahinipati, J., Mishra, S., Aggarwal, K., Jhajharia, S., Parida, P., Sahu, D., & Pradhan, T. (2023). Artificial Intelligence in Medical Education. *The Journal of International Medical Research, 1*(3), 87–91. DOI: 10.4103/jimr.jimr_17_23

Acut, D. P., Gamusa, E. V., Pernaa, J., Yuenyong, C., Pantaleon, A. T., Espina, R. C., Sim, M. J. C., & Garcia, M. B. (2025). AI Shaming Among Teacher Education Students: A Reflection on Acceptance and Identity in the Age of Generative Tools. In *Pitfalls of AI Integration in Education: Skill Obsolescence, Misuse, and Bias*. IGI Global., DOI: 10.4018/979-8-3373-0122-8.ch005

Acut, D. P., Malabago, N. K., Malicoban, E. V., Galamiton, N. S., & Garcia, M. B. (2024). "ChatGPT 4.0 Ghosted Us While Conducting Literature Search:" Modeling the Chatbot's Generated Non-Existent References Using Regression Analysis. *Internet Reference Services Quarterly, 29*(1), 27–54. DOI: 10.1080/10875301.2024.2426793

Alawneh, Y. J. J., Sleema, H., Salman, F. N., Alshammat, M. F., & Oteer, R. S., & ALrashidi, N. K. N. (2024). Adaptive Learning Systems: Revolutionizing Higher Education through AI-Driven Curricula. *2024 International Conference on Knowledge Engineering and Communication Systems (ICKECS), 1*, 1-5. https://doi.org/ DOI: 10.1109/ICKECS61492.2024.10616675

Almeida, R. S. d. (2023). Redefining Health Education in the Post-Pandemic World: How to Integrate Digital Technologies into the Curricula? In *Handbook of Research on Instructional Technologies in Health Education and Allied Disciplines*. IGI Global., DOI: 10.4018/978-1-6684-7164-7.ch001

As'ad, M. (2024). Intelligent Tutoring Systems, Generative Artificial Intelligence (AI), and Healthcare Agents: A Proof of Concept and Dual-Layer Approach. *Cureus*. Advance online publication. DOI: 10.7759/cureus.69710 PMID: 39308847

Aster, A., Laupichler, M. C., Rockwell-Kollmann, T., Masala, G., Bala, E., & Raupach, T. (2024). ChatGPT and Other Large Language Models in Medical Education — Scoping Literature Review. *Medical Science Educator, 35*(1), 1–13. DOI: 10.1007/s40670-024-02206-6 PMID: 40144083

Barwise, A. K., Curtis, S., Diedrich, D. A., & Pickering, B. W. (2024). Using Artificial Intelligence to Promote Equitable Care for Inpatients With Language Barriers and Complex Medical Needs: Clinical Stakeholder Perspectives. *Journal of the American Medical Informatics Association : JAMIA, 31*(3), 611–621. DOI: 10.1093/jamia/ocad224 PMID: 38099504

Boscardin, C. K., Gin, B., Golde, P. B., & Hauer, K. E. (2024). ChatGPT and Generative Artificial Intelligence for Medical Education: Potential Impact and Opportunity. *Academic Medicine*, *99*(1), 22–27. Advance online publication. DOI: 10.1097/ACM.0000000000005439 PMID: 37651677

Bozkurt, A., Xiao, J., Farrow, R., Bai, J. Y. H., Nerantzi, C., Moore, S., Dron, J., Stracke, C. M., Singh, L., Crompton, H., Koutropoulos, A., Terentev, E., Pazurek, A., Nichols, M., Sidorkin, A. M., Costello, E., Watson, S., Mulligan, D., Honeychurch, S., & Asino, T. I. (2024). The Manifesto for Teaching and Learning in a Time of Generative AI: A Critical Collective Stance to Better Navigate the Future. *Open Praxis*, *16*(4), 487–513. DOI: 10.55982/openpraxis.16.4.777

Buja, L. M. (2019). Medical Education Today: All That Glitters is Not Gold. *BMC Medical Education*, *19*(1), 1–11. DOI: 10.1186/s12909-019-1535-9 PMID: 30991988

Capuano, N., & Caballé, S. (2020). Adaptive Learning Technologies. *AI Magazine*, *41*(2), 96–98. DOI: 10.1609/aimag.v41i2.5317

Castro-Schez, J. J., Glez-Morcillo, C., Albusac, J., & Vallejo, D. (2021). An Intelligent Tutoring System for Supporting Active Learning: A Case Study on Predictive Parsing Learning. *Information Sciences*, *544*, 446–468. DOI: 10.1016/j.ins.2020.08.079 PMID: 32958966

Cervantes, J., Smith, B., Ramadoss, T., D'Amario, V., Shoja, M. M., & Rajput, V. (2024). Decoding Medical Educators' Perceptions on Generative Artificial Intelligence in Medical Education. *Journal of Investigative Medicine*, *72*(7), 633–639. DOI: 10.1177/10815589241257215 PMID: 38785310

Chen, Y., & Esmaeilzadeh, P. (2024). Generative AI in Medical Practice: In-Depth Exploration of Privacy and Security Challenges. *Journal of Medical Internet Research*, *26*, 1–19. DOI: 10.2196/53008 PMID: 38457208

Chowdhury, P. N., Vaish, A., Puri, B., & Vaishya, R. (2024). Medical Education Technology: Past, Present and Future. *Apollo Medicine*, *21*(4), 374–380. DOI: 10.1177/09760016241256202

Cook, D. A. (2024). Creating Virtual Patients Using Large Language Models: Scalable, Global, and Low Cost. *Medical Teacher*, *47*(1), 40–42. DOI: 10.1080/0142159X.2024.2376879 PMID: 38992981

Cox, G., Willmers, M., Brown, R., & Held, M. (2024). Learning along the Way: A Case Study on a Pedagogically Innovative Approach to Engage Medical Students in the Creation of Open Educational Resources Using ChatGPT. *Mousaion: South African Journal of Information Studies*, *42*(1), 1–21. DOI: 10.25159/2663-659X/15331

Cross, J. L., Choma, M. A., & Onofrey, J. A. (2024). Bias in Medical AI: Implications for Clinical Decision-Making. *PLOS Digital Health*, *3*(11), 1–19. DOI: 10.1371/journal.pdig.0000651 PMID: 39509461

Dai, C.-P., & Ke, F. (2022). Educational Applications of Artificial Intelligence in Simulation-Based Learning: A Systematic Mapping Review. *Computers and Education: Artificial Intelligence*, *3*, 1–17. DOI: 10.1016/j.caeai.2022.100087

Dao, X.-Q., Le, N.-B., & Nguyen, T.-M.-T. (2021). AI-Powered MOOCs: Video Lecture Generation. *Proceedings of the 2021 3rd International Conference on Image, Video and Signal Processing*, 95–102. https://doi.org/DOI: 10.1145/3459212.3459227

Dixon, D., Sattar, H., Moros, N., Kesireddy, S. R., Ahsan, H., Lakkimsetti, M., Fatima, M., Doshi, D., Sadhu, K., & Junaid Hassan, M. (2024). Unveiling the Influence of AI Predictive Analytics on Patient Outcomes: A Comprehensive Narrative Review. *Cureus*, *16*(5), e59954. DOI: 10.7759/cureus.59954 PMID: 38854327

Elendu, C., Amaechi, D. C., Okatta, A. U., Amaechi, E. C., Elendu, T. C., Ezeh, C. P., & Elendu, I. D. (2024). The Impact of Simulation-Based Training in Medical Education. *Revista de Medicina (São Paulo)*, *103*(27), 1–14. DOI: 10.1097/MD.0000000000038813 PMID: 38968472

Elhaddad, M., & Hamam, S. (2024). AI-Driven Clinical Decision Support Systems: An Ongoing Pursuit of Potential. *Cureus*, *16*(4), 1–9. DOI: 10.7759/cureus.57728 PMID: 38711724

Feigerlova, E., Hani, H., & Hothersall-Davies, E. (2025). A Systematic Review of the Impact of Artificial Intelligence on Educational Outcomes in Health Professions Education. *BMC Medical Education*, *25*(1), 1–18. DOI: 10.1186/s12909-025-06719-5 PMID: 39871336

Gantalao, L. C., Calzada, J. G. D., Capuyan, D. L., Lumantas, B. C., Acut, D. P., & Garcia, M. B. (2025). Equipping the Next Generation of Technicians: Navigating School Infrastructure and Technical Knowledge in the Age of AI Integration. In *Pitfalls of AI Integration in Education: Skill Obsolescence, Misuse, and Bias*. IGI Global., DOI: 10.4018/979-8-3373-0122-8.ch009

Garcia, M. B., Arif, Y. M., Khlaif, Z. N., Zhu, M., de Almeida, R. P. P., de Almeida, R. S., & Masters, K. (2024). Effective Integration of Artificial Intelligence in Medical Education: Practical Tips and Actionable Insights. In *Transformative Approaches to Patient Literacy and Healthcare Innovation* (pp. 1-19). IGI Global. https://doi.org/DOI: 10.4018/979-8-3693-3661-8.ch001

Garcia, M. B., de Almeida, R. P. P., Arif, Y. M., Miranda, J. P. P., Tavares, D. P., Tariq, M. U., de Almeida, R. S., & López, M. (2025). Technology-Enhanced Learning in Health Professions Education: Current Trends and Applications. In Jesus, Â. (Ed.), *Technological Approaches to Medical and Pharmaceutical Education* (pp. 455–488). IGI Global., DOI: 10.4018/979-8-3373-1127-2.ch013

Garcia, M. B., & Garcia, P. S. (2023). Intelligent Tutoring System as an Instructional Technology in Learning Basic Nutrition Concepts: An Exploratory Sequential Mixed Methods Study. In *Handbook of Research on Instructional Technologies in Health Education and Allied Disciplines*. IGI Global., DOI: 10.4018/978-1-6684-7164-7.ch012

Garcia, M. B., Garcia, P. S., Maaliw, R. R.III, Lagrazon, P. G. G., Arif, Y. M., Ofosu-Ampong, K., Yousef, A. M. F., & Vaithilingam, C. A. (2024). Technoethical Considerations for Advancing Health Literacy and Medical Practice: A Posthumanist Framework in the Age of Healthcare 5.0. In *Emerging Technologies for Health Literacy and Medical Practice*. IGI Global., DOI: 10.4018/979-8-3693-1214-8.ch001

Garcia, M. B., Rosak-Szyrocka, J., Yılmaz, R., Metwally, A. H. S., Acut, D. P., Ofosu-Ampong, K., Erdoğdu, F., Fung, C. Y., & Bozkurt, A. (2025). Rethinking Educational Assessment in the Age of Generative AI: Actionable Strategies to Mitigate Academic Dishonesty. In *Pitfalls of AI Integration in Education: Skill Obsolescence, Misuse, and Bias*. IGI Global., DOI: 10.4018/979-8-3373-0122-8.ch001

Genovese, A., Borna, S., Gomez-Cabello, C. A., Haider, S. A., Prabha, S., Forte, A. J., & Veenstra, B. R. (2024). Artificial Intelligence in Clinical Settings: A Systematic Review of Its Role in Language Translation and Interpretation. *Annals of Translational Medicine*, *12*(6), 1–16. DOI: 10.21037/atm-24-162 PMID: 39817236

Giannakos, M., Azevedo, R., Brusilovsky, P., Cukurova, M., Dimitriadis, Y., Hernandez-Leo, D., Järvelä, S., Mavrikis, M., & Rienties, B. (2024). The Promise and Challenges of Generative AI in Education. *Behaviour & Information Technology*, •••, 1–27. DOI: 10.1080/0144929X.2024.2394886

Gordon, M., Daniel, M., Ajiboye, A., Uraiby, H., Xu, N. Y., Bartlett, R., Hanson, J., Haas, M., Spadafore, M., Grafton-Clarke, C., Gasiea, R. Y., Michie, C., Corral, J., Kwan, B., Dolmans, D., & Thammasitboon, S. (2024). A Scoping Review of Artificial Intelligence in Medical Education: BEME Guide No. 84. *Medical Teacher*, *46*(4), 446–470. DOI: 10.1080/0142159X.2024.2314198 PMID: 38423127

Guraya, S. Y. (2024). Transforming Simulation in Healthcare to Enhance Interprofessional Collaboration Leveraging Big Data Analytics and Artificial Intelligence. *BMC Medical Education*, *24*(1), 941. Advance online publication. DOI: 10.1186/s12909-024-05916-y PMID: 39198809

Hale, J., Alexander, S., Wright, S. T., & Gilliland, K. (2024). Generative AI in Undergraduate Medical Education: A Rapid Review. *Journal of Medical Education and Curricular Development*, *11*, 1–15. DOI: 10.1177/23821205241266697

Han, Z., Battaglia, F., Udaiyar, A., Fooks, A., & Terlecky, S. R. (2024). An Explorative Assessment of ChatGPT as an Aid in Medical Education: Use It With Caution. *Medical Teacher*, *46*(5), 657–664. DOI: 10.1080/0142159X.2023.2271159 PMID: 37862566

Hanna, M. G., Pantanowitz, L., Jackson, B., Palmer, O., Visweswaran, S., Pantanowitz, J., Deebajah, M., & Rashidi, H. H. (2025). Ethical and Bias Considerations in Artificial Intelligence/Machine Learning. *Modern Pathology*, *38*(3), 1–13. DOI: 10.1016/j.modpat.2024.100686 PMID: 39694331

Hossain, E., Rana, R., Higgins, N., Soar, J., Barua, P. D., Pisani, A. R., & Turner, K. (2023). Natural Language Processing in Electronic Health Records in Relation to Healthcare Decision-Making: A Systematic Review. *Computers in Biology and Medicine*, *155*, 1–24. DOI: 10.1016/j.compbiomed.2023.106649 PMID: 36805219

Jackson, P., Ponath Sukumaran, G., Babu, C., Tony, M. C., Jack, D. S., Reshma, V. R., Davis, D., Kurian, N., & John, A. (2024). Artificial Intelligence in Medical Education - Perception Among Medical Students. *BMC Medical Education*, *24*(1), 1–9. DOI: 10.1186/s12909-024-05760-0 PMID: 38172860

Janumpally, R., Nanua, S., Ngo, A., & Youens, K. (2024). Generative Artificial Intelligence in Graduate Medical Education. *Frontiers in Medicine*, *11*, 1–9. DOI: 10.3389/fmed.2024.1525604 PMID: 39867924

Jin, Q., Chen, F., Zhou, Y., Xu, Z., Cheung, J. M., Chen, R., Summers, R. M., Rousseau, J. F., Ni, P., Landsman, M. J., Baxter, S. L., Al'Aref, S. J., Li, Y., Chen, A., Brejt, J. A., Chiang, M. F., Peng, Y., & Lu, Z. (2024). Hidden Flaws Behind Expert-Level Accuracy of Multimodal GPT-4 Vision in Medicine. *npj. Digital Medicine*, *7*(1), 1–6. DOI: 10.1038/s41746-024-01185-7 PMID: 38172429

Kabudi, T., Pappas, I., & Olsen, D. H. (2021). AI-Enabled Adaptive Learning Systems: A Systematic Mapping of the Literature. *Computers and Education: Artificial Intelligence*, *2*, 100017. DOI: 10.1016/j.caeai.2021.100017

Khojasteh, L., Kafipour, R., Pakdel, F., & Mukundan, J. (2025). Empowering Medical Students With AI Writing Co-Pilots: Design and Validation of AI Self-Assessment Toolkit. *BMC Medical Education, 25*(1), 1–22. DOI: 10.1186/s12909-025-06753-3 PMID: 39891148

Khosravi, M., Zare, Z., Mojtabaeian, S. M., & Izadi, R. (2024). Artificial Intelligence and Decision-Making in Healthcare: A Thematic Analysis of a Systematic Review of Reviews. *Health Services Research and Managerial Epidemiology, 11*, 1–15. DOI: 10.1177/23333928241234863 PMID: 38449840

Kirch, S. A., & Sadofsky, M. J. (2021). Medical Education From a Theory–Practice–Philosophy Perspective. *Academic Pathology, 8*, 1–15. DOI: 10.1177/23742895211010236 PMID: 33959676

Krive, J., Isola, M., Chang, L., Patel, T., Anderson, M., & Sreedhar, R. (2023). Grounded in Reality: Artificial Intelligence in Medical Education. *JAMIA Open, 6*(2), 1–7. DOI: 10.1093/jamiaopen/ooad037 PMID: 37273962

Lajoie, S. P., & Gube, M. (2018). Adaptive Expertise in Medical Education: Accelerating Learning Trajectories by Fostering Self-Regulated Learning. *Medical Teacher, 40*(8), 809–812. DOI: 10.1080/0142159X.2018.1485886 PMID: 30033791

Lin, C.-C., Huang, A. Y. Q., & Lu, O. H. T. (2023). Artificial Intelligence in Intelligent Tutoring Systems Toward Sustainable Education: A Systematic Review. *Smart Learning Environments, 10*(1), 1–22. DOI: 10.1186/s40561-023-00260-y

Lin, H., & Chen, Q. (2024). Artificial Intelligence (AI) -Integrated Educational Applications and College Students' Creativity and Academic Emotions: Students and Teachers' Perceptions and Attitudes. *BMC Psychology, 12*(1), 1–16. DOI: 10.1186/s40359-024-01979-0 PMID: 39285268

Liu, L. (2025). AI and the Crisis of Legitimacy in Higher Education. *American Journal of STEM Education, 4*, 16–26. DOI: 10.32674/42qssk59

Lobo, M. D., Miravent, S., de Almeida, R. P. P., & Garcia, M. B. (2024). Advancing Precision in Physical Education and Sports Science: A Review of Medical Imaging Methods for Assessing Body Composition. In *Global Innovations in Physical Education and Health*. IGI Global., DOI: 10.4018/979-8-3693-3952-7.ch011

MAI. (2025). All-in-One VR & MR Anatomy and Acupuncture Platform. https://www.mai.ai/

Martin, F., Chen, Y., Moore, R. L., & Westine, C. D. (2020). Systematic Review of Adaptive Learning Research Designs, Context, Strategies, and Technologies from 2009 to 2018. *Educational Technology Research and Development*, *68*(4), 1903–1929. DOI: 10.1007/s11423-020-09793-2 PMID: 32837122

McGee, R. G., Wark, S., Mwangi, F., Drovandi, A., Alele, F., Malau-Aduli, B. S., & The, A. C. (2024). Digital Learning of Clinical Skills and Its Impact on Medical Students' Academic Performance: A Systematic Review. *BMC Medical Education*, *24*(1), 1–23. DOI: 10.1186/s12909-024-06471-2 PMID: 39696150

Mir, M. M., Mir, G. M., Raina, N. T., Mir, S. M., Mir, S. M., Miskeen, E., Alharthi, M. H., & Alamri, M. M. S. (2023). Application of Artificial Intelligence in Medical Education: Current Scenario and Future Perspectives. *Journal of Advances in Medical Education & Professionalism*, *11*(3), 133–140. DOI: 10.30476/jamp.2023.98655.1803 PMID: 37469385

Mirchi, N., Ledwos, N., & Del Maestro, R. F. (2020). Intelligent Tutoring Systems: Re-Envisioning Surgical Education in Response to COVID-19. *The Canadian Journal of Neurological Sciences*, *48*(2), 198–200. DOI: 10.1017/cjn.2020.202 PMID: 32907644

Mousavinasab, E., Zarifsanaiey, N., & Niakan Kalhori, R., S., Rakhshan, M., Keikha, L., & Ghazi Saeedi, M. (. (2018). Intelligent Tutoring Systems: A Systematic Review of Characteristics, Applications, and Evaluation Methods. *Interactive Learning Environments*, *29*(1), 142–163. DOI: 10.1080/10494820.2018.1558257

Mustafa, M. Y., Tlili, A., Lampropoulos, G., Huang, R., Jandrić, P., Zhao, J., Salha, S., Xu, L., Panda, S., Kinshuk, , López-Pernas, S., & Saqr, M. (2024). A Systematic Review of Literature Reviews on Artificial Intelligence in Education (AIED): A Roadmap to a Future Research Agenda. *Smart Learning Environments*, *11*(1), 1–33. DOI: 10.1186/s40561-024-00350-5

Narayanan, S., Ramakrishnan, R., Durairaj, E., & Das, A. (2023). Artificial Intelligence Revolutionizing the Field of Medical Education. *Cureus*. Advance online publication. DOI: 10.7759/cureus.49604 PMID: 38161821

Naveen, P., & Trojovský, P. (2024). Overview and Challenges of Machine Translation for Contextually Appropriate Translations. *iScience*, *27*(10), 1–25. DOI: 10.1016/j.isci.2024.110878 PMID: 39391737

Nguyen, T. (2024). ChatGPT in Medical Education: A Precursor for Automation Bias? *JMIR Medical Education*, *10*, e50174. DOI: 10.2196/50174 PMID: 38231545

Nissen, L., Rother, J. F., Heinemann, M., Reimer, L. M., Jonas, S., & Raupach, T. (2025). A Randomised Cross-Over Trial Assessing the Impact of AI-Generated Individual Feedback on Written Online Assignments for Medical Students. *Medical Teacher*, •••, 1–7. DOI: 10.1080/0142159X.2025.2451870 PMID: 39831699

Ogden, K., Kilpatrick, S., & Elmer, S. (2023). Examining the Nexus Between Medical Education and Complexity: A Systematic Review to Inform Practice and Research. *BMC Medical Education*, *23*(1), 1–15. DOI: 10.1186/s12909-023-04471-2 PMID: 37408005

PCS. (2025). PCS: Patient Communication Simulators. https://www.pcs.ai/alex/

Pirri, C., Stecco, C., Porzionato, A., Boscolo-Berto, R., Fortelny, R. H., Macchi, V., Konschake, M., Merigliano, S., & De Caro, R. (2021). Forensic Implications of Anatomical Education and Surgical Training With Cadavers. *Frontiers in Surgery*, *8*, 1–10. DOI: 10.3389/fsurg.2021.641581 PMID: 34250002

Potter, L., & Jefferies, C. (2024). Enhancing Communication and Clinical Reasoning in Medical Education: Building Virtual Patients With Generative AI. *Future Healthcare Journal*, *11*, 100043. DOI: 10.1016/j.fhj.2024.100043

Preiksaitis, C., & Rose, C. (2023). Opportunities, Challenges, and Future Directions of Generative Artificial Intelligence in Medical Education: Scoping Review. *JMIR Medical Education*, *9*, 1–13. DOI: 10.2196/48785 PMID: 37862079

Resnik, D. B., & Hosseini, M. (2024). The Ethics of Using Artificial Intelligence in Scientific Research: New Guidance Needed for a New Tool. *AI and Ethics*, •••, 1–23. DOI: 10.1007/s43681-024-00493-8 PMID: 40337745

Riddle, E. W., Kewalramani, D., Narayan, M., & Jones, D. B. (2024). Surgical Simulation: Virtual Reality to Artificial Intelligence. *Current Problems in Surgery*, *61*(11), 1–55. DOI: 10.1016/j.cpsurg.2024.101625 PMID: 39477664

Saleem, N., Mufti, T., Sohail, S. S., & Madsen, D. Ø. (2024). ChatGPT as an Innovative Heutagogical Tool in Medical Education. *Cogent Education*, *11*(1), 1–10. DOI: 10.1080/2331186X.2024.2332850

Satapathy, P., Hermis, A. H., Rustagi, S., Pradhan, K. B., Padhi, B. K., & Sah, R. (2023). Artificial Intelligence in Surgical Education and Training: Opportunities, Challenges, and Ethical Considerations – Correspondence. *International Journal of Surgery*, *109*(5), 1543–1544. DOI: 10.1097/JS9.0000000000000387 PMID: 37037597

Schubert, T., Oosterlinck, T., Stevens, R. D., Maxwell, P. H., & van der Schaar, M. (2025). AI Education for Clinicians. *EClinicalMedicine*, *79*, 1–7. DOI: 10.1016/j.eclinm.2024.102968 PMID: 39720600

Serrano, D. R., Luciano, F. C., Anaya, B. J., Ongoren, B., Kara, A., Molina, G., Ramirez, B. I., Sánchez-Guirales, S. A., Simon, J. A., Tomietto, G., Rapti, C., Ruiz, H. K., Rawat, S., Kumar, D., & Lalatsa, A. (2024). Artificial Intelligence (AI) Applications in Drug Discovery and Drug Delivery: Revolutionizing Personalized Medicine. *Pharmaceutics*, *16*(10), 1–27. DOI: 10.3390/pharmaceutics16101328 PMID: 39458657

Singh, N., Gunjan, V. K., & Nasralla, M. M. (2022). A Parametrized Comparative Analysis of Performance Between Proposed Adaptive and Personalized Tutoring System "Seis Tutor" With Existing Online Tutoring System. *IEEE Access : Practical Innovations, Open Solutions*, *10*, 39376–39386. DOI: 10.1109/ACCESS.2022.3166261

Stretton, B., Kovoor, J., Arnold, M., & Bacchi, S. (2024). ChatGPT-Based Learning: Generative Artificial Intelligence in Medical Education. *Medical Science Educator*, *34*(1), 215–217. DOI: 10.1007/s40670-023-01934-5 PMID: 38510403

Strielkowski, W., Grebennikova, V., Lisovskiy, A., Rakhimova, G., & Vasileva, T. (2024). AI-Driven Adaptive Learning for Sustainable Educational Transformation. *Sustainable Development*. Advance online publication. DOI: 10.1002/sd.3221

Sun, W., Jiang, X., Dong, X., Yu, G., Feng, Z., & Shuai, L. (2024). The Evolution of Simulation-Based Medical Education Research: From Traditional to Virtual Simulations. *Heliyon*, *10*(15), 1–14. DOI: 10.1016/j.heliyon.2024.e35627 PMID: 39170203

Tang, Y. M., Chau, K. Y., Kwok, A. P. K., Zhu, T., & Ma, X. (2022). A Systematic Review of Immersive Technology Applications for Medical Practice and Education - Trends, Application Areas, Recipients, Teaching Contents, Evaluation Methods, and Performance. *Educational Research Review*, *35*, 1–22. DOI: 10.1016/j.edurev.2021.100429

Thomae, A. V., Witt, C. M., & Barth, J. (2024). Integration of ChatGPT Into a Course for Medical Students: Explorative Study on Teaching Scenarios, Students' Perception, and Applications. *JMIR Medical Education*, *10*, 1–10. DOI: 10.2196/50545 PMID: 39177012

Vaughn, J., Ford, S. H., Scott, M., Jones, C., & Lewinski, A. (2024). Enhancing Healthcare Education: Leveraging ChatGPT for Innovative Simulation Scenarios. *Clinical Simulation in Nursing*, *87*, 101487. DOI: 10.1016/j.ecns.2023.101487

Xia, Q., Weng, X., Ouyang, F., Lin, T. J., & Chiu, T. K. F. (2024). A Scoping Review on How Generative Artificial Intelligence Transforms Assessment in Higher Education. *International Journal of Educational Technology in Higher Education, 21*(1), 40. Advance online publication. DOI: 10.1186/s41239-024-00468-z

Xiao, J., Bozkurt, A., Nichols, M., Pazurek, A., Stracke, C. M., Bai, J. Y. H., Farrow, R., Mulligan, D., Nerantzi, C., Sharma, R. C., Singh, L., Frumin, I., Swindell, A., Honeychurch, S., Bond, M., Dron, J., Moore, S., Leng, J., van Tryon, P. J. S., & Themeli, C. (2025). Venturing into the Unknown: Critical Insights into Grey Areas and Pioneering Future Directions in Educational Generative AI Research. *TechTrends*. Advance online publication. DOI: 10.1007/s11528-025-01060-6

Yang, Y.-Y., & Shulruf, B. (2019). An Expert-Led and Artificial Intelligence System-Assisted Tutoring Course to Improve the Confidence of Chinese Medical Interns in Suturing and Ligature Skills: A Prospective Pilot Study. *Journal of Educational Evaluation for Health Professions, 16*, 7. DOI: 10.3352/jeehp.2019.16.7 PMID: 30986892

Yazdani, S., & Abardeh, M. H. (2019). Five Decades of Research and Theorization on Clinical Reasoning: A Critical Review. *Advances in Medical Education and Practice, 10*, 703–716. DOI: 10.2147/AMEP.S213492 PMID: 31695548

Zarei, M., Eftekhari Mamaghani, H., Abbasi, A., & Hosseini, M.-S. (2024). Application of Artificial Intelligence in Medical Education: A Review of Benefits, Challenges, and Solutions. *Medicina Clínica Práctica, 7*(2), 1–5. DOI: 10.1016/j.mcpsp.2023.100422

Zhai, C., Wibowo, S., & Li, L. D. (2024). The Effects of Over-Reliance on AI Dialogue Systems on Students' Cognitive Abilities: A Systematic Review. *Smart Learning Environments, 11*(1), 1–37. DOI: 10.1186/s40561-024-00316-7

Zidoun, Y., & Mardi, A. E. L. (2024). Artificial Intelligence (AI)-Based Simulators Versus Simulated Patients in Undergraduate Programs: A Protocol for a Randomized Controlled Trial. *BMC Medical Education, 24*(1), 1–7. DOI: 10.1186/s12909-024-06236-x PMID: 39501219

KEY TERMS AND DEFINITIONS

Artificial Intelligence: The simulation of human intelligence processes by machines to perform tasks such as learning, reasoning, and problem-solving.

ChatGPT: A conversational AI developed by OpenAI that generates human-like responses using large language models.

Generative AI: A type of artificial intelligence that creates new content—such as text, images, or audio—based on learned data patterns.

Large Language Models: Advanced AI systems trained on massive text datasets to understand and generate natural language with contextual accuracy.

Medical Education: The structured process of teaching and learning that prepares individuals for medical practice through knowledge acquisition and skill development.

Medical Training: The practical component of medical education involving clinical experience, simulations, and supervised patient care.

Medicine: The science and practice of diagnosing, treating, and preventing illness to improve health and well-being.

Chapter 6
Impact of Wearable Technology on Medical Education

Pandimurugan Vellaisamy
https://orcid.org/0000-0003-4766-996X
Acharya University, Karakul, Uzbekistan

Sajeer Karattil
https://orcid.org/0009-0007-1224-8555
University of Technology and Applied Sciences, Oman

Mohammed Mubarak Mohammed Al Araimi
https://orcid.org/0000-0002-4697-2214
University of Technology and Applied Sciences, Oman

V. Rajaram
https://orcid.org/0000-0002-7023-8327
SRM Institute of Science and Technology, India

B. Balakiruthiga
https://orcid.org/0000-0002-2037-8524
SRM Institute of Science and Technology, India

Angayarkanni S. A.
https://orcid.org/0000-0001-5140-7925
SRM Institute of Science and Technology, India

Baiju B. V.
https://orcid.org/0000-0001-8221-5483
Vellore Institute of Technology, India

ABSTRACT

Health Information Technology (HIT) along with the Internet of Medical Things (IoMT) employs wearable technology to monitor diseases through its capability to prevent medical mistakes from occurring. The devices track vital signs which medical professionals use for precise treatment decisions through real-time data transmission. IoT-driven medical devices improve telehealth service delivery as well as enhance patient monitoring functions. Virtual and augmented reality powers educational

DOI: 10.4018/979-8-3373-1519-5.ch006

wearables to assist medical student surgical training as well as human anatomy education. Research professionals obtain immediate biological feedback through their diagnostic work and clinical preparation. Wearable technology enhances healthcare operations through its support of educational initiatives and research activities which lead to better medical discoveries today and in upcoming years.

1. INTRODUCTION TO WEARABLES FOR MEDICAL EDUCATION

Modern technology becomes a cornerstone in medical education which improves student and professional acquisition and application of medical knowledge and its practice. Wearable devices prove essential for modernizing three main educational areas: clinical teaching procedures and simulation practices and student-directed educational assignments (Ali et al., 2025; Long & Chung, 2021). Medical institutions that implement wearable technology enable medical students to transition from classroom learning to clinical practice more easily which raises their preparedness for actual medical situations. The transformation of medical instruction occurs because medical stakeholders use technology embedded on their bodies that enables these educational and healthcare modifications.

1.1 Types of Wearables in Medical Education

The traditional medical education model uses lectures and textbooks that get followed by clinical education while training students. The emerging use of wearable technology creates a modern solution for medical skill advancement. The combination of smartwatches and AR headsets and biometric sensors allows medical students to access dynamic physiological information which expands their knowledge of nursing procedures. Students can use Microsoft HoloLens AR devices to examine 3D body models while conducting virtual cutups without needing physical cadaver specimens (Arivu et al., 2018). Students benefit from virtual medical practice through contemporary wearable devices that improve their understanding of complex topics and develop necessary spatial skills required for surgical work and clinical responsibilities. The figure 1 below displays different forms of wearable technology which medical education employs.

1.1.1 Smartwatches and Fitness Trackers

The Apple Watch along with Fitbit models provide users access to monitor their vital health statistics including heart rate measurements and ECG recordings and oxygen saturation numbers. Real-time tracking functions of these devices show medical learners detailed patient information so that they can practice translating scientific measurements into practical patient settings.Fitness monitoring devices aid students in learning about wellness connections between lifestyle elements and help them control persistent illnesses (Lakshminarayana et al., 2025; Wanjari & Patil, 2016). With wearable technology students obtain skills to detect medical conditions early since they learn how to identify abnormal patterns in patient-generated information.

1.1.2 Augmented Reality (AR) and Virtual Reality (VR) Headsets

The immersive medical simulation experiences are delivered by Microsoft HoloLens together with Oculus Quest devices. Users who employ AR overlays in their system can see anatomical structures plus practice surgical procedures to advance their medical training and provide procedural guidance. Records demonstrate that Virtual Reality (VR) teaching methods enhance knowledge understanding by 75% more effectively than traditional learning methods (Sun et al., 2025; Oh et al., 2025). The utilization of AR and VR tools by students results in better hand-eye coordination together with enhanced spatial awareness which leads to superior medical procedure performance. Through technological integration educational systems enable medical students and instructors to work together thereby establishing convenient worldwide medical education programs.

1.1.3 Smart Glasses

The hands-free system, Google Glass, helps health workers access electronic health records (EHRs) and watch live surgeries for educational purposes. These remote mentoring tools make medical training between students and their mentors possible by enabling immediate expert feedback. The real-time information overlays of smart glasses provide elevated medical simulations, leading to superior accuracy and precision in training protocols.

1.1.4 Wearable Biosensors

Patients receive real-time physiological data from devices, including continuous glucose monitors (CGMs) and wearable ECG patches. Evaluating patient biometrics by students and clinicians strengthens their diagnostic and monitoring competencies. Biosensors serve personal medicine through treatment response monitoring, which delivers training opportunities for medical students on precision healthcare and variable intervention approaches.

Figure 1. Types of wearable devices in the Medical Field

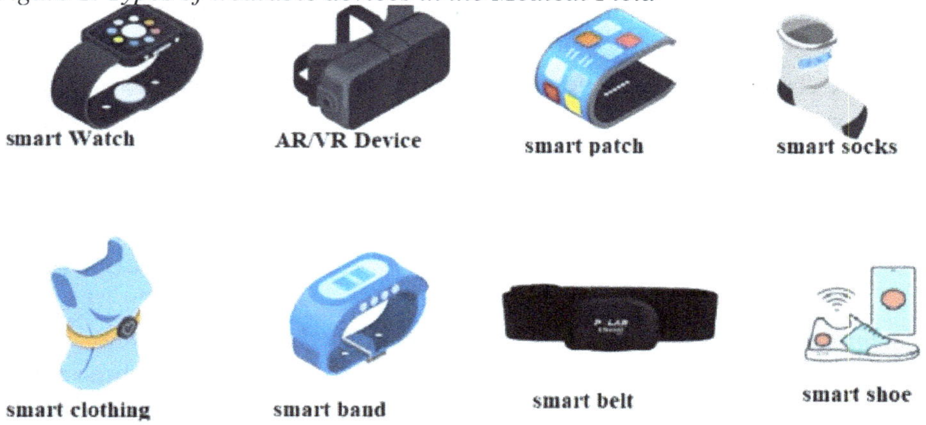

1.1.5 Haptic Feedback Devices

Medical students can experience textures alongside resistance and pressure during simulations through haptic glover and simulator tools. The training tools offer real-life procedure simulations, which improve students' precision and hand-eye coordination. Haptic feedback allows students to practice their suturing and laparoscopic surgery skills without exposing them to safety risks.

1.2 Benefits of Wearables in Medical Education

Wearable technology significantly enhances medical education by accelerating learning, increasing patient engagement, and strengthening clinical skills among healthcare providers. Key benefits include:

Augmented and virtual reality headsets allow students to safely practice medical procedures in a risk-free environment, helping them develop the competence needed to treat real patients (Powell, 2017). These simulations reduce the likelihood of errors in actual clinical settings by providing realistic and repeatable training experiences. Devices like smart glasses enable students to observe real-time procedures and engage in virtual consultations, expanding medical education beyond traditional classrooms. This advanced technology fosters adaptive learning environments and connects students with a global network of peers and mentors. Remote mentorship offers invaluable expert insights from professionals around the world. Training with wearable devices familiarizes students with clinical monitoring equipment, enhancing their ability to deliver effective patient care. This hands-on approach improves decision-making by providing students with the knowledge and skills to monitor disease progression and determine optimal treatment strategies. Using AR and smart glasses, clinicians can access clinical data and procedural guidelines in real time during patient care. This hands-free approach improves operational efficiency and supports fast-paced clinical environments, ensuring that medical education and patient care proceed seamlessly (Zhu et al., 2014).

Wearable technology transforms medical education by delivering realistic learning programs, storage capabilities, and distant collaborative opportunities between students. The future of medical training based on wearable technology adoption will build better clinical competency for healthcare providers while simultaneously ensuring enhanced patient outcomes. Educational wearables show continuous development toward interactive data-based learning, increasing access for upcoming healthcare students worldwide.

A visual representation shows how medical education adopts various wearable devices for their purposes. Various wearable technologies demonstrate their benefits toward improving medical training and patient care practices through this distribution, as shown in Figure 2.

Figure 2. WearablesDevices used in Medical Field

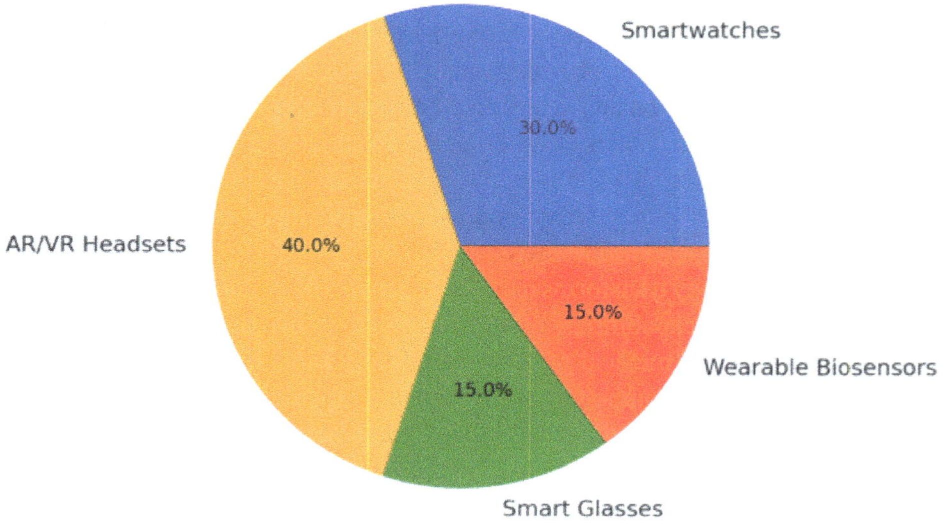

2. METHODOLOGY IN DATA COLLECTION AND ANALYSIS

This chapter adopts a narrative review approach, using sources from various medical databases ICMR, ICD, ISIC. Relevant literature from 2022–2025 was retrieved using MeSH/DeCS terms such as "wearable devices," "medical education," and "AR/VR simulation." Inclusion focused on peer-reviewed articles related to wearable technology in healthcare training. Data were thematically analyzed to highlight applications, benefits, and challenges.

2.1 Role of Wearable Technology in Medical Education

The educational environment of medicine now relies heavily on real-time data visualization to reach its maximum potential in hands-free student learning. Augmented reality (AR) headsets, smart glasses, and smartwatches help medical student's access straightforward data during medical procedures (Vallurupalli et al., 2013). The devices display real-time patient information, including vital signs, ima, ging scans, and electronic health records, to students who maintain uninterrupted contact with the patient. The technology enhances decision-making during critical situations in surgery suites and emergency departments (Zhang et al., 2019). Students who access real-time visual data displays acquire better insights about medical responses and bodily transformations, enhancing their education and producing superior clinical results (Izard et al., 2018). Instructors who implement these technologies with medical training programs enable collaborative learning through the ability to provide immediate educational support as they view displayed data information in real-time. Academic professionals who teach surgery use AR annotation features to show students critical anatomical parts through interactive educational experiences (Sui et al., 2023).

2.1.1 Real-Time Data Visualization

Instructors who implement these technologies with medical training programs enable collaborative learning through the ability to provide immediate educational support as they view displayed data information in real-time. Academic professionals who teach surgery use AR annotation features to show students critical anatomical parts through interactive educational experiences (Sui et al., 2023).

Combining haptic feedback features in bright gloves enables students to sense simulated patient reactions, improving their education (Chen et al., 2022). The training gloves simulate resistance during simulated needle procedures, while pressure applications would allow trainees to practice delicate operations safely. Real-time data visualization will emerge as essential for medical education because of evolving wearable technology development, transforming student information usage and clinical procedure execution (Fariah et al., 2024).

2.1.2 Remote Learning and Telemedicine

Utilizing wearable technology has completely changed the methods of remote education delivery and telemedical care in medical student training programs. Virtual reality (VR) and AR-enabled glasses enable students to engage in live surgical procedures remotely, regardless of location (Arch Virtual, 2018). Live surgical techniques become accessible for learners who can observe details of procedures and exchange real-time questions with instructors even when they cannot physically be present in operating rooms. Virtual simulations let medical students develop complex medical skills through safe practice simulations. Through VR platforms, medical education incorporates high-risk situations like cardiac arrests and emergency trauma, which enables students to improve their critical thinking capabilities and decision-making competencies (Mahato et al., 2024). The simulations let learners advance in difficulty levels so their expertise develops step by step.

2.1.3 Use Cases of Virtual Simulations in Medical Training

Here are some of the use cases of virtual simulation in Medical Training,

- Medical students receive training in cardiac arrest response through a VR simulation that puts them in realistic cardiac arrest situations for implementing CPR and defibrillation while following ACLS protocols and evaluating their performance based on timing and technique precision (Pankajavalli & Karthick, 2020). Students undergo experiences of critical emergency cases, which include treatment of gunshot wounds and auto accident injuries alongside battlefield trauma situations. The trainee must evaluate the patient's status and select treatment immediate actions before performing procedures, including intubations and haemorrhage control (Garcia & Almeida, 2024).
- Virtual reality platforms allow students to practice laparoscopic procedures, orthopaedic surgeries, and neurosurgical techniques. The simulation systems come with haptic feedback components that deliver touch sensations that resemble operating-room conditions.

Wearable devices enable medical trainees to perform remote medical consultations hands-free, which allows them to assist in patient diagnosis and treatment. Smart glasses technology allows distant specialists to supervise students during medical operations through live interactive instructions. During worldwide health emergencies, the proven value of this training strategy emerges since in-person instruction becomes restricted. Figure 3 shows how medical science uses wearable technology to deliver various devices to improve healthcare monitoring and treatment procedures. Smartwatches and biosensors, such as small implantable and adhesive devices, constantly monitor heart rate, blood oxygen levels, and physical activity levels. Surgeons obtain live procedural information through augmented reality-capable smart glasses as their operation assistant system.

Wearable ECG monitoring devices appear as chest patches to identify abnormal heartbeat patterns, and bright rings measure sleep activities, stress levels, and heart rate variation. EEG headbands worn by patients deliver neurological data through their brain waves to monitor neurological health, and robotic prosthetics benefit from AI systems that enhance mobility for people who have undergone amputation. Insulin pumps attached to patients' bodies help diabetic patients receive precise insulin amounts, while bright clothing with sensor systems track body positions, muscle movements, and respiratory activities. Medical rehabilitation therapy benefits from haptic feedback gloves that produce simulated touch sensations, a vital advancement in modern healthcare practice.

2.1.4 Accessibility for Disabled Students

Wearable technology allows medical education to become more inclusive toward disabled students through its innovative designs. Traditional medical training environments often present challenges for individuals with mobility impairments or other physical limitations. Disabled students experiencing barrier-free educational activities can now learn hands-free through wearable devices, voice-controlled systems, and haptic feedback instruments. Students can practice advanced medical procedures using augmented and virtual reality simulation platforms that function without physical movement. The limited mobility of a student does not limit their ability to exploit AR glasses with built-in eye tracking that lets them conduct virtual surgical tasks by making visual selections instead of handling controls manually. AI-powered wearable technology assists visually impaired students through audio visualization of visual information, which helps them understand medical images, al diagrams, and social videos.

3. IMPACT OF WEARABLE TECHNOLOGY ON CLINICAL TRAINING AND PATIENT CARE

3.1 Improved Clinical Decision-Making

Patients in medical school learn theory before gaining only limited time under direct clinical supervision. Modern wearable technology assists medical trainees by boosting their ability to make better decisions. The devices are additional sensing instruments, delivering urgent health information that unifies classroom lessons with hands-on clinical understanding. Wearable technology facilitates ongoing data acquisition during learning sessions, helping students build better clinical reasoning abilities for improved data-based patient care methods (Al-Shaqi et al., 2021; Patel et al., 2021).

3.1.1 Real-Time Monitoring and Data Analysis for Enhanced Learning

The use of wearable devices allows students in medical studies to gather biometric measurements that standard methods typically cannot acquire in real time. The students receive non-stop monitoring of vital signs such as heart rate variability, blood oxygen levels, and blood pressure modulations (Davoudi et al., 2022). The consistent flow of patient data based on real-time monitoring enables students to understand complex patient physiology changes in diverse medical situations to study physiological responses. Mobile application technologies permit students to superimpose their diagnostic findings onto patient documentation and medical standards, improving their symptom interpretation skills while helping them predict potential medical issues.

Tracking real-time bodily responses by medical monitoring systems is an essential educational tool to develop students' diagnostic abilities and decision-making competencies (Punj et al., 2025; Ghavami Hosein Pour et al., 2025). Figure 3 shows the Flow of Real-Time Monitoring and Data Analysis for Enhanced Learning.

Figure 3. Flow of Real-Time Monitoring and Data Analysis for Enhanced Learning

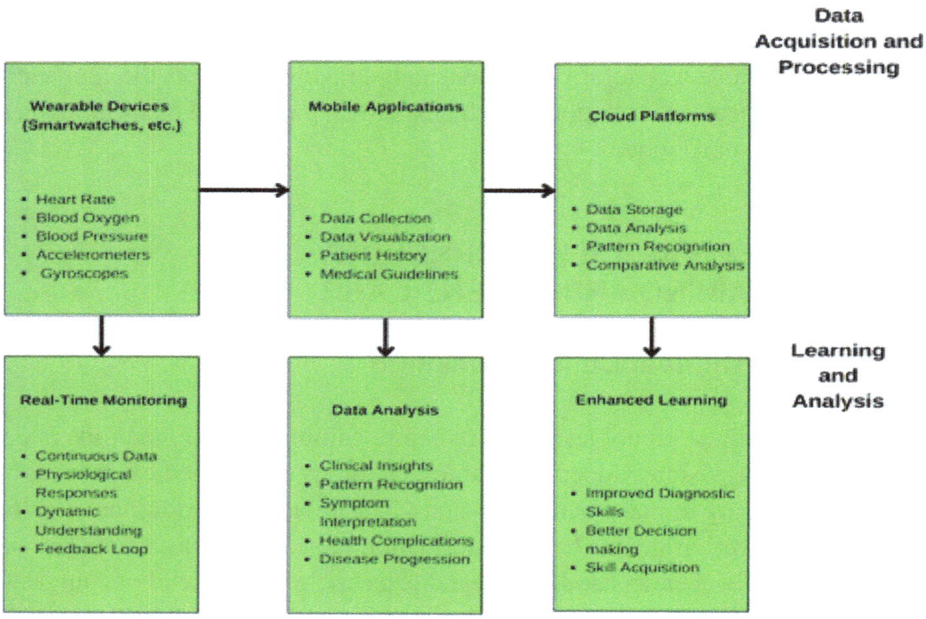

3.1.2 Case-Based Learning Through Wearable-Integrated Simulations

Wearable technology enhances medical education simulation learning through its fundamental role in training curriculums. The inclusion of wearable sensors within simulation manikins lets instructors establish authentic scenarios, which makes students interpret realistic physiological data through clinical decision-making (Hurst et al., 2020). Simulations designed for various medical fields let students develop their response abilities by managing emergency incidents, treating chronic conditions, and treating patients after surgery.

Figure 4. Case-Based Learning Through Wearable-Integrated Simulations

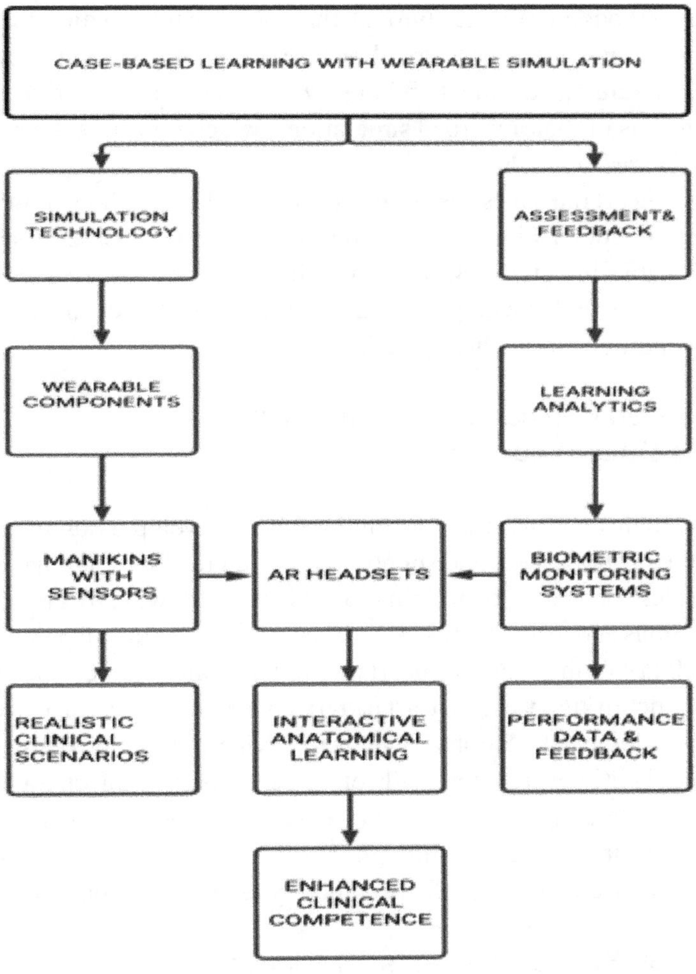

Students use augmented reality innovative headsets to view anatomical structures in 3-dimensional shapes when they perform virtual investigations followed by surgical procedure practice (Georgieva-Tsaneva et al., 2025). By combining digital learning with wearable technology, students learn advanced medical subjects while improving their spatial understanding and fine motor skills (Patel et al., 2021).

The training tools enable students to experience interactive learning activities, which improve their education through applied practice and thus prepare them for clinical scenarios. The educational sensors used on students provide monitoring functions by assessing psychological activity and physical body responses during training sessions.

Teaching methods are adjusted through this collected information so trainees can acquire competencies vital for hospital operational areas. Students develop superior critical pressure management abilities by receiving customized feedback from assessment results of their recorded simulations, which improves their approach to patient care (Harari et al., 2016).

Monitoring heart rate and stress levels reveals to educators how trainees respond in demanding situations. Figure 4 shows the flow diagram of Case-Based Learning Through Wearable-Integrated Simulations.The recorded data enables instructors to develop personalized teaching strategies, which prepare students to manage the demanding conditions of medical practice.

3.1.3 Enhanced Clinical Competency through Continuous Data Exposure

Digital analytics and wearable technology help develop assessment tools that evaluate student achievement and supply customized feedback. Online medical education provides specialization training to students worldwide by providing access to expert surgeons and teaching professionals across all regions (Ferrier et al., 2022; Perle et al., 2025). Using wearable heart monitors, medical students gain first-hand knowledge of identifying various heart pattern abnormalities, cardiac irregularities, and other physiological deviations. With these devices, educational instructors help students build their interpretation skills of authentic patient information, strengthening their diagnostic capability and clinical understanding. Students develop better patient-oriented care knowledge through their ability to monitor extended patient data patterns and see treatment effects on bodily responses throughout time.

3.1.4 Decision Support Systems for Clinical Reasoning Development

AI capabilities in wearable devices go beyond data acquisition by improving clinical diagnosis decisions. Digital systems that evaluate current patient data help trainees get therapy recommendations while enhancing their healthcare management skills proactively (Patel et al., 2021). AI-driven wearable applications help form differential diagnoses by matching real-time patient measurements versus large medical databases to suggest patient diagnoses and treatment plans to students. The advanced wearable monitoring devices track minor body alterations to allow training students to identify upcoming medical concerns early. Exposure to this technology drives therapeutic development toward proactive healthcare practices, which enables future medical professionals to deliver precision-based treatments and preventive care at early stages. These tools help hospitals develop an early-warning system that notifies clinicians about patient health changes to enhance medical results and decrease healthcare resource costs.

3.2 Better Patient Interaction and Communication

A healthcare organization depends on effective communication because it shapes patient health results and their experience. The medical encounter is transforming because wearable technology increases patient access and helps healthcare providers across different languages while improving information transfer in clinical settings (Al-Shaqi et al., 2021). The increasing number of digital health tools provides medical professionals more chances to offer personalized care, strengthening their patient relationships and boosting treatment plan adherence.

3.2.1 Smart Glasses for Enhanced Medical Rounds and Patient Care

Medical professionals now use smart glasses to transform patient interactions and procedures for completing clinical rounds. The hands-free devices allow immediate access to patient databases, test outcomes, and medical imaging studies, which supports healthcare providers in staying connected with their patients during their work (Sezer & Gül, 2024). Smart glasses and electronic health records enable physicians to find current patient histories and treatment plans without stopping their patient consultation (Greenhalgh et al., 2021).

In hospital settings, doctors use smart glasses for remote consultations so that specialists can guide their junior doctor trainees during actual patient examinations. Trainees benefit from utilizing these devices to watch surgical procedures through their own eyes, which provides them with crucial operational knowledge and decision-making strategies. During live consultations, the immediate partnership between seasoned physicians and trainees helps students learn better and leads to correct and accurate patient care decisions.

3.2.2 Real-time Language Translation Wearables for Cross-Cultural Communication

Healthcare encounters that feature language barriers create problems of ineffective communication, which results in delayed medical diagnosis and reduces the quality of patient treatment. Compact translation equipment functions as badges or innovative earpiece components automatically detecting spoken words for instant real-time translation services (Araujo et al., 2024). The medical tools mentioned here allow doctors to maintain a precise dialogue that requires no third-party interpreter while safeguarding patient privacy and creating superior healthcare interactions. Modern medical education and patient care undergo rapid changes through wearable technology because it provides real-time data collection mechanisms alongside decision-making aids and solves communication challenges (Babu et al., 2024; Wang et al., 2023). The next generation of healthcare professionals will attain better outcomes in clinical care because they acquire these technological advancements during their training and practice (Ashraf et al., 2022). Medical trainees and experienced practitioners will gain access through future wearable device innovation to advanced tools that boost patient care and educational quality. Table 1 shows the Comparative Overview of Language Translation Devices in Healthcare.

Table 1. Comparative Overview of Language Translation Devices in Healthcare

Device	FormFactor	Languages Supported	Key Features	Benefits in Healthcare
Fujitsu Speech Translator	Badge-styledevice	Multiple global languages	Hands-free, auto-detects pause, instant translation	Preserves confidentiality, reduces miscommunication
Pocketalk Translator	Handheld/portable	84+languages	Two-way audio & text translation, AI-powered	Improves patient-provider interaction
Google Pixel Buds	Smart earpiece	40+ languages	Real-time speech-to-text and translation via smartphone	Hands-free, supports direct doctor-patient dialogue
Vuzix M400 Smart Glasses	Wearable smart glasses	Multiple languages	Augmented reality interface, real-time subtitles	Ideal for rounds & remote consultations

4. CHALLENGES AND ETHICAL CONSIDERATIONS

4.1 Data Privacy and Security Concerns

With the increasing adoption of wearable devices in medical education and practice, data privacy and security concerns have become paramount. Wearable technology collects vast amounts of sensitive patient data, including real-time physiological metrics, electronic health records, and video recordings of medical procedures. If not properly secured, this data is susceptible to breaches, unauthorized access, and cyberattacks (Tang, 2022). The transmission of patient data over wireless networks poses additional security risks. Medical institutions must implement robust encryption and secure communication channels to prevent data interception. Additionally, students and educators using wearable devices must be trained in best practices for data security, such as using strong authentication measures and regularly updating software to patch vulnerabilities (Patel et al., 2015).

4.1.1 Risks Associated with Patient Data Storage and Transmission

Another challenge is the storage of wearable-generated data. Medical institutions must adopt cloud-based solutions with end-to-end encryption to ensure patient information remains secure. Furthermore, data access controls must be strictly enforced, granting access only to authorized personnel. Biometric authentication methods, such as fingerprint and facial recognition, can add an extra layer of security to prevent unauthorized data access.

4.1.2 Compliance with HIPAA and GDPR Regulations

To mitigate data privacy risks, wearable technology in medical education must adhere to regulatory frameworks such as the Health Insurance Portability and Accountability Act (HIPAA) in the United States and the General Data Protection Regulation (GDPR) in the European Union. These regulations mandate strict guidelines for handling, storing, and transmitting patient information, ensuring that personal data is protected and used ethically (Piwek et al., 2016).

Medical institutions incorporating wearable technology must establish compliance protocols, such as obtaining informed consent from patients before recording or transmitting their data. Additionally, anonymization and data minimization techniques should be employed to reduce the risk of exposure in a breach. By adhering to these regulatory standards, educators and students can use wearable devices responsibly while upholding ethical medical practices.

4.1.3 Ethical Implications of Wearable Technology in Medical Education

Beyond regulatory compliance, the ethical implications of wearable technology in medical education must be carefully considered. Additionally, there is a risk of over-reliance on technology in medical training. While wearables provide invaluable learning opportunities, they should complement, rather than replace, traditional hands-on training methods. Striking a balance between technology-driven education and direct patient interaction is essential to ensure students develop the clinical skills and empathy required in medical practice.Another ethical challenge is the potential bias in AI-driven wearable devices (Hong et al., 2025). By addressing these challenges and ethical considerations, the integration of wearable technology in medical education can be optimized to enhance learning outcomes while safeguarding patient rights and data security.

4.1.4 Sample use case for Wearable techniques

Educational applications of wearable technology serve as the primary use case in medical education. The medical education sector experiences transformation through wearable devices, including smart glasses, AR headsets, OVEs, VRs, and emulators because they provide real-time data visualization, remote capabilities, and haptic feedback. These technological tools advance medical student and instructor skills and healthcare institution capabilities with interactive simulation and remote surgical abilities and abilities to develop skills. The research illustrates the connections between device applications and stakeholders. The dataset presents how different wearable devices interact with medical education applications through their connections with healthcare field stakeholders. Table 2 consists of entities that contain device entities together with application entities and stakeholder entities.

Table 2. Various Wearable Technologies in Medical field

Id	Label	Type
1	Smart Glasses	Device
2	AR Headsets	Device
3	Smart Gloves	Device
4	VR Simulations	Application
5	Remote Surgery	Application
6	Medical Students	Stakeholder

continued on following page

Table 2. Continued

Id	Label	Type
7	Instructors	Stakeholder
8	Hospitals	Stakeholder
9	Real-Time Data Display	Feature
10	Haptic Feedback	Feature

Table 3. Relationship between the Mechanisms

Source Mechanism	Target Mechanism	Relation Exists	Cost or Weight
1	4	Permits	1
1	5	Permits	1
2	9	Supports	1
3	10	Integrates with	1
4	6	Trains	2
5	7	Assists	2
6	8	Collaborates with	1
7	4	Uses	1
8	2	Implements	1

Figure 5. Visualization of weights in technology network

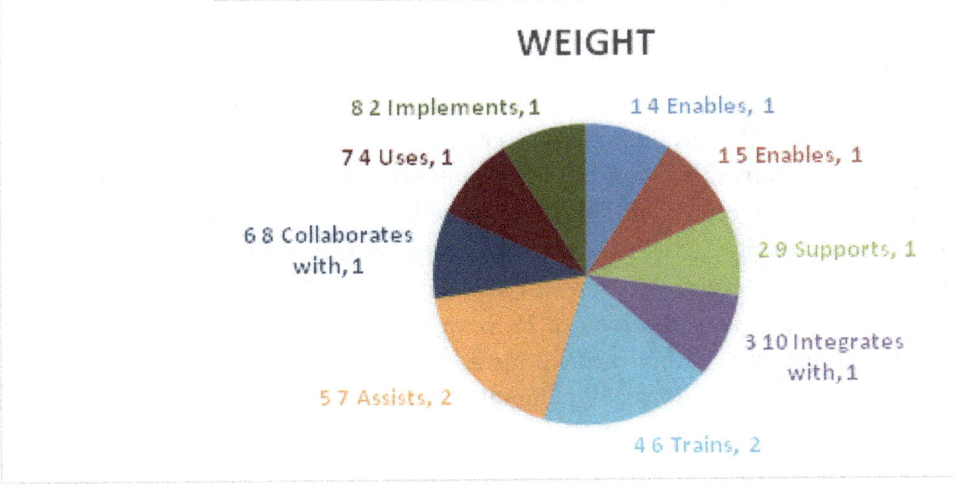

The connectivity between the devices based on their relationship ensures that each device relates to another based on the application.

Inference from the Figure 5: Relationship Weights in Wearable Technology Network

1. **Weight Distribution of Relationships:** The presented network graph shows the weights of relationships in wearable technology. Weight measurements between 0 and 2 are shown on the axis that stands for weight values. Different relationship weights, including “Enables,” “Supports,” “Trains,” “Assists,” and others, are shown along the X-axis. This graph shows count values through its label positions, which might represent the number of connections for each type.
2. **Key Observations:** Wearable technology relationships with “Trains” and “Assists” hold the most significant weight factor compared to other network connections. The stakeholders exhibit an average level of interaction with technology, which may stem from institutional collaborations with technology vendors. “Implements” has the lowest weight (~0.8). The low implementation weight suggests technical or financial barriers that impede system deployment.
3. **Implications:** Wearable technology demonstrates optimal utility in training and assistance functions because medical education greatly profits from immersive learning modalities (including AR/VR and haptic gloves) (Mohammed, Li, & Liu, 2024). Technology is an enabler in supporting medical education, among the other essential factors shaping its outcome. Low “Implementation” weight indicates adoption barriers exist to overcome before implementing these strategies (cost barriers, institutional obstacles, and limitations for accessibility).

4.2 High Costs and Accessibility Issues

In the field of medical education Wearable technology has an excellent potential to make transformations. It delivers immersive learning experience with personalized feedback, thereby improving competency. Although wearables offer wide scope of development and enhances learning efficiency, the main challenge is the huge implementation cost of them. Yet these hurdles pose additional hurdles that could further enhance existing inequalities between medical education institutions, students who can access the newest tools, and those who are left out of the loop (Georgieva-Tsaneva, Serbezova, & Beloeva, 2025). In this section, I outline the financial constraints within medical institutions in adopting wearable technology and discuss the implications of the digital divide regarding equitable access to such resources.

4.2.1 Financial constraints of medical institutions in adopting wearable technology.

With financial support from educational and government institutions it can be helpful in integrating the wearable technology into the education system. Investments should not only cover initial software and hardware implementation costs, but also recurring costs such as updates, maintenance, faculty training and support. This is the major threat for developing countries and are with financial constraints.

1. **Initial Investment Costs:** However, such costly wearable devices for medical education (such as advanced VR/AR headsets, haptic gloves, etc.) can be out of reach for medical education labs. Most high-fidelity VR/AR systems need expensive hardware and software packages. Substantial investment is also made in Haptic gloves to develop tactile feedback for real-life surgical simulations. In addition to that, there is an investment in the infrastructure designed to host such technologies as high-power computers, high-speed internet connectivity, and laboratory spaces.
2. **Ongoing Operational Costs:** Medical facilities need funds to continuously operate their wearable technology devices after buying them. This includes:
   a. The wearable technology platforms depend on updated software licenses, creating repeated costs for medical offices.
   b. Medical facilities must budget for standard equipment lifespan maintenance plus repairs when their wearable devices need technical work.
   c. Education institutions must be having domain experts to handle the issues with hardware md software then and there, to reduce the failure time.
3. **Impact on Institutional Budgets:** Medical institutions suffering from tight budgets find these expenses too heavy to handle. The need to spend more on technology prompts medical schools to make hard choices that impact other essential aspects of their education system. Developing countries' medical institutions struggle to adopt technology because of their limited budgets, increasing the educational resource gap between these nations (Ferrier, Lee, Mbuli, & James, 2022).
4. **Potential Mitigation Strategies:** While the financial challenges are significant, several strategies can help mitigate the burden on medical institutions:
   - **Phased Implementation:** Institutions can adopt a stage wise evolutionary approach to implementing wearable technology, starting with a pilot program or focusing on areas where the impact is likely to be most significant. This allows for more manageable investment and an opportunity to assess technology's effectiveness before scaling up.

- **Consortium Purchasing:** Medical institutions can collaborate to purchase wearable technology in bulk, potentially negotiating discounted prices from vendors. This collective bargaining power can significantly reduce the cost per institution.
- **Open-Source Alternatives:** Exploring and utilizing open-source software and hardware solutions can reduce reliance on expensive proprietary systems, lowering initial and ongoing costs.

4.2.2 The Digital Divide and Unequal Access to Technological Resources

The digital divide blocks the fair use of wearable technology in medical education because medical schools work with restricted budgets. The digital divide refers to the gap between individuals, households, businesses, and geographic areas at different socioeconomic levels with regard 1 to their access to information and communication technologies (ICTs) and their use of the Internet (Shcherbina et al., 2017). The digital divide makes people without proper technology access experience unequal chances to use wearable devices for medical education.

1. **Disparities in Infrastructure and Connectivity:** Most wearable technology applications need internet access because their functions depend on cloud-based systems and instant data transfer. Medical facilities in remote areas and their students struggle with poor internet service because it prevents them from joining VR/AR simulations and learning from a distance using wearable digital tools. Those without decent digital infrastructure at their location suffer from severe connectivity problems.
2. **Unequal Distribution of Devices:** Despite their financial resources, institutions cannot always provide equal access to students who need wearable technology. Your chances to use technology for learning depend strongly on where you live, your financial status, and school rules. Students from low-income homes lack personal access to devices that they cannot afford, and those enrolled in resource-limited schools encounter restricted shared device limits. Impaired resource distribution worsens the difference between students based on their socioeconomic background.
3. **Lack of Digital Literacy and Skills:** People need basic digital comprehension and technology skills to use wearable technology effectively. People who need help using technology find it hard to use and teach with wearables when they do not know how to use them properly. Students who cannot use technology will not adopt available wearable tools. Different levels of digital literacy depend

on age group, background, and income level, which makes some students more limited than others.

4. **Implications for Equity and Inclusion:** Wearable technology creates major differences between medical education students and hurts their chances of being equally included. Students who cannot use high-tech resources fall behind classmates who have access to these tools for hands-on learning. The unequal use of medical education innovations prevents students from underprivileged areas from getting equal education benefits. Students who lack digital access contribute less to building healthcare practice methods that accept diverse cultures.
5. **Strategies to Bridge the Digital Divide:**
    1. Several parties must cooperate to provide all people equal access to digital wearables and bridge the internet gap.
    2. The government must invest in digital projects to reach remote regions and provide schools with affordable devices.
    3. Military hospitals should establish written rules that boost student and faculty access to wearable technology by sharing medical equipment for free and creating technology support areas plus digital learning sessions.
    4. Establishing links with community groups and libraries helps students from poor backgrounds gain digital literacy skills through technology resources.

Overall, the high costs associated with wearable technology and the pervasive digital divide pose significant challenges to its widespread and equitable adoption in medical education. Addressing the financial constraints institutions face and implementing strategies to bridge the digital divide are crucial steps towards ensuring that all medical students, regardless of their socioeconomic background or geographic location, can benefit from these innovative tools (Mendes et al., 2024). Only through concerted efforts to overcome these hurdles can the full potential of wearable technology to revolutionize medical education and improve healthcare outcomes be realized for all.

4.3 Ethical Implications

Medical students will learn better and hone their skills while gaining customized training through wearable technology in medical studies. However, the benefits of current technology require us to confront important moral issues before we can use them appropriately. Our analysis will examine how medical students must agree to wearables while training and how well AI-powered medical tools share their solutions with users.

4.3.1. Consent and Transparency in Wearable Technology Use During Medical Training

When students learn with wearable technology, their personal body and performance data become visible to the training program. Students need to understand and agree to use their personal data, while school leaders need to explain clearly how they use these data. Ethical conduct in education depends on this practice.

1. **Informed Consent:** The ethical practice of data collection requires a clear patient understanding of how their medical data will be used and protected. When students use wearable technology for medical training, they need a complete understanding of these three key points.
    a. The form lists all data types, including heart rate, sleep measurements, stress data and performance results that the wearable device monitors.
    b. Students need to know what purposes their gathered data helps achieve. They need to know if their data will serve multiple functions, including evaluating their performance and teaching skills, scientific research, or training progress development.
2. **Transparency:** Transparency goes hand in hand with informed consent. Educational institutions must be transparent about their policies and procedures regarding the use of wearable technology. This includes:
    a. Medical training facilities should develop detailed guidelines that explain how and what wearable technology is used during student training. Students and teachers should have easy access to all policies related to wearable technology use.
    b. Students and their faculty must have straightforward ways to ask questions about personal data protection rules when using wearable technology in their medical studies.
    c. Medical institutions should transform raw student data into anonymized groups to shield individual privacy when research teams use data for medical school evaluation.

Challenges and Considerations

Medical training facilities should develop detailed guidelines that explain how and what wearable technology is used during student training (Steinhubl, Muse, & Topol, 2015). Students and teachers should have easy access to all policies related to wearable technology use.

1. Students and their faculty must have straightforward ways to ask questions about personal data protection rules when using wearable technology in their medical studies.
2. Medical institutions should transform raw student data into anonymized groups to shield individual privacy when research teams use data for medical school evaluation.
3. Our organization will have teams check data collection and use activities often to confirm that these practices meet our ethical policies and standards.

4.3.2. Potential Bias in AI-Powered Diagnostic Tools Integrated into Wearables

Wearable technology uses artificial intelligence to share real-time monitoring feedback, customized help, and medical coaching during training. Using AI in medical education can help learning, but it introduces a possible bias risk that creates unfair test results and extends healthcare inequalities.

1. **Sources of Bias in AI:** AI systems develop biases because data problems exist in several areas, including
   a. A healthcare AI system becomes biased during training when it handles patient populations that do not match the full range of patient diversity. This causes AI systems to misdiagnose patients and give wrong medical recommendations to specific groups.
   b. Bias may exist within AI algorithms at different stages during creation and use, even when training data remains neutral. These problems arise because of how we select features for our model, plus our preferences when designing its structure and learning processes.
2. **Implications for Medical Training:**
   a. Medical training faces major problems because AI diagnostic systems in wearables tend to produce unfair results.
   b. The system gives students unfair results because it displays biased judgments against members of specific groups and patient populations that are not present in its training data.
   c. Something missing from AI in diagnosis can spread medical stereotypes to the future healthcare workforce.
3. **Mitigating Bias in AI for Medical Training:** Addressing the risk of bias in AI-powered diagnostic tools requires a multi-faceted approach:
   a. Trainers must feed AI models abundant patient data showing all specific population types to reduce bias.

b. Fairness metrics and adversarial training techniques help medical educators find and correct unfairness in their AI programs.
c. Developing AI systems that show how they make decisions lets educators and students see into the system to find bias problems.

Medical schools must handle the ethical aspects of using wearable technology with students before moving forward. Students need to know how their data will be collected and handled before these actions start to trust and maintain personal privacy (Chen et al., 2022). Good medical education requires us to find and reduce bias in AI-powered tools built into wearables to create just results and sustain professional development.

5. FUTURE PROSPECTS OF WEARABLE TECHNOLOGY IN MEDICAL EDUCATION

The merging of artificial intelligence with machine learning technology in wearable devices transforms medical education practice standards for the better. The progression of educational technology in educational technology brings essential alterations to how medical knowledge will be acquired through educational practices (Liu et al., 2021). Integrating artificial intelligence technology with wearable devices creates individualized learning modules that also provide developmental student tracking and complex clinical training systems for enhancing healthcare education (Rodríguez-Fernández et al., 2021).

5.1 AI and Machine Learning Integration

Medical training benefits significantly from integrating artificial intelligence technology with machine learning capabilities delivered by wearable devices. End-to-end education transitioned from traditional classroom methods to student-specific training models because of technological achievements that produce personalized academic delivery. Medical training results in higher achievements for students who show excellent educational performance.

5.1.1 AI-Driven Personalized Learning Experiences

Medical school training programs become achievable because student performance analytics combine with wearable devices that track student behaviours. Educational systems combine student-generated behaviour records and performance outcome data to generate specific educational paths that align with academic targets. Educational institutions achieve their best educational success through personalized methods to develop future clinical practitioners.

AI-based personalized learning delivers its three vital aspects through these specific points:

- Understanding gaps within students can be detected through monitoring devices that measure their heart rate variability, pupil dilation, and electrodermal activity. Teaching professionals receive direct feedback that helps them supply vital help to students during their most urgent learning moments.
- Teachers obtain AI-mediated automatic material adjustment features through process automation and format conversion to manage speed and complexity dimensions based on individual student learning requirements. The system improves medical subject memorization by operating at individual student knowledge levels to enhance their focus.

5.1.2 Predictive Learning Analytics for Educational Progress

The convergence of machine learning algorithms with wearable devices helps generate performance predictions and detects vulnerable students while recommending customized help that prevents clinical problems from developing. Medical and educational institutions benefit from these capabilities because they shift their learning approach from a reactive model to a proactive model, which lets educators address problems during an early stage before they develop into major concerns.

Learning analytics deployments use three main applications:

The system uses predictive analytics by detecting minor academic warning signs to provide timely counselling services (Swan, 2012). The timely recognition of academic challenges becomes fundamental to prevent students' backward strides so they stay on target for academic success.

Wearable technology evaluates biological signatures and behavioural patterns to project future medical skill capabilities. Educational institutions can use monitoring data to develop specialized training curricula and help students learn appropriate skills.

Through AI monitoring of physiological factors, including cortisol levels and sleep patterns, the system identifies students who face stress-related burnout dangers. Programs addressing these students can be initiated for their welfare and academic achievement.

5.1.3 Enhanced Simulation Fidelity Through AI Integration

AI boosts simulation-based education by developing heightened, realistic, interactive, and adaptable training situations. Through its connection with wearable devices, AI creates simulations replicating student behaviour in an advanced interactive learning environment.

Innovative wearable technology's assessment abilities enable users to attain quantitative benchmarks through data collection of their simulated motions and physiological information (Tonino, 2019). The tool directly provides feedback to students to allow them to enhance their performance techniques.

Smart glasses and headsets enable medical students to participate in augmented reality training programs that provide hands-free immersive practice for real medical procedures. Working with this technology lets students gain practical training experience in controlled clinical areas to prepare them for actual medical cases (Dodds, 2020).

5.1.4 Future Developments in AI-Powered Education

Machine learning linked to AI technologies reveals promising educational applications with increasing sophistication during future developments. Future Medicine education technology will probably involve wearable AI systems that will enhance educational experiences while creating bespoke learning approaches and engaged student participation (Aquino et al., 2018). AI runs predictive genomic models that enable educators to predict medical course directions toward precision medicine while forecasting patient health developments and therapeutic response patterns (Mahato, Pathak, Sweta, & Choubey, 2024). The combined curriculum allows students to acquire contemporary educational information and health education competencies of tomorrow. Educational strategies receive brain-activity-specific information through brain-computer interface analysis to enhance learning methods (Stansfield et al., 2016). Technology indicates it can contribute to enhanced educational results by creating educational approaches based on separate cognitive processes.

5.1.5 Ethical Considerations and Implementation Challenges

Implementing AI-integrated wearable technology in medical education requires addressing serious ethical matters and technical obstacles because this technology holds tremendous potential for educational development (Miller & Johnson, 2022). Managing these issues enables learning institutions to establish a more secure and equalized learning space that delivers better results.

Data Privacy and Security

Among the most critical matters is protecting data security and privacy. Wearable medical educational devices gather large quantities of private student data, including their physical and biological health information (Singh et al., 2023). Data collection makes student performance and learningbehaviour analysis possible, which presents serious protected information risks when data management is inadequate (Pankajavalli & Karthick, 2020).

Wearable devices in medical education require institutions to build strong data management policies to solve their concerns. These policies should include:

Students require precise information about collected data and its use together with their informed consent before any data collection process starts. The organization follows legal and ethical standards such as GDPR and HIPAA to maintain compliance with data protection laws. The protection of student data alongside its security needs to be prioritized because it builds essential trust relationships between educational organizations and their student population.

Assessment and Validation

AI-enhanced medical education tools demonstrate potential value to the field, although their usefulness needs sustained evaluation processes (Evans et al., 2022). These technologies should demonstrate their contribution to developing clinical competencies and maintaining knowledge levels (Wilson & Carter, 2023).

AI-Integrated Wearable Technology in Medical Education: Ethical Considerations and Implementation Challenges

AI-Integrated Wearable Technology in Medical Education: Ethical Considerations and Implementation Challenges.

The essential elements for assessment include:

Machine learning tools need continuous assessments to evaluate student outcomes for performance measurement and tool advancement detection.

The system needs to establish feedback platforms accessible to students and instructors, which will evaluate learning tool effectiveness and overall utility.

Integration with Traditional Methods

The practical implementation of AI training methods must coexist with proven educational practices to uphold complete educational practices. The medical education discipline benefits from the learning advancements of AI and wearable technology systems yet continues to require fundamental teaching practices. AI-Integrated Wearable Technology in Medical Education: Ethical Considerations and Implementation Challenges, shown in Figure 6.

Considerations for integration include

Educators should build hybrid educational structures that unite artificial intelligence solutions with established instructional procedures for better student learning. The institution should provide training programs that enable teachers to integrate educational technologies with standard teaching methods.

Figure 6. AI-Integrated Wearable Technology in Medical Education: Ethical Considerations and Implementation Challenges

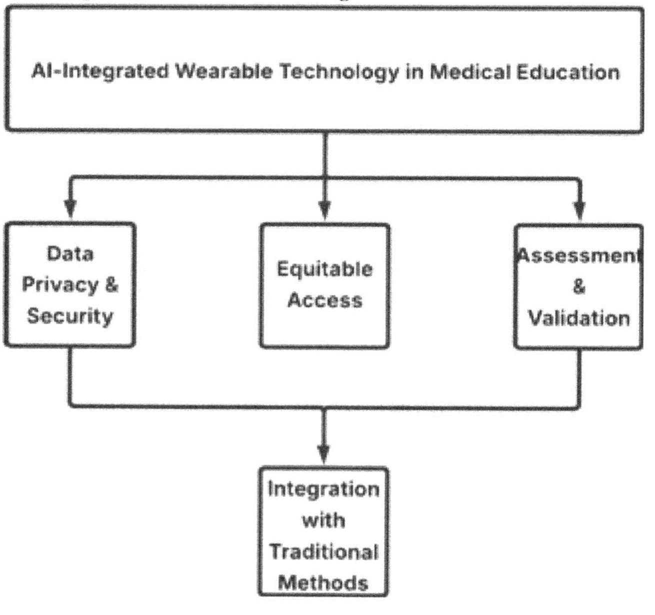

The curriculum needs adaptation to accept emerging technologies while maintaining fundamental educational principles. The most successful educational approach in clinical preparation for students uses strategically organized combinations of advanced and conventional teaching methods to deliver complete curricula.

5.2 Enhancements in Augmented Reality

Users can mingle simulated three-dimensional content with their actual surroundings while using immersive interactive features because of emerging artificial reality technology. The technology which operates through smartphones and tablets and dedicated devices enhances educational delivery and practical learning sessions. The gaming and entertainment sector first adopted AR technology but it has since started to grow popular with multiple industries including healthcare along with retail, marketing, education and military applications and tourism and automotive manufacturing and architecture and engineering (Garcia & Almeida, 2024).

Research on AR in medical education examines how this technology affects students' progression through their courses as well as their academic performances. The foundation of AR educational practices focuses on three main objectives which are streamlining complex subject matter entry points and enhancing understanding abilities among students while enhancing their learning experience. Medical students benefit from AR through three learning advantages which enhance their theoretical concepts while improving practical capabilities and developing interpersonal relationship skills (Singh & Ali, 2025). Three notable AR applications namely HoloHuman, OculAR SIM and HoloPatient focus specifically on medical education enhancement.

The main difference between AR and virtual reality centers on how they integrate digital components because AR combines virtual aspects with actual reality while virtual reality creates an entirely artificial world. The classification of mixed reality (MR) expands into two distinct areas which acknowledge AR and MR together as related technologies. Researches recognized this classification system more than 25 years ago when they started studying related concepts in a unified field.

5.2.1 Improving Student Engagement and Learning Outcomes through AR-Based Medical Education Programs

The Main Goals of AR-Based Learning

1. **Simplify the Delivery of Complex Information:** The complex information breakdown capabilities of AR present conceptual information through visual and reactive elements, which simplifies educational learning.
2. **Advance Communication Skills:** Professional team interaction improves thanks to simulation-based collaboration and instant performance feedback while using these techniques.
3. **Enhance Sense of Reality:** AR enables the creation of combined virtual-real-world experiences, which strengthen learning effects.

5.2.2 Benefits of AR-Based Surgeries and Diagnostics

- Students get to train for complex surgical procedures in virtual reality workflows leading up to actual patient procedures.
- Students understand anatomical relationships better because visualizing organs and tissues in three dimensions improves their academic learning.
- An AR-based safe environment enables learning through failure because it offers an opportunity to learn without facing repercussions, which promotes experimental methods.
- Remote Learning Capabilities: Facilitates access to expert guidance and surgical demonstrations from anywhere.

Figure 7. Role of AR/VR in the Medical field

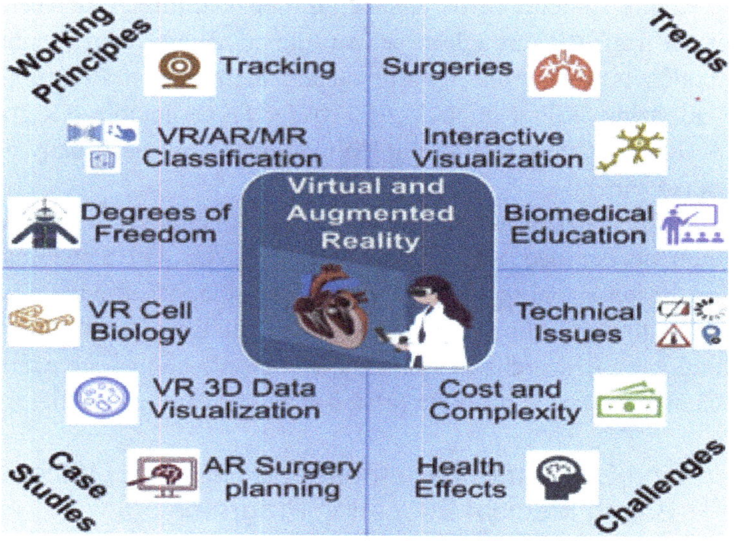

Healthcare professionals can experience interactive surgical training using HoloLens and Mixed-Reality Headsets that deliver real-time educational resources.The diagnostic process receives assistance through AR-enabled smart Glasses, which display patient information during examinations, as shown in Figure 7.

Mobile AR Applications: Deliver interactive case studies and anatomy exploration tools.

Both tactile feedback features allow surgical simulators to attain higher realism levels through touch-based responses. AR and VR integrate seamlessly with healthcare systems through digital radiology imaging, a crucial healthcare sector trend. Medical devices in this sector have experienced rising approvals due to this trend. The devices must complete a complete regulatory process that examines their safety operations and standard compliance before market availability (Shafik, 2024). AR devices for routine medical work must be certified as medical devices before entering the market.

5.3 Expansion of Remote Learning in Medical Education

Distance learning in medical education allows students from all regions to study at leading institutions and interact with their faculty staff remotely. Hands-on training receives additional support from advanced technologies implementing virtual reality (VR), augmented reality (AR) and wearable devices. The combination of broadcast surgery streams and artificial intelligence-based simulations allows learners to participate in genuine time-oriented instructional activities. Collaborating remotely enables students to perform international research and analyze cases worldwide. Flexible internet-based medical courses allow students from remote areas to access the education they need.

5.3.1 Key Aspects of Remote Learning in Medical Education

Remote learning through technology has transformed medical education into a universal opportunity for students to gain high-quality training. The advancement of digital technology enables students to watch virtual lectures aside from joining interactive simulations and accessing top medical specialists from various countries for collaboration. Through wearable devices, students gain better hands-on education experiences through artificial intelligence (AI) and virtual reality (VR) applications, which help connect classroom learning with clinical practice. Medical education benefits from increasing flexibility, and people worldwide can collaborate more through innovations in education. The progressive development of technology will determine how remote education becomes a fundamental component of how doctors receive their training.

1. **Global Access to Expertise & Institutions:**
    - Cross-cultural learning and Diversity elements teach students global healthcare systems and international medical practice examples, enabling them to develop worldwide medical perspectives.
    - Remote students can interact with famous medical experts from top fields through video guest lectures and virtual mentorship meetings with Nobel laureates and specialists.

- Advanced online resources offer virtual dissection laboratories besides clinical simulations and interactive anatomy software through interactive virtual labs and simulations.
- The combination of live and autonomous learning lets medical personnel develop additional skills while maintaining work-and-study balance.
- Medicine students benefit from remote education since standardized medical training delivers uniform educational content to students across countries and nations.
- Students gain the opportunity to join distant research initiatives because leading global institutions allow them to participate in distance learning.
- Online education decreases the expenses of attending elite medical institutions by removing the barriers of relocation costs, thus providing accessible elite medical education.

2. **Wearable Technology Enhancing Practical Training:** The practical value of theoretical knowledge is established through wearables, which bridge theory with real-world implementation. These devices include:
   - Microsoft HoloLens and other Augmented Reality (AR) Headsets provide medical students with visualization capabilities for anatomy studies, virtual dissection experiences, and 3D model interactions.
   - Haptic feedback gloves and bright touch technology allow medical learners to sense different physical properties through their hands during procedures such as suturing and physical examinations.
   - Bio-sensors and smartwatches are wearables remotely monitoring student analysis of current patient health indicators.
3. **Interactive & Immersive Learning Experiences:**
   - VR Medical Simulations provides virtual reality technology, including Touch Surgery and Osso VR platforms, allowing students to practice surgical techniques without risk.
   - Medical institutions provide live surgical broadcasts for student observation and direct questions to the operating surgeons during scheduled sessions.
   - Virtual patient systems with artificial intelligence automation produce chatbots and simulated patients to enhance student diagnostic capabilities.
4. **Collaboration & Knowledge Sharing:**
   - Medical conferences and symposiums become accessible to participants through virtual participation methods.
   - Student and professional researchers can collaborate for global research studies and clinical trial work from remote locations.

- Through remote learning, access allows students from underprivileged regions to obtain high-end medical education.

5. **Challenges & Solutions:**
   - Lack of hands-on experience- Integration of AR/VR simulations & remote proctoring of practical exams.
   - Digital divide & access to technology- Investment in affordable devices & infrastructure for remote areas
6. **Future of Remote Medical Education:** Medical remote learning will improve its efficiency combined with increasing technological advancement. Future trends include:
   - The AI technology will automatically customize educational materials based on students' developmental levels and learning approaches.
   - 5G and edge computing technologies will escalate network performance, enhancing remote surgical operations and educational training through live sessions.
   - Medical training will achieve its best results through training models that combine traditional clinical practice with digital simulation programs.

CONCLUSION

Medical education based on wearable technology significantly improves academic learning activities while building better clinical practitioner skills and fast data collection for medical decisions. Smartwatches, augmented reality (AR) headsets, and biosensors enable students to learn medical knowledge by permitting virtual simulation training and distance learning programs. The innovations better medical diagnosis capabilities while protecting patient safety through error prevention. Medical education faces various challenges regarding wearable technology due to its high costs together with accessibility issues, data security concerns, and ethical implications. This technology's full potential requires strategic deployment, proper regulation, and equal technology availability to handle and overcome existing difficulties. Wearable medical devices incorporating artificial intelligence (AI) and machine learning will enhance the personalization of medical education while maximizing student-learning effectiveness and producing better healthcare results in the future. Wearable technology maintains its fundamental position as an essential medical education tool in establishing the future of clinical education by embracing theoretical-to-practical knowledge gaps.

REFERENCES

Ali, A. S. M., Ali, S., Ziaullah, K., Joo, M.-I., & Kim, H.-C. (2025). *IoMT and blockchain synergy: A novel approach to health data validation and storage*. IEEE., DOI: 10.1109/ACCESS.2025.3555289

Araujo, A. A. C., Gardim, L., Salma, J., Stephen, T., Santos, S. S. D., Silva, Í. R., Godoy, S., & Mendes, I. A. C. (2024). Advancing nursing education through wearable electronic devices: A scoping review. *Nurse Education in Practice*, *79*, 104075. DOI: 10.1016/j.nepr.2024.104075 PMID: 39068061

Arch Virtual. (2018, August 21). Virtual reality medical simulation: 7 ways VR is revolutionizing healthcare training. *Arch Virtual*. https://archvirtual.com/2018/08/21/vr-medical-simulation-7-ways/

Arivu, S. A., Amutha, R., Muthumeenakshi, K., & Edna, E. N. (2018). Design of smart vest to monitor physical activities of children. In *2018 Fourth International Conference on Advances in Electrical, Electronics, Information, Communication and Bio-Informatics (AEEICB)* (pp. 1–4). IEEE. DOI: 10.1109/AEEICB.2018.8480993

Babu, M., Lautman, Z., Lin, X., Sobota, M. H. B., & Snyder, M. P. (2024). Wearable devices: Implications for precision medicine and the future of health care. *Annual Review of Medicine*, *75*(1), 401–415. DOI: 10.1146/annurev-med-052422-020437 PMID: 37983384

Chen, M., Wang, R., Zhou, Y., He, Z., Liu, X., He, M., & Tao, G. (2022). Digital medical education empowered by intelligent fabric space. *National Science Open*, *1*(1), 20220011. DOI: 10.1360/nso/20220011

Chen, M., Wang, R., Zhou, Y., He, Z., Liu, X., He, M., & Tao, G. (2022). Digital medical education empowered by intelligent fabric space. *National Science Open*, *1*(1), 20220011. DOI: 10.1360/nso/20220011

Chu, S. L., Garcia, B. M., & Rani, N. (2023, November). Research on wearable technologies for learning: A systematic review. [). Frontiers Media SA.]. *Frontiers in Education*, *8*, 1270389.

Fariah, F., Mahato, S., Pattanaik, C. R., & Mohanty, S. N. (2024). Application of wearable devices in the medical domain. In *Reconnoiter*. Taylor & Francis., DOI: 10.1201/9781003401841-7

Ferrier, B., Lee, J., Mbuli, A., & James, D. A. (2022). Translational applications of wearable sensors in education: Implementation and efficacy. *Sensors (Basel)*, *22*(4), 1675. DOI: 10.3390/s22041675 PMID: 35214578

Ferrier, B., Lee, J., Mbuli, A., & James, D. A. (2022). Translational applications of wearable sensors in education: Implementation and efficacy. *Sensors (Basel), 22*(4), 1675. DOI: 10.3390/s22041675 PMID: 35214578

Garcia, M. B., & Almeida, R. P. P. (2024). *Emerging technologies for health literacy and medical practice*. IGI Global., DOI: 10.4018/979-8-3693-1214-8

Georgieva-Tsaneva, G., Serbezova, I., & Beloeva, S. (2025). Application of virtual reality, artificial intelligence, and other innovative technologies in healthcare education (nursing and midwifery specialties): Challenges and strategies. *Education Sciences, 15*(1), 11. DOI: 10.3390/educsci15010011

Ghavami Hosein Pour, B., Karimian, Z., & Hatami Niya, N. (2025). A narrative review of advancing medical education through technology: The role of smart glasses in situated learning. *BMC Medical Education, 25*(1), 359. DOI: 10.1186/s12909-025-06949-7 PMID: 40065257

Harari, G. M., Lane, N. D., Wang, R., Crosier, B. S., Campbell, A. T., & Gosling, S. D. (2016). Using smartphones to collect behavioral data in psychological science. *Perspectives on Psychological Science, 11*(6), 838–854. DOI: 10.1177/1745691616650285 PMID: 27899727

Hong, H., Dai, L., & Zheng, X. (2025). Advances in wearable sensors for learning analytics: Trends, challenges, and prospects. *Sensors (Basel), 25*(9), 2714. DOI: 10.3390/s25092714 PMID: 40363153

Izard, S. G., Juanes, J. A., García Peñalvo, F. J., Estella, J. M. G., Ledesma, M. J. S., & Ruisoto, P. (2018). Virtual reality as an educational and training tool for medicine. *Journal of Medical Systems, 42*(3), 1–5. DOI: 10.1007/s10916-018-0900-2 PMID: 29392522

Lakshminarayana, S., Ranganatha, M., Sun, Y., & Park, H. (2025). Smartphone enabled wearable diabetes monitoring system. *IEEE Access : Practical Innovations, Open Solutions, 13*, 52324–52333. DOI: 10.1109/ACCESS.2025.3552731

Long, N. M. H., & Chung, W.-Y. (2021). Wearable noninvasive glucose estimation based on multi-wavelength reflective photoplethysmography. In *2021 IEEE Photonics Conference (IPC)* (pp. 1–2). IEEE. DOI: 10.1109/IPC48725.2021.9592997

Mahato, S., Pathak, L. K., Sweta, S., & Choubey, D. K. (2024). Wearable smart technologies. In *Changing the future of healthcare*. Taylor & Francis., DOI: 10.1201/9781003388845-11

Mendes, I. A. C., Gardim, L., Salma, J., Stephen, T., Santos, S. S. D., Silva, Í. R., Godoy, S., & Araújo, A. A. C. (2024). Advancing nursing education through wearable electronic devices: A scoping review. *Nurse Education in Practice*, *79*, 104075. DOI: 10.1016/j.nepr.2024.104075 PMID: 39068061

Mohammed, A., Li, S., & Liu, X. (2024). Exploring the potentials of wearable technologies in managing vestibular hypofunction. *Bioengineering (Basel, Switzerland)*, *11*(7), 641. DOI: 10.3390/bioengineering11070641 PMID: 39061723

Oh, K., Choi, J. K., Park, H., & Lee, S. (2025). Personalized ensemble based stress detection using wearable sensor data. In *2025 27th International Conference on Advanced Communications Technology (ICACT)* (pp. 470–475). IEEE. DOI: 10.23919/ICACT63878.2025.10936652

Pankajavalli, P. B., & Karthick, G. S. (Eds.). (2020). *Incorporating the Internet of Things in healthcare applications and wearable devices*. IGI Global., DOI: 10.4018/978-1-7998-1090-2

Patel, M. S., Asch, D. A., & Volpp, K. G. (2015). Wearable devices as facilitators, not drivers, of health behavior change. *Journal of the American Medical Association*, *313*(5), 459–460. DOI: 10.1001/jama.2014.14781 PMID: 25569175

Perle, J. G., Chandran, D. N., Brezler, E., Coleman, M., Deziel, J., Nahhas, P., McDonald, G., & Jent, J. F. (2025). Technology-enhanced practice competencies: Scoping review and novel model development. *Frontiers in Digital Health*, *7*, 1571518. DOI: 10.3389/fdgth.2025.1571518 PMID: 40352328

Piwek, L., Ellis, D. A., Andrews, S., & Joinson, A. (2016). The rise of consumer health wearables: Promises and barriers. *PLoS Medicine*, *13*(2), e1001953. DOI: 10.1371/journal.pmed.1001953 PMID: 26836780

Powell, K. R. (2017). Patient-perceived facilitators of and barriers to electronic portal use: A systematic review. *CIN: Computers, Informatics. Computers, Informatics, Nursing*, *35*(11), 565–573. DOI: 10.1097/CIN.0000000000000377 PMID: 28723832

Punj, A., Negassa, A., Gutierrez, A. K., Ch'en, P., & Jariwala, S. (2025). Technology enhanced medical education using smart glasses for oral and dental examinations: An observational pilot study. *BMC Medical Education*, *25*(1), 252. DOI: 10.1186/s12909-025-06853-0 PMID: 39962453

Sezer, H., & Gül, A. (2024). Health sciences students' perspectives on metaverse and digital technology use: Cross-sectional descriptive study. *BMC Nursing*, *23*(1), 656. DOI: 10.1186/s12912-024-02309-w PMID: 39278911

Shafik, W. (2024). Wearable medical electronics in artificial intelligence of medical things. In *Artificial Intelligence of Medical Things*. Taylor & Francis., DOI: 10.1201/9781003370321-2

Shcherbina, A., Mattsson, C. M., Waggott, D., Salisbury, H., Christle, J. W., Hastie, T., Wheeler, M. T., & Ashley, E. (2017). Accuracy in wrist-worn, sensor-based measurements of heart rate and energy expenditure in a diverse cohort. *Journal of Personalized Medicine*, *7*(2), 3. DOI: 10.3390/jpm7020003 PMID: 28538708

Singh, V. K., & Ali, Z. (2025). *Design and Simulation of Wearable Antennas for Healthcare*. IGI Global. https://www.igi-global.com/book/design-simulation-wearable-antennas-healthcare/338208

Steinhubl, S. R., Muse, E. D., & Topol, E. J. (2015). The emerging field of mobile health. *Science Translational Medicine*, *7*(283), 283rv3. Advance online publication. DOI: 10.1126/scitranslmed.aaa3487 PMID: 25877894

Sui, A., Sui, W., Liu, S., & Rhodes, R. (2023). Ethical considerations for the use of consumer wearables in health research. *Digital Health*, *9*, 20552076231153740. Advance online publication. DOI: 10.1177/20552076231153740 PMID: 36756643

Sun, L., He, L., Han, L., Yu, B., & Lin, J. (2025). Self-powered piezoelectric wearable sensor with motion recognition capability. *IEEE Sensors Journal*, *25*(9), 14760–14769. Advance online publication. DOI: 10.1109/JSEN.2025.3549451

Swan, M. (2012). Health 2050: The realization of personalized medicine through crowdsourcing, the quantified self, and the participatory biocitizen. *Journal of Personalized Medicine*, *2*(3), 93–118. DOI: 10.3390/jpm2030093 PMID: 25562203

Tang, Y. M., Chau, K. Y., Kwok, A. P. K., Zhu, T., & Ma, X. (2022). A systematic review of immersive technology applications for medical practice and education: Trends, application areas, recipients, teaching contents, evaluation methods, and performance. *Educational Research Review*, *35*, 100429. DOI: 10.1016/j.edurev.2021.100429

Tonino, R., Larimer, K., Eissen, O., & Schipperus, M. R. (2019). Remote Patient Monitoring in Adults Receiving Transfusion or Infusion for Hematological Disorders Using the VitalPatch and accelerateIQ Monitoring System: Quantitative Feasibility Study. *Journal of Medical Internet Research*, *22*(7), e15103. DOI: 10.2196/15103 PMID: 31789596

Vallurupalli, S., Paydak, H., Agarwal, S. K., Agrawal, M., & Assad-Kottner, C. (2013). Wearable technology to improve education and patient outcomes in a cardiology fellowship program: A feasibility study. *Health and Technology*, *3*(4), 267–270. DOI: 10.1007/s12553-013-0065-4

Wang, X., Young, G. W., Iqbal, M. Z., & Guckin, C. M. (2023). The potential of extended reality in rural education's future – perspectives from rural educators. *Education and Information Technologies*, *29*(7), 8987–9011. DOI: 10.1007/s10639-023-12169-7

Wanjari, N. D., & Patil, S. C. (2016). Wearable devices. In *2016 IEEE International Conference on Advances in Electronics, Communication and Computer Technology (ICAECCT)* (pp. 287–290). IEEE. DOI: 10.1109/ICAECCT.2016.7942600

Zhang, Z., Cajochen, C., & Khatami, R. (2019). Social jetlag and chronotypes in the Chinese population: Analysis of data recorded by wearable devices. *Journal of Medical Internet Research*, *21*(6), e13482. DOI: 10.2196/13482 PMID: 31199292

Zhu, E., Hadadgar, A., Masiello, I., & Zary, N. (2014). Augmented reality in healthcare education: An integrative review. *PeerJ*, *2*, e469. DOI: 10.7717/peerj.469 PMID: 25071992

Chapter 7
Mobile Learning in Medical Education

Pudasaini Pramila
https://orcid.org/0000-0003-4950-9855
Life Skills Education, Nepal

Ioannis Adamopoulos
https://orcid.org/0000-0002-4942-7123
School of Public Health, University of West Attica, Greece

Alisha Rijal
https://orcid.org/0000-0002-6605-1199
Yeti Health Science Academy, Nepal

ABSTRACT

Mobile learning (mLearning) is revolutionizing medical education with its flexibility, accessibility, and interactive features. This chapter identifies gaps in integrating mLearning into curricula, focusing on challenges like digital distractions, usability, and cost. Using PRISMA 2020 guidelines, it reviews literature from Scopus, Medline, PubMed, and Web of Science. Findings highlight benefits like enhanced engagement and clinical reasoning through gamified tools but note challenges like high costs and limited patient interaction. Recommendations include blended learning, collaboration, and theories like SDT and CLT to boost motivation and efficiency. The chapter emphasizes further research to optimize mLearning for improved global healthcare education.

DOI: 10.4018/979-8-3373-1519-5.ch007

INTRODUCTION

Mobile learning (mLearning) has emerged as a transformative innovation in medical education, offering unparalleled accessibility, flexibility, and interactivity. Rooted in Alan Kay's concept of the "Dynabook" (1972), mLearning has evolved into an essential tool for 21st-century education, enabling students to access resources on smartphones and tablets anytime and anywhere (Walsh, 2015). This approach promotes self-directed learning and supports knowledge retention, essential in the ever-evolving field of medicine (Kalantarion et al., 2022). Incorporating mobile applications, such as virtual patient simulations and gamified platforms, mLearning fosters critical skills like clinical reasoning and decision-making, addressing limitations in traditional resource availability (Scherr et al., 2023; Watari et al., 2020). Moreover, during global disruptions such as the COVID-19 pandemic, mobile apps have proven to sustain learner engagement and confidence, offering a flexible solution to disrupted educational norms (Alsharif et al., 2024). In developing regions, mobile apps like Medscape and digital medical dictionaries bridge educational gaps, making vital learning materials more accessible (Gavali et al., 2017). Despite these advantages, challenges persist. Issues such as app usability, screen size limitations, internet access, and digital distractions can hinder mLearning's effectiveness (Ahmady et al., 2024). Addressing these barriers requires integrating Self-Determination Theory (SDT) and Cognitive Load Theory (CLT) to optimize learning experiences by enhancing intrinsic motivation and managing cognitive demands (Kusurkar et al., 2011; Sweller, 1988). For mLearning to achieve its full potential, structured implementation within the medical curriculum, along with teacher collaboration and blended learning approaches, is critical (Kilag et al., 2023). With innovation and strategic adoption, mLearning is poised to revolutionize medical education, meeting the demands of modern healthcare and ensuring meaningful, lifelong learning for students globally.

The integration of mLearning into medical education has transformed the way medical students and professionals access information, acquire skills, and engage in continuous learning. This evolution reflects broader technological advancements and a shift towards more flexible, accessible, and learner-centered educational paradigms. Early development and adoption of the concepts of m-learning were proposed by computer scientist Alan Kay in the 1970s. Kay proposed the "Dynabook," a portable computer intended to facilitate learning anywhere. Although the Dynabook was never realized, it laid the foundation for future m-learning innovations (Kay, A. C., 1972). A consideration of historical and cultural events influencing mLearning traces its origins far back, even before Gutenberg's printing press or the Industrial Revolution. While these milestones enabled the mobile age, recent history has uniquely shaped m-learning. This chapter explores the separation of "mobile" and "learning" before detailing their interconnection, establishing mLearning as a distinct, emerging field (Crompton, 2019). At this time, there is no definitive definition of m-learning. If terms like distance education serve as an indication, it is probable that there will not be a lasting definition of m-learning for a long time to come. In January 2005, Laouris & Eteokleous (2014) noted this uncertainty. While m-learning is a powerful tool with the potential to bridge divides, its transformative impact requires more than just technology access. Visionary leadership, strategic planning, scientific theories, robust methodologies, and unwavering commitments are critical for turning this potential into reality. The optimistic promises of technology to address illiteracy and economic challenges must be tempered with practical insights. Real-world success demands integrating holistic approaches that address socio-political, educational, and economic contexts. Thus, mlearning is a catalyst, but its true power lies in the collective effort to drive sustainable changes (Crompton, 2019; Eteokleous, 2016; Laouris & Eteokleous, 2014). An article by Traxler (2005) has proposed an excellent document of some of the most important international conferences, highlighting m-learning as a new, evolving concept, potentially a subset of e-learning. It explores definition challenges through research and case studies from the UK and beyond. Like other areas, m-learning is gaining power in medical education. In this instance, an article by Walsh (2015) noted that m-learning has significantly advanced medical education, offering accessibility, cost efficiency, and interactive, contextual learning. Likewise, another review by Kalantarion, M., et al. (2022) highlighted the growing role of m-learning in medical education, particularly after the COVID-19 pandemic. It critically examines eight models and introduces a comprehensive m-learning framework, emphasizing key elements: stakeholders, interaction, and technology. The models account for essential influences such as mobiquette, legitimacy, and awareness, offering valuable insights for effective m-learning implementation in medical education. Additionally, another study by Chase et al. (2018) revealed the impact of m-learning devices, such as tablets and smartphones, on medical students during clinical rotations. The results suggest that m-learning devices positively affect students' perceptions of efficiency in their work. However, internet access limitations hinder optimal usage. Students prefer using the devices during downtime rather than as part of their clinical learning. Overall, the study supports the feasibility of m-learning devices in clinical education but emphasizes the need for universal internet access to maximize their potential.

Importance of Mobile Learning in Education, Including Pedagogical Concerns

Mobile learning refers to a range of terms and expressions such as mobile education" and education on the move." In the field of education, thousands of courses are available via mobile terminals. Some institutions have begun offering educational certificates to learners upon the successful completion of specific educational or instructional activities conducted via mobiles (Alshurideh et al. 2023). A majority of educational enthusiasts strongly believe in the advantages of mobile learning in education; it is a tool for guided learning outside the classroom that allows users to benefit greatly from the urban space and its services, digitized heritage, and shared experiences. Mobile learning, as an evolutionary step in e-learning, is opportunistic, flexible, and substantially enhances the process of learning. It is like e-learning but makes the process of learning more interactive, convenient, and integrated (Akour et al. 2021). Over the years, there has been a significant change in the learning methodologies. Initially, it was just limited to instructor-focused learning on one side, then it moved to collaborative learning, web-based learning, and blended learning. The technological developments and the increased access by the learners have made mobile learning a possibility (Rahiem, 2020). Mobile learning comes in different forms, such as apps, virtual environments, and social media. But when do we actually have to move from e-learning to m-learning? We move from e-learning to mobile learning when the learning need does not warrant a traditional class setup, it does not need highly clinical learning, job resources are the key training, or we are purely revising things (Hosen et al. 2021). Mobile learning is important for mostly two reasons: participants and the economy. Several studies reported that today's students and teachers have changed significantly in their use of new technologies. Technologies like smartphones and laptops are not stand-alone technologies. They are characterized by their ability to be connected with the world (Cranfield et al. 2021). Tablets, smartphones, and other mobile gadgets are now prevalent in today's society; the excitement surrounding contemporary technologies lies in the affordance they provide to move beyond the traditional classroom. Today's mobile learning can be best described as learning on the move (Tlili et al. 2022). It leverages the capability of computer technologies, the internet, and web applications reminiscent of e-learning. The typical methods of contemporary *m-learning* deliver a learning *module*, resource, or assessment to a mobile device that 'accompanies' the learner, who can access it at various chosen locations (Elfirdoussi et al. 2020). In education, *m-learning* is playing a critical part in the way teaching and training are being developed, offered, and conducted (Martens et al. 2021). Provides students of different levels of maturity with a variety of tools to support their pedagogy and other aspects of student life; however, the accessibility, ease of use, and convenience of this kind of initiative must be weighed against the dangers and technical difficulties (Doyumgaç et al., 2021). A number of privacy issues could also be encountered when using mobile devices (Al-Emran et al. 2020). Some advantages of mobile learning are listed here; first, and probably foremost, is the matter of time that mobile learning provides (Sophonhiranrak, 2021). Generally speaking, mobile learning allows learners to study at their own pace and according to their own schedule; as a result, a perfect match between learners' cognitive performance and learning material can be achieved (Hattie et al., 2023; McClure & Williams, 2021). This elemental necessity for meaningful learning is increasingly felt to be lacking in the narrowly specified curricula of local elementary and secondary educational institutions (Al-Shamsi et al. 2020; Saikat et al. 2021). Secondly, mobile learning can bridge geographical gaps and offer educational possibilities where there are geographical limitations and the absence of a local population that prefers to learn in traditional educational settings (Curum & Khedo, 2021; Hwang & Chang, 2021). Moreover, it contributes to both increasing and widening skills (Kearney et al., 2020; Chen & Tsai, 2021; Jeong, 2022).

Exploring the Significance of Mobile Learning in Transforming Traditional Medical Education

The initiation of mobile learning (mLearning) has revolutionized education across various disciplines, including medical education. With the widespread use of smartphones, tablets, and other portable devices, mLearning has emerged as a vital component complementing traditional teaching methods. This transformation is driven by the increasing demand for flexibility, convenience, and innovative approaches to learning. Mobile learning provides unique opportunities to enhance the teaching and learning process by enabling access to educational resources anytime, anywhere. This is particularly significant in the dynamic and demanding field of medical education. By integrating digital technologies into the curriculum, mLearning offers tools such as e-books and interactive applications. It supports self-directed learning, improves knowledge retention, and enhances clinical decision-making skills. For instance, a study by Inzunza et al. (2023) highlighted the transformative potential of mobile learning through gamification and virtual assistance in anatomy education. Conducted across two Chilean universities with 131 participants, the study demonstrated that gamified components effectively addressed challenges such as limited access to cadaveric materials, improving student engagement and academic performance. Additionally, predictive recommendations from virtual assistants identified areas for improvement, paving the way for adaptive, AI-driven, personalized learning scenarios in future medical education. Similarly, a study by Alsharif et al. (2024) emphasized the critical role of mLearning in traditional medical education during the COVID-19 pandemic. Mobile learning apps became essential tools for e-learning, addressing the need for flexibility and accessibility among Egyptian medical students at Menoufia University. The study revealed a significant increase in app usage during and after the lockdown. Confidence in mLearning grew, with 81.3% of students during the lockdown and 88.1% post-lockdown finding mobile apps flexible and effective learning methods. However, challenges such as a lack of app knowledge remained barriers to optimal utilization in medical education. Medical education apps are versatile tools that facilitate communication and learning. According to Remtulla (2020), the development of mobile medical apps has expanded the potential of smartphones in healthcare, enhancing learning, diagnosis, and decision-making. These apps serve as valuable supplements to traditional learning environments, providing medical students with convenient access to up-to-date medical information and expertise. In developed countries, a UK survey by Frederick et al. (2012) found that mobile learning is revolutionizing traditional medical education, with widespread smartphone usage among medical students (79%) and faculty (74.8%). Apps were frequently used for clinical decision-making, diagnosis, and drug references. Participants emphasized the potential of mobile tools to enhance education and improve patient care, highlighting the need for innovative medical apps to meet educational and clinical demands. Similarly, Wallace et al. (2012) explored the integration of mobile devices like iPhones in medical education. Over 85% of participants, including students and faculty, used mobile devices for information management, communication, and time management. While these tools improved learning flexibility and patient care, challenges such as distractions and privacy concerns underscored the need for structured guidance in their implementation. In developing countries like India, a study by Gavali et al. (2017) examined smartphone usage as a learning tool among 446 medical students. The study found a 96% ownership rate, with Android dominating (72.4%), followed by iPhones (13%). Popular apps included Medscape, anatomy apps, and medical dictionaries, which facilitated learning and provided instant access to resources. Over 90% of students felt technologically skilled, while 79.4% supported integrating smartphones into the MBBS curriculum. Hence, integration of mobile learning into medical education offers immense potential to transform traditional teaching methods. By addressing challenges such as accessibility and engagement, mLearning enhances self-directed learning, clinical decision-making, and knowledge retention. However, overcoming barriers like lack of app knowledge and distractions is crucial to fully realize its benefits. With continued innovation and structured implementation, mLearning can play a pivotal role in shaping the future of medical education.

Simulation and Clinical Scenario Training for Medical Students Using Devices

Simulation and clinical scenario training through mobile devices have revolutionized medical education by providing interactive, accessible, and cost-effective learning opportunities. Mobile-based simulation tools allow students to engage with realistic patient scenarios, hone decision-making skills, and practice clinical procedures in a safe environment. These tools foster experiential learning and bridge the gap between theoretical knowledge and practical application. A study by Scherr et al. (2023) highlights that simulation training using tools like ChatGPT bridges the gap between preclinical knowledge and clinical application. ChatGPT's interactive simulations, such as advanced cardiac life support and sepsis management, enable students to practice diagnostic and therapeutic decision-making in lifelike scenarios. These simulations provide accessible, adaptable, and cost-effective learning experiences, enhancing medical education while addressing resource disparities. Similarly, a study by Watari et al. (2020) examined the use of Virtual Patient Simulations (VPSs) as a novel approach to medical education. This study, involving 169 fourth-year medical students, assessed the impact of a two-hour VPS session using a pre-post experimental design. Results revealed significant improvements in clinical reasoning ($p < 0.001$) and knowledge ($p = 0.003$) scores, demonstrating the potential of VPSs to enhance decision-making skills without direct lecturer supervision. These findings support integrating VPS programs into medical curricula to foster clinical competence and better prepare students for real-world healthcare challenges. Furthermore, Datta et al. (2012) emphasized that simulation and clinical scenario training have revolutionized medical education by offering immersive, hands-on learning while avoiding real-life risks. This approach enhances cognitive, psychomotor, and affective skills, focusing on patient safety, autonomy, and error management. By mimicking real-world complexities, simulation promotes experiential learning, teamwork, and crisis resource management. It benefits undergraduate teaching, postgraduate training, continuing medical education, and specialized fields such as disaster and military trauma management.

Theoretical Perspectives

Mobile Learning and Self-Determination Theory (SDT) in Medical Education

Self-Determination Theory (SDT), developed by Edward Deci and Richard Ryan, is one of the major motivational theories in psychology. SDT research has been conducted in many areas, including education and healthcare, but its application in medical education is relatively rare. Intrinsic motivation (IM) and autonomous self-regulation for learning are positively associated with academic performance and well-being. Autonomy-supportive teaching stimulates the development of IM and autonomous self-regulation in learning. Successes and failures in many elements of medical education can be understood from the perspective of SDT (Kusurkar et al., 2011). Self-Determination Theory (SDT) is vital in understanding the relationship between mobile learning and medical education (Ahmady et al., 2024). SDT highlights key variables such as autonomy, relatedness, and competence, which significantly enhance engagement, academic performance, and psychological empowerment in medical students (Kusurkar et al., 2011). This framework supports autonomy by allowing students to learn at their own pace and access resources, quizzes, and simulations anytime and anywhere (Davies, 2024). For example, tools like virtual anatomy models or diagnostic case studies help students build competence by providing immediate feedback, fostering mastery of complex concepts. Relatedness is supported through collaborative learning approaches, such as team-based discussions, which cultivate empathy-driven learning and foster a sense of community and shared purpose among students (Ahmady et al., 2024; Davies, 2024). Moreover, mobile platforms designed with SDT principles reduce extrinsic pressures and instead create meaningful, intrinsic motivations. By aligning learning opportunities with the values of medical education, students feel empowered to practice and explore, resulting in greater academic performance and personal growth. Features such as gamified progress tracking further enhance engagement and motivation (Williams & Ryan, 2018). By integrating SDT into mobile learning, this approach not only complements traditional medical education but also empowers students with flexibility, self-directed learning opportunities, and improved psychological well-being, ultimately enriching their overall educational experience.

Cognitive Load Theory and Mobile Learning in Medical Education

Cognitive Load Theory (CLT), proposed by Sweller (1988), offers a framework for designing mobile learning tools that manage the mental effort required by medical students. In medical education, where students must learn vast and complex materials, it is essential to present content in ways that reduce extraneous cognitive load while optimizing germane load, which contributes to meaningful learning (Young et al., 2014).A study by Gutierrez et al. (2023) highlighted that mobile learning can apply CLT by breaking content into smaller, manageable segments. Using preparatory online modules in simulation-based education optimizes cognitive load by increasing intrinsic and germane load while reducing extraneous load. This enhances performance, as evidenced by higher scores in OSCE assessments among postgraduate medical trainees. For example, instructional videos had a significant impact on increasing cognitive load and motivation. Instructional videos featuring only the instructor's hands and watched in laboratory settings proved to be more effective. Based on these findings, the study provided important directions for future research and practice. Applying CLT and optimizing video design for mobile medical education can enhance outcomes and balance cognitive demands. A study by Leppink and Ph (2017) concluded that the introduction of CLT in medical education has advanced both fields. While challenges remain in distinguishing cognitive load types, CLT's application in medical education promotes further research, fostering excitement and motivation within the educational community.

Technology Acceptance Model (TAM) and Its Role in Mobile Applications for Medical Education

The integration of different technologies, particularly mobile applications, is an emerging trend in medical education. The TAM supports this application because it explains how users accept and use technology (Davis et al., 1989). TAM consists of two variables:

Perceived usefulness: Mobile applications in medical education are simple to use and do not require extensive experience. Most medical students are already familiar with digital tools, making these applications highly beneficial.

Perceived Ease of Use: Mobile applications allow students to access different apps and software efficiently, enhancing their learning experiences. The ease of use contributes to the effective utilization of mobile technology in medical education.

Overall, m-learning applications are highly useful, and many students suggest that their adoption has a significant impact on learning. Hence, mobile applications are widely accepted in medical education. However, certain social factors may influence students' attitudes, as their perceptions derive their actions and behaviors. To foster the wise use of mobile applications in medical education, these factors must be carefully considered.

The Role Of Emotional Intelligence And Digital Intelligence

Another important framework in this context is Emotional Intelligences(EI) and Digital Intelligence (DI), studied by Danila Goleman, and others researchers' encompasses a broad set of skills and competencies required to navigate digital environment, EI, on the other hand, plays a crucial in performances, as individuals with high EI tend to achieve better results(Cobb & Mayer, 2000).Since medical students frequently interact with patients and cross-disciplinary teams, they need to develop EI, DI and Human intelligences (HI) to enhances their academic success and well-being. Essential personal skills such as self- awareness, self- managements and social skills are necessary to navigate both medical practices and digital learning environment effectively.

Student-Centered Learning Theory

Student-centered learning emphasizes tailoring educational experiences to the needs, preferences, and goals of students, fostering autonomy and active engagement. In mobile application adoption for medical education, this theory highlights how apps empower students to manage their learning pace, access diverse resources, and participate in collaborative activities (Kerimbayev et al., 2023; Mustapa et al., 2022). Research indicates that mobile learning enhances problem-solving skills and critical thinking, crucial for medical students (Kerimbayev et al., 2023). Furthermore, it supports personalized learning pathways, enabling students to revisit complex medical concepts as needed. Mobile applications exemplify student-centered learning by integrating multimedia content, assessments, and feedback mechanisms, making them effective tools for medical education (Kerimbayev et al., 2023; Traxler, 2015).

METHODOLOGY

Research-Design

This Book chapter explores the review study uses a systematic reviews design guided by the PRISMA 2020 guidelines (Page et al., 2021) to examine the existing state of oral health education and the impact of mobile learning in medical education. The design approach ensures transparency and rigor in examining relevant literature, focusing on understanding key approaches to medical education and mobile learning within the digital landscape.

Search Strategy

A structured search strategy was employed to examine studies from various databases, adhering to the PRISMA approach. Key terms related to mobile learning, medical education, clinical reasoning, blended learning, and digital distraction were used. The review aims to provide a comprehensive analysis of the literature, focusing on the purposes of the approaches and their effectiveness in improving medical education through mobile learning.

Study Selection

The study selection process was based on inclusion and exclusion criteria to ensure relevance and quality. Inclusion criteria focused on studies exploring the role of mobile learning in medical education, particularly in the context of clinical reasoning and self-directed learning. Independent reviewers evaluated the selected studies to assess their relevance and quality, ensuring that only studies meeting the defined criteria were included in the review.

Data Synthesis

Data synthesis involved summarizing key findings from the selected studies to explore evidence-based approaches and best practices for integrating mobile learning into medical education. This synthesis aimed to identify themes related to behavior changes, student engagement, technology acceptance, and self-directed learning. The goal is to provide actionable insights and suggestions for stakeholders, including policymakers, educators, technology developers, and students, on enhancing mobile learning in medical education to improve healthcare services and educational outcomes. Figure 1 shows the research of the literature reviews PRISMA flow diagram of this book chapter study.

Figure 1. Research methods of Book Chapter study, PRISMA flow Diagram.

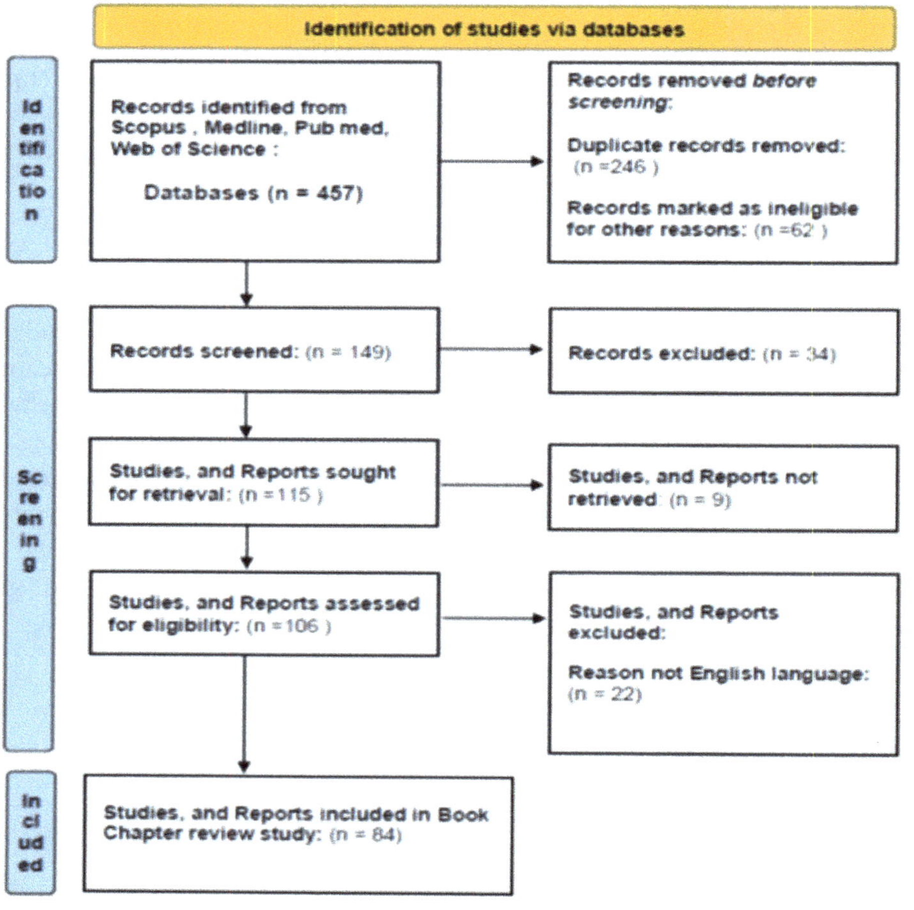

DISCUSSION

Trends of Mobile Practice in Medical Education

Mobile e-learning practices in medical education exhibit innovative approaches across different countries. For example, the flipped classroom model, widely adopted in vocational and higher education, involves asynchronous study of multimedia content and synchronous learner-centered activities like collaborative learning, problem-solving, and discussion. Studies such as those on medical terminology courses in Turkey explore the effectiveness of the flipped classroom model in a fully online medical terminology course within a vocational college program. Learners engage with interactive multimedia content asynchronously and participate in synchronous activities like collaborative learning and problem-solving. Academic achievement, system usability, and learner perception highlighted that time investment and the perception of deep learning were key factors in success, though issues with time expectations, instructional material, and guidelines were noted (Tekin et al., 2020). In India, mobile learning practices in medical education show how smartphones are revolutionizing medical education by enhancing access to study materials, videos, updates, and research tools. They provide portable, easy-to-use devices that aid in note-taking, literature reviews, and data collection (Chandra et al., 2019). In China, mobile technology plays a crucial role in enhancing medical education and healthcare. With nearly 1 billion mobile phone subscribers, mobile tools improve patient-provider communication, health education, and public health campaigns. Controlled studies and public health reports indicate that mobile interventions significantly improve health outcomes, highlighting the need for further research to refine and expand mobile health applications (Corpman, D. W., 2013). Likewise, another study by Mahmood (2019) reveals that 73.2% of doctors in the Department of Pediatrics at the University of the Witwatersrand, Johannesburg, South Africa, use medical apps multiple times a day. The most commonly used apps include reference tools (81.7%), diagnostic tools (58.17%), and decision-making support tools (43.79%). Doctors rely on peer recommendations, app credibility, functionality, and usability when selecting apps for clinical practice.

Best Practices in Mobile Learning in Medical Education Worldwide

A rapid increase in the use of mobile devices, most noticeably mobile phones and tablet computers, has been seen worldwide in the last three or four years, in particular regarding internet and application use. The competitive market, where devices have increased storage, processing power, screen size, and an ever-growing offer of applications specific to areas of interest, brings more usefulness to users Sophonhiranrak, 2021). Medical education is a relevant area of interest since continuous studying habits, viewing reference textbooks or medical journal articles, in addition to mono/sub-specialty-related apps, can take full advantage of mobile solutions. Mobile use, coupled with new specialization trends and an increasing knowledge base, is leading to a significant use of mobile solutions in education and medical services worldwide El-Sofany & El-Haggar, 2020). Medical students use technologies for searching or consulting specific study content during small lectures and, more specifically, for solving cases during clinical or similar activities. Also, the educational environments evolve through the combination of information and communication technologies, pedagogical theories, and educational technology strategies by means of blended learning. Problems and solutions are also advanced Nikolopoulou, 2020). Medical education has long been engaged in exploring and exploiting the potential of this technology in the undergraduate teaching of pre-clinical and clinical subjects. Mobile devices are essential instruments used by students and staff in learning, teaching, assessment, and research activities Klimova & Polakova, 2020). Teachers and students who chose to share research on and use mobile devices in undergraduate medical education resent original contributions in the form of educational research, educational policies, educational experiences, and pedagogical reflections explaining a multitude of novel strategies, models, techniques, and challenges Alghazi et al., 2021). The main purpose of this section of the chapter in this book is to stimulate further interaction and collaboration of teachers regarding blended-styled learning of higher education medical students, after acknowledging the benefits of designing situations for connected students throughout their studies Tkachuk et al. 20200). Finally, may researchers also improve the correlations of machine learning, which is considered one of the most significant techniques associated with medical learning in diagnostic methods of COVID-19 and impact issues on public hygiene in public health services (Adamopoulos et al., 2022; Adamopoulos et al., 2023; Thapa et al., 2024; Mijwil et al., 2024).

Issues, Problems, and Their Contribution to Mobile Learning in Medical Education

Mobile learning, or m-learning, becomes more and more important all over the world, including in medical education. It offers sufficient flexibility and open related aspects and options in timing, location, and content; there are many things, particularly conventional ones, that need to be memorized (Krishnamurthy et al. 2022). Technical skills that should follow some details in a given sequence, some episodes should be learned and repeated several times so that the trainee can learn from their mistakes, the learners are always eager to get an answer as soon as possible or to have an accurate reference available at all times (Ngenzi et al., 2021). The use of learning cards as an m-learning system helped the trainees to cover such situations; the results of evaluations indicate that the learners support the use of mobile phones and social networks to support learning and to be used all the time (Curum & Khedo, 2021). The use of mobile learning facilitated knowledge acquisition and skills development, encouraged the practice of medical students in family medicine, and more initiatives are needed to launch research and development of m-learning in medical education (Criollo-Cet al. 2021; Burgess et al., 2020; Jumreornvong et al., 2020).

Thinking about the future of education is absent from the dialogue about the future of health and health care. Medical education is changing in an age of information technology. Health care, something for which society is clamoring, continues to be an arena of resistance to innovation and change (Gaur et al. 2020). The development and delivery of education every year place more reliance on computers and internet access. Networks should be blended with other traditional learning technologies, including simulations, distance learning, e-learning lectures, classes, and others. This is because education is a continuously changing discipline, influenced by new state-of-the-art accelerations, social, and cultural values (Alsoufi et al. 2020). The internet and all kinds of web have helped in capacity-building activities globally, including in healthcare and many others, letting them be involved in the ensuing technological revolution of soft technology and advanced features of connectivity. Many universities are trying to adopt mobile learning technology and also develop supporting infrastructure (Binks et al. 2021). It is always common for an educated physician to be acknowledged in the generations of ancient civilizations. In fact, interest in this digital training has penetrated almost all developed countries in Asia, Europe, the USA, and others (Al-Balas et al. 2020). Features have been enhanced for college students, postgraduates, and experts, and for all hospital staff regardless of their grade and rank (Wilcha, 2020).

Although the majority agree that mobile learning is a flexible way of learning, they also acknowledge that these apps cannot be solely relied upon during medical study. Issues such as not knowing which apps to use, limited internet access, and high costs were the main obstacles preventing students from using the apps more widely (Alsharif et al., 2024). Additionally, 37.2% expressed concerns that smartphone use might reduce patient interaction. The study highlighted the potential of smartphones in medical education but called for further research on their impact on students' academic performance (Gavali et al., 2017). Other challenges include cost, dependency, distractions, and health concerns. Despite these issues, students show a positive attitude toward smartphone use, suggesting that mLearning has great potential if effectively implemented in medical curricula.

Linkages with Similar Themes: Medical Education, Sustainable Development, and 21st-Century Skills

Interdisciplinary approaches enhance understandings of complex contemporary issues; linking medical education and sustainable development goals can be seen as interdisciplinary (Meschede, 2020). This exploration links medical education with the international policy focus on sustainable development, which has increasing emphasis in global institutional policy contexts but which has been largely overlooked in relation to medical education (Chaleta et al., 2021). Of the activities that are associated with medical education, the general capabilities that are identified as fundamental or 21st-century skills are seen as aligning particularly well with the development of an extended understanding of sustainable development goals and can be considered a key part of a new professionalism that is essential for the delivery of healthcare in the contemporary world (Hsiao & Su, 2021; Chankseliani & McCowan, 2021). The activity focus is designed to start the conversation or development of innovative curricula reflecting the needs of the future relating to professional skills and personal attributes. Medical skills, leadership, community engagement, and citizenship to build better understanding through mapping of pedagogic methods to desirable outcomes and theories underpinning them that demonstrate how pedagogic enhancements can lead to capabilities (Kulkov et al. 2024). With respect to the deepest underpinning capabilities, the work provokes reflection upon the drivers and motivations for inspirational graduate outcomes and also upon ideas from parallel education policy contexts (Bahroun et al., 2023). Link to a forward-looking, collective impact or system change perspective that can inform and drive change in the development of teaching and learning environments. Approaches best suited to address the future desired substantive change both for the regulatory bodies and individuals who are to ensure the robustness and fairness of health professional practice, and for the end-users (Hsiao & Su, 2021). Accomplishments in this proposed work will help to build a community of practice that can commit to addressing the future challenges with structures to support that work (Pandey et al., 2022; Lee et al., 2021).

Integration with Curriculum, Teacher Training, and the Entire Medical Education System

The educational model based on the full incorporation of the student within the framework of student learning recognizes the importance of aligning the curriculum, teacher training, and the whole system; all of them pose a critical approach capable of bringing innovation to the field. They also acknowledge the importance of collective work (Baker et al. 2021). Fragmenting the system of education reform, a common vision and work moving towards the understanding of training and medical education at different levels will help to continue supporting the success of students; the implementation of policies in one area or another may have different speeds. The challenges to collective action in the curriculum and medical education may be complex, but the opportunities available to us in the form of possibilities to act and innovate are numerous (Kilag et al. 2023). The potential provided by the critical analysis developed in favor of a more balanced concession, and policy-makers and any other stakeholders interested in improvement and the leading changes in medical education, these teaching professionals come to education from the direction of modern healthcare needs with the same intention: to contribute to the field with greater expertise in terms of promoting and achieving meaningful training (MacPhail et al. 2023). Although there is no magic formula for curricular medicine, universities in general and health sciences in particular face the challenge of integrating educational innovation and research for contribution; the synthesized can represent the basis for developing the pilot and other assessments: a research qualification approach to verifying the implications of the actions developed as a result of the consensus launched (Kilag et al. 2023). The perspective and research experience from the seminar series on the future of day-to-day legal education plan for educational research to identify possible issues and themes of great interest to educators and students and invite them to write or present at the conference (Loughlin et al. 2021). Through the collaboration and identification of the above, the approach to access and change was discussed in the public forum, making a significant contribution in a number of areas, raising the profile of the partnership between the medical school, the legal record, and this kind of engagement (Atuhurra & Kaffenberger 2022). The approach adopted had the added benefit of learning from the varied experiences of all parties. This report brings the much closer potential of the various disciplines and their high level of commitment by the health sciences in supporting the main goal of the medical school and to reflect the values we collectively hold (Martinez, 2022).

Table 1. Comparative between traditional learning and mobile application-based learning (modern) in medical education

Traditional Learning	Mobile Application-Based Learning
Accessibility and Flexibility	
Requires physical presence, scheduled classes, and institutional attendance, limiting access for remote learners.	Allow learners to access content anytime and anywhere, enhancing convenience and supporting flexible, on-demand education.
Learning Engagement and Interaction	
Often lecture-based with limited interaction, which can hinder students' engagement and deeper learning.	Incorporate multimedia, quizzes, gamification, and peer collaboration to improve engagement and perceived depth to boost interactivity and learner motivation.
Content Delivery and Updates	
Relies on textbooks and printed material that may become outdated and are harder to revise frequently.	Whereas smartphones provide apps for diagnostics, references, and decision-making support, enhancing practical application during learning
Pedagogical Innovation and Blended Strategies	
Traditional one-way information delivery	Mobile learning supports blended learning by integrating digital content, interactive pedagogy, and instant updates.

continued on following page

Table 1. Continued

Traditional Learning	Mobile Application-Based Learning
Challenges and Digital Davide	
Traditional methods are consistent.	Mobile learning faces challenges like app selection, internet issues, and screen fatigue, though it still garners students' support.

Smart Learning: Smart Mobile Apps in Healthcare

Mobile applications have become an essential part of medical education and other education, especially in the context of modern digital learning. Everywhere and everyone seems to be talking about mobile applications, and their presence in medical education is growing rapidly. Due to increasing complexity in medical topics, rising healthcare costs, and inequality in access to treatment and services, mobile applications are emerging as innovative solutions. In many regions—especially rural and underserved areas—access to healthcare and education remains limited. However, mobile technology offers a promising alternative that bridges this gap. These apps are increasingly available even in developing nations, offering accessibility and affordability. Numerous studies suggest that mobile applications are among the best tools for promoting awareness, preventive healthcare, and early detection services. They are user-friendly, low-cost, and require minimal training, making them suitable for the general population. With the rise of artificial intelligence, there is potential for automation to replace or reduce the workload of medical and educational professionals by more than 50%. Despite this, traditional educational approaches still hold value. Medical professionals can benefit by learning and updating their skills through digital tools and mobile applications, ensuring they remain relevant and effective in a rapidly evolving digital world. To support this transition, strategies are needed to cultivate skills, motivation, and engagement using modern theories and practices. If medical professionals can adopt positive perceptions toward technology, they can enhance learning, connect with broader communities, and support underserved populations. This contributes to skill development, especially the essential 21st-century skills needed in today's digital landscape. These skills include digital literacy, emotional intelligence, motivation, and the ability to engage effectively in both personal and professional contexts. They help individuals adapt to digital environments, boost learning outcomes, and foster social connections. However, challenges remain. Evidence shows that without attention to self-care—such as proper sleep, exercise, and social support—even the most advanced tools can fall short. Educators and medical professionals must prioritize personal and social well-being to maintain physical, mental, and emotional fitness. Therefore, integrating mobile applications into education and healthcare must be balanced with human-centered approaches to ensure holistic well-being in the digital age.

Smart Skills, Smart Systems

The smart medical career signifies a futuristic model of healthcare integration, where smart medical specialists are prepared with digital learning, clinical proficiency, and emotional intelligence (EI). With the spread of mobile applications, medical experts now have prompt access to updated clinical strategies, drug databases, diagnostic tools, and telemedicine service area. This mobile-based prototypical foster continuous learning, real-time communication, and modified service delivery. Smartphones act as portable helpers, enabling medical scholars and specialists to engage in flipped classrooms, mobile learning modules, virtual simulations, social media, text messaging, group messaging, and decision-support structures. AI-powered investigative tools, screening, e-prescriptions, communication with service providers and stakeholders, remote monitoring, medical awareness, health promotion services, electronic health records, surveys, and medical research enhance the accuracy, efficiency, and accessibility of care, even in underserved regions. This embryonic ecosystem aligns with sustainable development goals, promoting equitable healthcare and problem-solving skills, critical thinking, and creativity in medical education. Though, for such a system to be real, integration with medical curricula, teacher training, and supportive infrastructure is vital. This confirms that specialists are not just technology users but critical thinkers and empathetic caregivers in the digital land.

Ethical Reflections of M-learning in Medical Education

M-learning in medical education raises numerous ethical attentions related to equity, professional accountability, and patient confidentiality. While mobile devices increase access to knowledge and foster self-directed education, ethical worries emerge concerning the digital divide. Scholars with inadequate access to smartphones or tablets face inequalities. Further worries include privacy, data safety, permission, distraction, misrepresentation, screen time(ST), academic honesty, competence, equity, plagiarism, dependence, prejudice, theft, surveillance, correctness, abuse, misuse, and discretion (Chandra et al., 2019).Additionally, overreliance on mobile apps for clinical decision-making might negotiation the development of critical reasoning and diagnostic services, raising worries about the depth and incorporation of medical training (Tekin et al., 2020). Ethical observes also request that students using mobile devices in clinical settings preserve strict privacy of patient data, safeguarding compliance with privacy guidelines. In South Africa, where 73.2% of pediatric doctors often use medical apps, the status of app reliability, data security, and ethical usage is manifest (Mahmood, 2019). Mobile learning settings must be planned with robust ethical strategies that report informed app use, data safety, and equitable access. Eventually, integrating m-learning ethically necessitates institutional accountability to safeguard students are digitally cultured, professionally accountable, and reinforced by inclusive, ethical, and protected educational systems.

CONCLUSION

In conclusion, this book chapter explores how mobile learning (mLearning) has emerged as a transformative tool in medical education, offering unprecedented opportunities for flexible, accessible, and engaging learning experiences. The integration of mobile technologies such as smartphones and tablets has enabled medical students to access educational resources anytime and anywhere, fostering self-directed learning and enhancing knowledge retention. mLearning has proven particularly beneficial in dynamic fields like medicine, where staying updated with the latest developments and clinical practices is crucial. Through the use of virtual patient simulations, gamified applications, and other innovative tools, students can improve their clinical reasoning and decision-making skills while overcoming traditional resource limitations.

Despite its advantages, there are challenges associated with mLearning, such as app usability, screen size limitations, and potential digital distractions. The cost of mobile devices and internet access, especially in low-resource settings, can also hinder its widespread adoption. Furthermore, while mobile learning enhances engagement and academic performance, an overreliance on digital tools could potentially reduce patient interaction and clinical exposure. To fully realize the potential of mLearning in medical education, there is a need for a systematic and strategic approach that aligns curriculum, teacher training, and institutional support. Collaborative efforts from educators, policymakers, and technology developers are essential to address the challenges and create an environment conducive to effective mLearning. By integrating mobile learning into the medical curriculum, fostering blended learning approaches, and ensuring the quality and usability of mobile apps, mLearning can significantly enhance the learning experience and contribute to the development of well-rounded, competent healthcare professionals. As technology continues to evolve, mLearning is poised to become an essential part of medical education worldwide, aligning with the demands of the 21st century.

Funding: This chapter received no specific funding.

Conflicts of Interest: The authors declare no conflicts of interest.

Acknowledgements: We would like to express our sincere gratitude to everyone who supported and inspired the completion of this chapter, especially for their direct and indirect contributions.

REFERENCES

Ahmady, S., Khajeali, N., Kohan, N., Zarei, A., Biswas, B., Barzegar, M., & Moghaddam, A. K. (2024). Medical students' perception of mobile learning during COVID-19 in Iran: A national study. *PLoS One*, *19*(10), e0308248. DOI: 10.1371/journal.pone.0308248 PMID: 39423220

Akour, I., Alshurideh, M., Al Kurdi, B., Al Ali, A., & Salloum, S. (2021). Using machine learning algorithms to predict people's intention to use mobile learning platforms during the COVID-19 pandemic: Machine learning approach. *JMIR Medical Education*, *7*(1), e24032. DOI: 10.2196/24032 PMID: 33444154

Al-Balas, M., Al-Balas, H. I., Jaber, H. M., Obeidat, K., Al-Balas, H., Aborajooh, E. A., Al-Taher, R., & Al-Balas, B. (2020). Distance learning in clinical medical education amid COVID-19 pandemic in Jordan: Current situation, challenges, and perspectives. *BMC Medical Education*, *20*(1), 1–7. DOI: 10.1186/s12909-020-02257-4 PMID: 33008392

Al-Emran, M., Arpaci, I., & Salloum, S. A. (2020). An empirical examination of continuous intention to use m-learning: An integrated model. *Education and Information Technologies*, *25*(4), 2899–2918. DOI: 10.1007/s10639-019-10094-2

Al-Shamsi, A., Al-Mekhlafi, A. M., Al Busaidi, S., & Hilal, M. M. (2020). The effects of mobile learning on listening comprehension skills and attitudes of Omani EFL adult learners. *International Journal of Learning. Teaching and Educational Research*, *19*(8), 16–39. DOI: 10.26803/ijlter.19.8.2

Alghazi, S. S., Kamsin, A., Almaiah, M. A., Wong, S. Y., & Shuib, L. (2021). For sustainable application of mobile learning: An extended UTAUT model to examine the effect of technical factors on the usage of mobile devices as a learning tool. *Sustainability (Basel)*, *13*(4), 1856. DOI: 10.3390/su13041856

Alsharif, M. A., Bahbah, A. A., Ghonaim, M. M., Omran, J. A., Rihan, M. M., Zayed, M. A., Tabour, M. S., Alwardany, M. H., & Aboshady, O. A. (2024). Usage and attitude of medical students towards mobile medical applications during and after COVID-19 lockdown: Repeated cross-sectional study. *BMC Medical Education*, *24*(1), 233. DOI: 10.1186/s12909-024-05216-5 PMID: 38438883

Alshurideh, M., Al Kurdi, B., Salloum, S. A., Arpaci, I., & Al-Emran, M. (2023). Predicting the actual use of m-learning systems: A comparative approach using PLS-SEM and machine learning algorithms. *Interactive Learning Environments*, *31*(3), 1214–1228. DOI: 10.1080/10494820.2020.1826982

Alsoufi, A., Alsuyihili, A., Msherghi, A., Elhadi, A., Atiyah, H., Ashini, A., Ashwieb, A., Ghula, M., Ben Hasan, H., Abudabuos, S., Alameen, H., Abokhdhir, T., Anaiba, M., Nagib, T., Shuwayyah, A., Benothman, R., Arrefae, G., Alkhwayildi, A., Alhadi, A., & Elhadi, M. (2020). Impact of the COVID-19 pandemic on medical education: Medical students' knowledge, attitudes, and practices regarding electronic learning. *PLoS One*, *15*(11), e0242905. DOI: 10.1371/journal.pone.0242905 PMID: 33237962

Atuhurra, J., & Kaffenberger, M. (2022). Measuring education system coherence: Alignment of curriculum standards, examinations, and teacher instruction in Tanzania and Uganda. *International Journal of Educational Development*, *92*, 102598. DOI: 10.1016/j.ijedudev.2022.102598

Bahroun, Z., Anane, C., Ahmed, V., & Zacca, A. (2023). Transforming education: A comprehensive review of generative artificial intelligence in educational settings through bibliometric and content analysis. *Sustainability (Basel)*, *15*(17), 12983. DOI: 10.3390/su151712983

Baker, L. R., Phelan, S., Woods, N. N., Boyd, V. A., Rowland, P., & Ng, S. L. (2021). Re-envisioning paradigms of education: Towards awareness, alignment, and pluralism. *Advances in Health Sciences Education : Theory and Practice*, *26*(3), 1045–1058. DOI: 10.1007/s10459-021-10036-z PMID: 33742339

Binks, A. P., LeClair, R. J., Willey, J. M., Brenner, J. M., Pickering, J. D., Moore, J. S., Huggett, K. N., Everling, K. M., Arnott, J. A., Croniger, C. M., Zehle, C. H., Kranea, N. K., & Schwartzstein, R. M. (2021). Changing medical education, overnight: The curricular response to COVID-19 of nine medical schools. *Teaching and Learning in Medicine*, *33*(3), 334–342. DOI: 10.1080/10401334.2021.1891543 PMID: 33706632

Boulos, M. N. K., Brewer, A. C., Karimkhani, C., Buller, D. B., & Dellavalle, R. P. (2014). Mobile medical and health apps: State of the art, concerns, regulatory control and certification. *Online Journal of Public Health Informatics*, *5*(3). Advance online publication. DOI: 10.5210/ojphi.v5i3.4814 PMID: 24683442

Castellano, M. S., Contreras-McKay, I., Neyem, A., Farfán, E., Inzunza, O., Ottone, N. E., del Sol, M., Alario-Hoyos, C., Alvarado, M. S., & Tubbs, R. S. (2024). Empowering human anatomy education through gamification and artificial intelligence: An innovative approach to knowledge appropriation. *Clinical Anatomy (New York, N.Y.)*, *37*(1), 12–24. DOI: 10.1002/ca.24074 PMID: 37453079

Chaleta, E., Saraiva, M., Leal, F., Fialho, I., & Borralho, A. (2021). Higher education and sustainable development goals (SDG)—Potential contribution of the undergraduate courses of the school of social sciences of the University of Évora. *Sustainability (Basel), 13*(4), 1828. DOI: 10.3390/su13041828

Chandra, A., Nongkynrih, B., & Gupta, S. K. (2019). Role of smartphone technology in medical education in India. *Indian Journal of Community and Family Medicine, 5*(2), 103–107. DOI: 10.4103/IJCFM.IJCFM_42_19

Chankseliani, M., & McCowan, T. (2021). Higher education and the sustainable development goals. *Higher Education, 81*(1), 1–8. DOI: 10.1007/s10734-020-00652-w PMID: 33173242

Chase, T. J., Julius, A., Chandan, J. S., Powell, E., Hall, C. S., Phillips, B. L., Burnett, R., Gill, D., & Fernando, B. (2018). Mobile learning in medicine: An evaluation of attitudes and behaviours of medical students. *BMC Medical Education, 18*(1), 1–8. DOI: 10.1186/s12909-018-1264-5 PMID: 29945579

Chen, C. H., & Tsai, C. C. (2021). In-service teachers' conceptions of mobile technology-integrated instruction: Tendency towards student-centered learning. *Computers & Education, 170*, 104224. https://doi.org/doi:10.1016/j.compedu.2021.104224

Cobb, C. D., & Mayer, J. D. (2000). Emotional intelligence. *Educational Leadership, 58*(3), 14–18. DOI: 10.2190/dugg-p24e-52wk-6cdg

Corpman, D. W. (2013). Mobile health in China: A review of research and programs in medical care, health education, and public health. *Journal of Health Communication, 18*(11), 1345–1367. DOI: 10.1080/10810730.2013.778370 PMID: 23915211

Cranfield, D. J., Tick, A., Venter, I. M., Blignaut, R. J., & Renaud, K. (2021). Higher education students' perceptions of online learning during COVID-19—A comparative study. *Education Sciences, 11*(8), 403. DOI: 10.3390/educsci11080403

Criollo-C, S., Guerrero-Arias, A., Jaramillo-Alcázar, Á., & Luján-Mora, S. (2021). Mobile learning technologies for education: Benefits and pending issues. *Applied Sciences (Basel, Switzerland), 11*(9), 4111. DOI: 10.3390/app11094111

Crompton, H. (2013). A historical overview of mobile learning: Toward learner-centered education. In Berge, Z. L., & Muilenburg, L. Y. (Eds.), *Handbook of mobile learning* (pp. 3–14)., https://www.academia.edu/5601076/A_historical_overview_of_mobile_learning_Toward_learner_centered_education

Curum, B., & Khedo, K. K. (2021). Cognitive load management in mobile learning systems: Principles and theories. *Journal of Computers in Education*, *8*(1), 109–136. DOI: 10.1007/s40692-020-00173-6

Datta, R., Upadhyay, K. K., & Jaideep, C. N. (2012). Simulation and its role in medical education. *Medical Journal, Armed Forces India*, *68*(2), 167–172. DOI: 10.1016/S0377-1237(12)60040-9 PMID: 24623932

Davies, E. (2024). Health simulation through the lens of self-determination theory — Opportunities and pathways for discovery. *Advances in Simulation (London, England)*, *9*(1), 31. DOI: 10.1186/s41077-024-00304-4 PMID: 39039553

Davis, F. D., Bagozzi, R. P., & Warshaw, P. R. (1989). User Acceptance of Computer Technology : A Comparison of Two Theoretical Models. *Management Science*, *35*(8), 982–1003. DOI: 10.1287/mnsc.35.8.982

Doyumgaç, I., Tanhan, A., & Kiymaz, M. S. (2021). Understanding the most important facilitators and barriers for online education during COVID-19 through online photovoice methodology. *International Journal of Higher Education*, *10*(1), 166–190. DOI: 10.5430/ijhe.v10n1p166

El-Sofany, H., & El-Haggar, N. (2020). The effectiveness of using mobile learning techniques to improve learning outcomes in higher education. https://doi.org/DOI: 10.3991/ijim.v14i08.13125

Elfirdoussi, S., Lachgar, M., Kabaili, H., Rochdi, A., Goujdami, D., & El Firdoussi, L. (2020). Assessing distance learning in higher education during the COVID-19 pandemic. *Education Research International*, *2020*(1), 8890633. DOI: 10.1155/2020/8890633

Gaur, U., Majumder, M. A. A., Sa, B., Sarkar, S., Williams, A., & Singh, K. (2020). Challenges and opportunities of preclinical medical education: COVID-19 crisis and beyond. *SN Comprehensive Clinical Medicine*, *2*(11), 1992–1997. DOI: 10.1007/s42399-020-00528-1 PMID: 32984766

Gavali, M. Y., Khismatrao, D. S., Gavali, Y. V., & Patil, K. B. (2017). Smartphone, the new learning aid amongst medical students. *Journal of Clinical and Diagnostic Research : JCDR*, *11*(5), JC05–JC08. DOI: 10.7860/JCDR/2017/20948.9826 PMID: 28658804

Gutierrez, G., Lunsky, I. O., Van Heer, S., Szulewski, A., & Chaplin, T. (2023). Cognitive load theory in action: E-learning modules improve performance in simulation-based education. A pilot study. *Canadian Journal of Emergency Medical Care*, *25*(11), 893–901. DOI: 10.1007/s43678-023-00586-z PMID: 37751082

Hattie, L. D., Sahlberg, C. W., & Comer, P. P. (2023). Impact of mobile learning apps on study habits and academic performance of college students in the United States: A review of literature. *Journal of Education*, *6*(3), 13–22. DOI: 10.53819/81018102t4182

Hosen, M., Ogbeibu, S., Giridharan, B., Cham, T. H., Lim, W. M., & Paul, J. (2021). Individual motivation and social media influence on student knowledge sharing and learning performance: Evidence from an emerging economy. *Computers & Education*, *172*, 104262. DOI: 10.1016/j.compedu.2021.104262

Hsiao, P. W., & Su, C. H. (2021). A study on the impact of STEAM education for sustainable development courses and its effects on student motivation and learning. *Sustainability (Basel)*, *13*(7), 3772. DOI: 10.3390/su13073772

Hwang, G. J., & Chang, S. C. (2021). Facilitating knowledge construction in mobile learning contexts: A bi-directional peer-assessment approach. *British Journal of Educational Technology*, *52*(1), 337–357. DOI: 10.1111/bjet.13001

Jang, H. W., & Kim, K. J. (2014). Use of online clinical videos for clinical skills training for medical students: Benefits and challenges. *BMC Medical Education*, *14*(1), 1–6. DOI: 10.1186/1472-6920-14-56 PMID: 24650290

Jeong, K. O. (2022). Facilitating sustainable self-directed learning experience with the use of mobile-assisted language learning. *Sustainability (Basel)*, *14*(5), 2894. DOI: 10.3390/su14052894

Jumreornvong, O., Yang, E., Race, J., & Appel, J. (2020). Telemedicine and medical education in the age of COVID-19. *Academic Medicine*, *95*(12), 1838–1843. DOI: 10.1097/ACM.0000000000003711 PMID: 32889946

Kalantarion, M., Sadoughi, M. M., Ahmady, S., Kallestrup, P., Katibeh, M., & Khajeali, N. (2022). Introducing a mobile learning model in medical education during COVID-19; a critical review. *Journal of Advances in Medical Education & Professionalism*, *10*(3), 145. DOI: 10.30476/JAMP.2022.93494.1534 PMID: 35910511

Kay, A. C. (2011). A personal computer for children of all ages. *Proceedings of the ACM Annual Conference*- Volume 1.https://doi.org/DOI: 10.1145/800193.1971922

Kearney, M., Burden, K., & Schuck, S. (2020). Theorising and implementing mobile learning. *Springer Nature*, *10*, 978–981.

Kerimbayev, N., Umirzakova, Z., Shadiev, R., & Jotsov, V. (2023). *A student - centered approach using modern technologies in distance learning : a systematic review of the literature*. Smart Learning Environments., DOI: 10.1186/s40561-023-00280-8

Kilag, O. K., Marquita, J., & Laurente, J. (2023). Teacher-led curriculum development: Fostering innovation in education. *Excellencia: International Multi-disciplinary Journal of Education (2994-9521), 1*(4), 223-237. https://multijournals.org/index.php/excellencia-imje/article/view/53

Kilag, O. K., Tokong, C., Enriquez, B., Deiparine, J., Purisima, R., & Zamora, M. (2023). School Leaders: The Extent of Management Empowerment and Its Impact on Teacher and School Effectiveness. *Excellencia: International Multi-disciplinary Journal of Education (2994-9521), 1*(1), 127-140. https://multijournals.org/index.php/excellencia-imje/article/view/13/12

Klimova, B., & Polakova, P. (2020). Students' perceptions of an EFL vocabulary learning mobile application. *Education Sciences, 10*(2), 37. DOI: 10.3390/educsci10020037

Krishnamurthy, K., Selvaraj, N., Gupta, P., Cyriac, B., Dhurairaj, P., Abdullah, A., Krishnapillai, A., Lugova, H., Haque, M., Xie, S., & Ang, E. T. (2022). Benefits of gamification in medical education. *Clinical Anatomy (New York, N.Y.), 35*(6), 795–807. DOI: 10.1002/ca.23916 PMID: 35637557

Kulkov, I., Kulkova, J., Rohrbeck, R., Menvielle, L., Kaartemo, V., & Makkonen, H. (2024). Artificial intelligence-driven sustainable development: Examining organizational, technical, and processing approaches to achieving global goals. *Sustainable Development (Bradford), 32*(3), 2253–2267. DOI: 10.1002/sd.2773

Laouris, Y., & Eteokleous, N. (2005, October). We need an educationally relevant definition of mobile learning. In *Proceedings of mLearn* (Vol. 2005).

Leppink, J. (2017). Cognitive load theory: Practical implications and an important challenge. *Journal of Taibah University Medical Sciences, 12*(5), 385–391. DOI: 10.1016/j.jtumed.2017.05.003 PMID: 31435268

Loughlin, C., Lygo-Baker, S., & Lindberg-Sand, Å. (2021). Reclaiming constructive alignment. *European Journal of Higher Education, 11*(2), 119–136. DOI: 10.1080/21568235.2020.1816197

MacPhail, A., Tannehill, D., Leirhaug, P. E., & Borghouts, L. (2023). Promoting instructional alignment in physical education teacher education. *Physical Education and Sport Pedagogy, 28*(2), 153–164. DOI: 10.1080/17408989.2021.1958177

Mahmood, S. (2019). *The use of medical apps amongst doctors working in the Department of Paediatrics and child health of the University of the Witwatersrand, in Johannesburg South Africa* (Doctoral dissertation, Faculty of Health Sciences, University of the Witwatersrand, Johannesburg). https://wiredspace.wits.ac.za/server/api/core/bitstreams/740ff759-0b0a-4b0a-b1ec-0f3a231ec26a/content

Martens, T., Beck, R. W., Bailey, R., Ruedy, K. J., Calhoun, P., Peters, A. L., Pop-Busui, R., Philis-Tsimikas, A., Bao, S., Umpierrez, G., Davis, G., Kruger, D., Bhargava, A., Young, L., McGill, J. B., Aleppo, G., Nguyen, Q. T., Orozco, I., Biggs, W., & Balo, A.MOBILE Study Group. (2021). Effect of continuous glucose monitoring on glycemic control in patients with type 2 diabetes treated with basal insulin: A randomized clinical trial. *Journal of the American Medical Association*, *325*(22), 2262–2272. DOI: 10.1001/jama.2021.7444 PMID: 34077499

Martinez, C. (2022). Developing 21st century teaching skills: A case study of teaching and learning through project-based curriculum. *Cogent Education*, *9*(1), 2024936. DOI: 10.1080/2331186X.2021.2024936

McClure, C., & Williams, P. (2021). Gather. town: An opportunity for self-paced learning in a synchronous, distance-learning environment. *Compass (Eltham)*, *14*(2). Advance online publication. DOI: 10.21100/compass.v14i2.1232

Meschede, C. (2020). The sustainable development goals in scientific literature: A bibliometric overview at the meta-level. *Sustainability (Basel)*, *12*(11), 4461. DOI: 10.3390/su12114461

Mijwil, M. (2024). M., Adamopoulos, I., & Pudasaini, P. (2024). Machine learning Helps in Quickly Diagnosis Cases of "New Corona". *Mesopotamian Journal of Artificial Intelligence in Healthcare*, *16–19*. Advance online publication. DOI: 10.58496/MJAIH/2024/003

Mustapa, M., Shaharuddin, S., Wisman, M., Hamid, A., Noorul, N., & Mohamed, S. (2022). Student-Centred Approach in Medical Education : A Review of the Teaching- Student - Centred Approach In Medical Education : A Review of the Teaching - Learning Activities and the Perceptions of Educators on the Students Engagement and Performance At the Faculty of Medicine and Defence Health. *National Defence University of Malaysia.*, (May). Advance online publication. DOI: 10.4103/aihb.aihb

Ngenzi, J. L., Scott, R. E., & Mars, M. (2021). Information and communication technology to enhance continuing professional development (CPD) and continuing medical education (CME) for Rwanda: A scoping review of reviews. *BMC Medical Education*, *21*(1), 245. DOI: 10.1186/s12909-021-02607-w PMID: 33926419

Nikolopoulou, K. (2020). Secondary education teachers' perceptions of mobile phone and tablet use in classrooms: Benefits, constraints and concerns. *Journal of Computers in Education, 7*(2), 257–275. DOI: 10.1007/s40692-020-00156-7

Pandey, N., de Coninck, H., & Sagar, A. D. (2022). Beyond technology transfer: Innovation cooperation to advance sustainable development in developing countries. *Wiley Interdisciplinary Reviews. Energy and Environment, 11*(2), e422. DOI: 10.1002/wene.422

Payne, K. F. B., Wharrad, H., & Watts, K. (2012). Smartphone and medical related App use among medical students and junior doctors in the United Kingdom (UK): A regional survey. *BMC Medical Informatics and Decision Making, 12*(1), 1–11. DOI: 10.1186/1472-6947-12-121 PMID: 23110712

Rahiem, M. D. (2020). The emergency remote learning experience of university students in Indonesia amidst the COVID-19 crisis. *International Journal of Learning. Teaching and Educational Research, 19*(6), 1–26. DOI: 10.26803/ijlter.19.6.1

Remtulla, R. (2020). The present and future applications of technology in adapting medical education amidst the COVID-19 pandemic. *JMIR Medical Education, 6*(2), e20190. DOI: 10.2196/20190 PMID: 32634107

Saikat, S., Dhillon, J. S., Wan Ahmad, W. F., & Jamaluddin, R. A. D. (2021). A systematic review of the benefits and challenges of mobile learning during the COVID-19 pandemic. *Education Sciences, 11*(9), 459. DOI: 10.3390/educsci11090459

Scherr, R., Halaseh, F. F., Spina, A., Andalib, S., & Rivera, R. (2023). ChatGPT interactive medical simulations for early clinical education: Case study. *JMIR Medical Education, 9*, e49877. DOI: 10.2196/49877 PMID: 37948112

Sophonhiranrak, S. (2021). Features, barriers, and influencing factors of mobile learning in higher education: A systematic review. *Heliyon, 7*(4), e06696. Advance online publication. DOI: 10.1016/j.heliyon.2021.e06696 PMID: 33869873

Suliman, M. A. E.. (2024). Medical student's acceptance of mobile learning: Integrating TAM model with perceived reusability. *Education and Information Technologies, 1*(24). Advance online publication. DOI: 10.1007/s10639-024-12917-3

Sweller, J. (1988). Cognitive Load During Problem Solving. *Effects on Learning., 285*, 257–285. DOI: 10.1207/s15516709cog1202

Tekin, P., Ilgaz, H., Adanır, G., Yıldırım, D., & Gülbahar Güven, Y. (2020). Flipping e-learning for teaching medical terminology: A study of learners' online experiences and perceptions. *Online Learning : the Official Journal of the Online Learning Consortium, 24*(2), 76–93. DOI: 10.24059/olj.v24i2.2030

Ten Cate, O. T. J., Kusurkar, R. A., & Williams, G. C. (2011). How self-determination theory can assist our understanding of the teaching and learning processes in medical education. AMEE guide No. 59. *Medical Teacher*, *33*(12), 961–973. DOI: 10.3109/0142159X.2011.595435 PMID: 22225433

Tkachuk, V., Yechkalo, Y., Semerikov, S., Kislova, M., & Hladyr, Y. (2020, October). Using mobile ict for online learning during covid-19 lockdown. In *International Conference on Information and Communication Technologies in Education, Research, and Industrial Applications* (pp. 46-67). Cham: Springer International Publishing. DOI: 10.1007/978-3-030-77592-6_3

Tlili, A., Huang, R., Shehata, B., Liu, D., Zhao, J., Metwally, A. H. S., Wang, H., Denden, M., Bozkurt, A., Lee, L.-H., Beyoglu, D., Altinay, F., Sharma, R. C., Altinay, Z., Li, Z., Liu, J., Ahmad, F., Hu, Y., Salha, S., & Burgos, D. (2022). Is Metaverse in education a blessing or a curse: A combined content and bibliometric analysis. *Smart Learning Environments*, *9*(1), 1–31. DOI: 10.1186/s40561-022-00205-x

Traxler, J. (2005, June). Defining mobile learning. In IADIS international conference mobile learning (Vol. 261, p. 266).

Wallace, S., Clark, M., & White, J. (2012). 'It's on my iPhone': Attitudes to the use of mobile computing devices in medical education, a mixed-methods study. *BMJ Open*, *2*(4), e001099. DOI: 10.1136/bmjopen-2012-001099 PMID: 22923627

Walsh, K. (2015). Mobile learning in medical education. *Ethiopian Journal of Health Sciences*, *25*(4), 363–366. DOI: 10.4314/ejhs.v25i4.10 PMID: 26949301

Watari, T., Tokuda, Y., Owada, M., & Onigata, K. (2020). The utility of virtual patient simulations for clinical reasoning education. *International Journal of Environmental Research and Public Health*, *17*(15), 5325. DOI: 10.3390/ijerph17155325 PMID: 32722097

Wilcha, R. J. (2020). Effectiveness of virtual medical teaching during the COVID-19 crisis: Systematic review. *JMIR Medical Education*, *6*(2), e20963. DOI: 10.2196/20963 PMID: 33106227

Williams, G. C., Saizow, R. B., & Ryan, R. M. (1999). The importance of self-determination theory for medical education. *Academic Medicine*, *74*(9), 992–995. DOI: 10.1097/00001888-199909000-00010 PMID: 10498090

Young, J. Q., Van Merrienboer, J., Durning, S., & Ten Cate, O. (2014). Cognitive load theory: implications for medical education: AMEE Guide No. 86. *Medical Teacher*, *36*(5), 371–384. DOI: 10.3109/0142159X.2014.889290 PMID: 24593808

KEY TERMS AND DEFINITIONS

Mobile Learning (m-Learning): Use of mobile devices for a flexible, location-independent medial learning experience.

Flipped Classroom: Learners study content asynchronously, then apply knowledge through active collaboration.

Medical Apps: Smartphone-based tools supporting diagnostic, references, and clinical decision-making tasks.

Blended Learning: An education approach combining online resources with face-to-face medical instruction.

Digital Health Education: Teaching healthcare skills using digital tools, improving public health knowledge.

21st Century Skills: Core competencies like communication, collaboration, and problem-solving for medical professionals.

Curriculum Integration: Embedding mobile learning tools systemically within structural mediation education programs.

Chapter 8
3D Printing Revolutionizing Rural Dental Care: Empowering Healthier Smiles

Mariya Dimitrova
https://orcid.org/0000-0003-2444-2471
Department of Prosthetic Dentistry, Faculty of Dental Medicine, Medical University of Plovdiv, Bulgaria

ABSTRACT

3D printing, or additive manufacturing, is transforming dentistry by enabling precise, affordable, and localized production of dental devices. Using a layer-by-layer process with materials like resins and metals, it creates prosthetics, orthodontic devices, and surgical guides, improving workflows and patient care. In rural areas, where economic and infrastructure barriers limit access to specialized dental care, 3D printing offers a revolutionary solution. By enabling on-site production of custom devices, it reduces costs, shortens treatment times, and bridges the gap between rural and urban healthcare. Successful cases in India, Sub-Saharan Africa, and Southeast Asia highlight its potential to empower local providers and improve accessibility. However, challenges like high startup costs, limited materials, and training requirements hinder broader adoption. Future advancements, including AI integration and improved materials, could overcome these barriers.3D printing promises equitable, high-quality dental care by decentralizing production and improving access.

DOI: 10.4018/979-8-3373-1519-5.ch008

1. INTRODUCTION

3D printing has transformed healthcare, especially in dentistry, by revolutionizing patient care, particularly in rural areas where access to specialized services can be limited. What was once seen as a futuristic idea is now a practical and affordable way to create accurate, customized dental devices. This advancement has increased the efficiency and accessibility of dental care, benefiting both urban and rural populations (Tian et al., 2021; Della Bona et al., 2021). In cities, 3D printing has optimized workflows and improved patient outcomes (Khorsandi et al., 2021). In contrast, in rural areas, it addresses challenges like long travel distances and financial burdens by allowing for on-site production of prosthetics and minimizing the need for distant laboratories (Al Hamad et al., 2022).

To better integrate 3D printing into the historical context of dentistry, it's essential to trace the evolution from early manual methods to digital techniques like CAD/CAM, and then into the rise of 3D printing as a transformative technology. Understanding the progression from traditional prosthetic fabrication to the advanced digital manufacturing processes available today can help highlight the significant impact 3D printing has had in revolutionizing dental care.

Traditional Dental Prosthetics: A Brief History

1. Early Beginnings (Pre-20th Century):
   - The origins of dental prosthetics date back to ancient civilizations, where rudimentary dentures were created from materials like ivory, wood, and gold. These prosthetics were often custom-made but lacked precision and durability.
   - In the 18th century, advancements included the creation of dentures using porcelain, which were more functional than their predecessors but still had limitations in terms of fit and comfort.
2. **20th Century: The Rise of Modern Techniques**:
   - **Early 1900s**: The invention of dental materials such as acrylic resins significantly improved the quality of dentures. At this point, manual techniques like wax modeling and the use of molds were common.
   - **1960s–1970s**: Introduction of more advanced materials, including metal alloys and ceramics, alongside improved techniques for creating crowns, bridges, and implants. However, many steps still involved manual labor and time-consuming processes.
3. **1980s–1990s: The Dawn of Digital Dentistry**:
   - **CAD/CAM (Computer-Aided Design/Computer-Aided Manufacturing)** technology began to emerge. The first CAD/CAM

system, introduced by Dr. François Duret in the 1980s, enabled dentists to design prosthetics digitally and manufacture them using milling machines. This was a significant step toward reducing manual labor and improving the precision of dental restorations.

- **Rapid Prototyping** techniques like stereolithography (SLA) also emerged in the 1990s, helping to create prototypes and custom dental parts more quickly.

The Introduction and Evolution of 3D Printing in Dentistry

1. **Early 2000s: The First Uses of 3D Printing**:
   - By the early 2000s, 3D printing began to gain traction in various fields, including dentistry. Initial applications were focused on creating prototypes, surgical guides, and custom implants.
   - **Stereolithography (SLA)** and **Fused Deposition Modeling (FDM)**, two prominent 3D printing techniques, were utilized to create more accurate dental prosthetics with reduced lead times compared to traditional methods.
2. **Mid 2000s – 2010s: Expanding Applications and Materials**:
   - As 3D printing technology advanced, it became capable of producing full dental restorations, including crowns, bridges, and dentures, using biocompatible materials. This revolutionized the customization of dental prosthetics and made the process more efficient.
   - The **introduction of dental-specific 3D printers** and materials, such as resins and metal powders, allowed for better integration with traditional prosthetic workflows, making it easier for dental professionals to offer customized treatments.
3. **2010s: 3D Printing and Personalized Dentistry**:
   - **Personalized dental care** became a major focus, with the ability to print prosthetics tailored to a patient's exact specifications. Digital impressions and scans combined with 3D printing created a seamless workflow, reducing human error and speeding up production times.
   - The development of more **biocompatible materials** for use in 3D printing further increased its role in permanent dental restorations, like crowns, bridges, and even orthodontic devices.
4. **2020s: Continued Innovation and Integration**:
   - By the 2020s, 3D printing in dentistry had become an integral part of the industry. Innovations included **3D-printed implants, orthodontic aligners**, and **surgical guides** tailored to the individual patient.

- o **AI and machine learning** began to complement 3D printing in creating more efficient workflows, predictive models, and enhanced prosthetics.

How 3D Printing Fits into the Broader Evolution of Dentistry

- **Enhancing Precision**: The primary advantage of 3D printing over traditional methods is its ability to create highly precise, custom prosthetics based on digital scans of the patient's mouth. This marks a shift from manual molding to a more digital, accurate process.
- **Faster Production Times**: 3D printing significantly reduces the time needed to create prosthetics. Traditional methods could take several weeks, while 3D printing may only require a few days, improving patient turnaround.
- **Customization and Personalization**: 3D printing allows for personalized dental prosthetics that match the exact contours of a patient's mouth, leading to more comfortable and functional restorations.
- **Cost-Effectiveness**: In some cases, 3D printing can be more affordable than traditional methods, especially when factoring in the reduction in time and labor.

This chapter explores how 3D printing is transforming rural dentistry by making high-quality dental care more accessible. With the capability to produce prosthetics on-site and create portable dental solutions, this technology is fostering innovation in underserved communities (Yang et al., 2022). The discussion will focus on its cost-effectiveness, accuracy, and positive effects on rural areas, while also considering challenges such as the need for training, material availability, and the importance of collaboration (Goguta et al., 2021). Through case studies and insights into future trends, this chapter illustrates how 3D printing can help close healthcare gaps in rural regions (Chen et al., 2022). As a technology that builds objects layer by layer from digital designs, 3D printing has rapidly gained traction across various industries, including healthcare. In medicine, it has enabled the creation of personalized treatments, from prosthetic limbs to bioprinted tissues (Wuershing et al., 2022). Its affordability and adaptability make it especially valuable in resource-limited settings (Lee et al., 2022). In dentistry, 3D printing is transforming the production of prosthetics, surgical guides, and educational models by enhancing efficiency, precision, and overall patient outcomes (Valenti et al., 2022).

The 3D printing process in dentistry begins with a digital design, which is typically created using intraoral scanners, cone-beam computed tomography (CBCT), or other imaging technologies that capture highly detailed representations of a patient's oral structures (Della Bona et al., 2021). These digital impressions eliminate the need for conventional molds, reducing discomfort for patients while ensuring greater precision in dental restorations. Once the scan is obtained, computer-aided design (CAD) software is used to refine and optimize the model, ensuring it meets the necessary functional and aesthetic requirements (Figure 1).

Figure 1. Preparing the virtual model using CAD software (author's own clinical case).

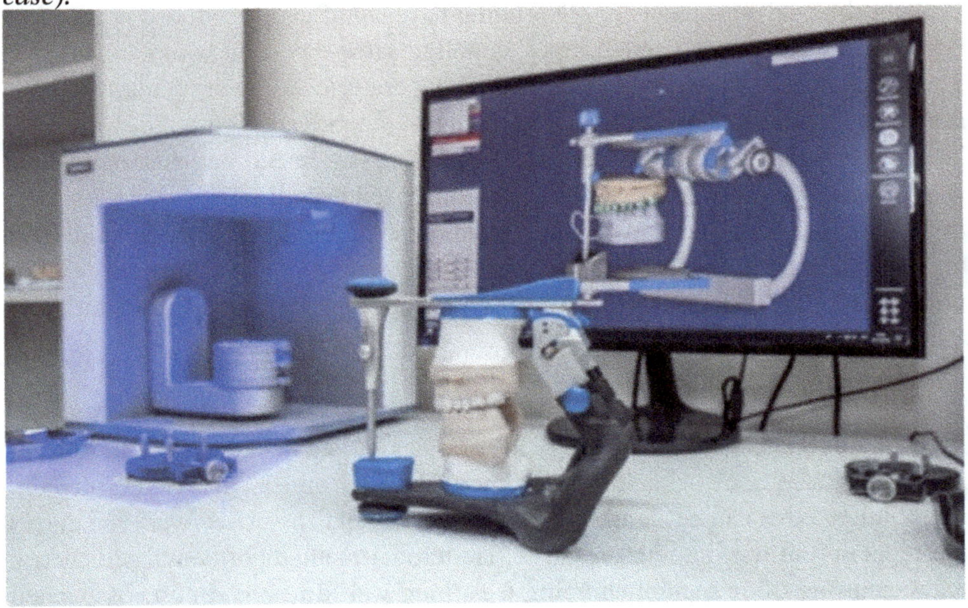

After finalizing the design, the model is converted into a format compatible with 3D printers, such as an STL (stereolithography) file. The digital model is then processed using slicing software, which divides it into ultra-thin horizontal layers, allowing the printer to build the object sequentially. Depending on the type of 3D printing technology used—such as stereolithography (SLA), digital light processing (DLP), fused deposition modeling (FDM), or selective laser sintering (SLS)—various materials, including dental resins, ceramics, polymers, and biocompatible metals, are utilized to create the final product (Goguta et al., 2021).

Once the object is printed, it undergoes essential post-processing steps to enhance its durability, functionality, and aesthetics. These steps may include washing, curing under ultraviolet (UV) light, polishing, and additional modifications such as staining or glazing to achieve a lifelike appearance. In cases involving metal-based restorations, sintering or heat treatment may be required to improve mechanical strength (Lee et al., 2022).

This approach to manufacturing allows for the creation of intricate, highly customized dental restorations that would be challenging or prohibitively expensive to produce using traditional methods (Muthu et al., 2021). Unlike conventional milling or casting techniques, which generate significant material waste, 3D printing is an additive process that builds structures layer by layer, minimizing excess material usage and contributing to more sustainable dental practices.

Over time, advancements in 3D printing have significantly reduced production costs and shortened turnaround times, enabling same-day or next-day treatments. This has decreased dependence on centralized laboratories, allowing dental clinics—especially in rural and resource-limited settings—to fabricate high-quality prosthetics and restorations on-site (Huang et al., 2022). As a result, patients experience shorter wait times, fewer dental visits, and improved overall satisfaction with their treatment outcomes. Additionally, the continuous evolution of printing materials and techniques is further enhancing the strength, biocompatibility, and longevity of 3D-printed dental products, paving the way for more efficient and accessible dental care.

- **Economic Feasibility of 3D Printing in Rural Dentistry**

Adopting 3D printing technology in rural dental practices involves an upfront investment in equipment such as 3D printers, digital scanners, and CAD software. These initial costs can be significant; however, they may be offset over time due to the reduction in outsourcing expenses. Traditional methods of dental prosthetics manufacturing often require shipping fees, long wait times, and costs associated with external laboratories, all of which can strain a rural practice. With 3D printing, dental professionals can produce crowns, dentures, bridges, and other prosthetics directly in their clinic, reducing reliance on third-party labs and cutting down the logistical challenges of rural dental care. Ongoing costs, including maintenance of the 3D printer and materials such as resins and filaments, must also be considered. While the materials for 3D printing may be more expensive than traditional dental materials, the overall long-term financial savings can be considerable. Faster turnaround times can lead to more efficient patient care, with higher patient throughput and fewer delays in treatment, contributing to improved practice revenue. Over time, these savings, combined with enhanced workflow efficiency, can make 3D printing a financially viable option for rural practices.

- **Legal and Regulatory Considerations**

One of the critical barriers to the widespread adoption of 3D printing in rural dentistry is the legal and regulatory landscape surrounding medical devices. Different countries and regions have stringent regulations governing the production and use of medical devices, including dental prosthetics. In many jurisdictions, dental prosthetics are classified as medical devices, which means they must adhere to rigorous standards for safety, quality, and efficacy. Regulatory bodies such as the FDA in the United States or the European Medicines Agency (EMA) in Europe enforce strict guidelines for the approval of medical devices, including those made through 3D printing technologies. These regulatory requirements can increase the complexity and cost of implementing 3D printing in rural dental practices. In some cases, specific certifications or quality control processes may be required for 3D-printed prosthetics before they can be legally used in patient care. These legal barriers could pose challenges for rural dental practices that have limited access to regulatory expertise or the resources necessary to navigate the approval process. Addressing these regulatory concerns and ensuring compliance will be key to ensuring that 3D printing technology can be safely and effectively integrated into rural dental care.

- **Training and Skill Development for Rural Dentists**

The successful integration of 3D printing technology into rural dental practices depends on the availability of comprehensive training and education programs for dental professionals. While 3D printing has the potential to revolutionize rural dentistry, it requires a skilled workforce capable of designing, operating, and maintaining 3D printers and using advanced digital tools like CAD software. The chapter should explore specific training programs or platforms designed to bridge the knowledge gap for rural dental professionals. These could include online courses, workshops, and continuing education programs offered by dental schools or professional organizations. Partnerships with universities or dental associations could be established to offer accessible training opportunities tailored to the needs of rural dentists. In addition to technical skills, training should also focus on the integration of 3D printing into everyday dental practices, helping professionals understand how the technology can improve patient care and practice efficiency.

- **Environmental Impact and Sustainability**

The environmental implications of using 3D printing in dentistry are an important consideration, particularly in rural settings with limited waste management infrastructure. One of the advantages of 3D printing over traditional dental manufacturing methods is its potential for material efficiency. Traditional prosthetic production processes often involve cutting away large amounts of material from a block to create the final product, generating significant waste. In contrast, 3D printing uses an additive process, where material is added layer by layer, minimizing waste. However, the materials used in 3D printing, such as resins, plastics, and metal powders, can still pose environmental challenges if not properly disposed of. It is important for rural dental practices to consider sustainable practices, such as recycling unused or excess materials, to reduce their environmental footprint. Additionally, adopting 3D printing could encourage more localized production of dental prosthetics, reducing the need for transportation and associated carbon emissions, which can be particularly beneficial in rural areas with long distances between practices and laboratories. By integrating sustainable practices and reducing material waste, 3D printing can offer both financial and environmental benefits to rural dental practices.

- **Integration with Remote Dental Services**

Integrating 3D printing with remote dental services presents a powerful solution for expanding access to high-quality dental care in rural areas. Tele-dentistry has gained momentum as a means of providing dental consultations and diagnostics remotely, but 3D printing takes this a step further by enabling the creation of custom dental prosthetics without requiring the patient to travel long distances. In rural settings, where access to dental care may be limited, 3D printing can be used to produce crowns, dentures, or orthodontic devices based on digital impressions sent remotely from a dentist's office. This technology enables virtual collaboration between dentists and dental labs or specialists in urban centers, improving the speed and efficiency of care. For rural patients, this could mean receiving a personalized dental prosthetic with minimal delay and without the need for multiple visits.

2. MAIN FOCUS OF THE CHAPTER

The main focus of this chapter is to explore the transformative role of 3D printing in rural dentistry. In many rural areas, dental practices face significant challenges, such as limited access to advanced equipment, long patient wait times, and difficulty obtaining custom dental prosthetics due to the geographical isolation of these communities. 3D printing offers a practical solution to these challenges by enabling the rapid production of high-quality, customized dental restorations, including crowns, bridges, dentures, and surgical guides, directly within the clinic. This technology can reduce dependency on external laboratories and specialists, improving both accessibility and cost-efficiency for patients. By providing a more precise, personalized approach to dental care, 3D printing enhances the speed and effectiveness of treatments, ultimately improving the quality of care in rural dental practices. The chapter highlights how this innovative technology is reshaping the future of dentistry in underserved areas, making essential dental services more accessible and affordable.

3. BACKGROUND

The advent of 3D printing has revolutionized modern dentistry by enhancing precision, improving patient care, reducing costs, and optimizing workflow efficiency. This cutting-edge technology has led to transformative changes across both urban and rural dental settings. In urban dentistry, practitioners benefit from its full capabilities, including advanced digital workflows, high-speed production, and innovative bioprinting applications. Meanwhile, rural regions stand to gain significantly through enhanced accessibility, affordability, and localized manufacturing of dental prosthetics. By narrowing the technological divide between these two settings, 3D printing plays a crucial role in creating a more inclusive and equitable oral healthcare system, ensuring that high-quality treatment is available to patients regardless of geographic location.

This chapter examines how 3D printing is redefining rural dentistry by enabling high-quality dental solutions in remote and underserved communities. With the ability to fabricate prosthetics on-site and support portable dental care initiatives, this technology is driving innovative advancements that address long-standing healthcare disparities (Yang et al., 2022). The discussion highlights key factors such as cost-effectiveness, precision, and overall benefits in rural regions, while also acknowledging challenges like the need for specialized training, material accessibility, and cross-sector collaboration (Goguta et al., 2021). Through real-world case studies and an exploration of future trends, this chapter showcases how 3D printing can help bridge critical healthcare gaps in rural areas (Chen et al., 2022).

Key Concepts of 3D Printing in Dentistry

3D printing, also known as additive manufacturing, is a revolutionary technique that constructs objects layer by layer from a digital model. This process has rapidly gained traction across multiple industries, particularly within the healthcare sector. In medicine, 3D printing has facilitated the development of personalized treatments, ranging from prosthetic limbs to bioprinted tissues (Wuershing et al., 2022). The affordability and adaptability of this technology make it especially valuable in resource-constrained environments (Lee et al., 2022).

In the field of dentistry, 3D printing has become an integral part of modern treatment planning and execution. The technology enables the fabrication of customized prosthetics, including crowns, bridges, dentures, and implants, with high levels of accuracy. It also facilitates the production of surgical guides and anatomical models used for educational and preoperative planning purposes (Valenti et al., 2022). The ability to generate complex designs with minimal waste makes 3D printing an efficient and sustainable alternative to conventional dental manufacturing methods.

The 3D printing workflow in dentistry typically begins with intraoral or extraoral digital scanning, which captures precise details of a patient's dental structures. This digital model is then processed through computer-aided design (CAD) software, where it is refined and optimized for printing. Once finalized, the design is sliced into layers and sent to a 3D printer, which constructs the object using various dental-compatible materials, such as resins, ceramics, or biocompatible polymers. Post-processing techniques, including curing and polishing, are applied to enhance strength, durability, and esthetic appeal (Chen et al., 2022).

Advancements in 3D printing have significantly lowered production costs and expedited treatment timelines, reducing reliance on centralized laboratories. As a result, patients can receive customized dental restorations in a matter of hours rather than weeks, leading to greater convenience and improved satisfaction (Vaz & Kumar, 2021). By integrating 3D printing into routine dental practice, clinics can streamline workflows, minimize material waste, and offer more affordable and accessible dental care.

Tele-Dentistry

Tele-dentistry leverages digital technology to provide remote dental care, consultations, and education, helping to bridge the gap in access to dental services, particularly in rural communities.

With an adoption rate of 40%, tele-dentistry is the most widely used digital dental service in rural areas.

This high percentage reflects its ability to overcome geographical barriers and provide accessible care where in-person visits may not be feasible.

Digital Imaging

Digital imaging involves advanced imaging technologies that capture highly detailed visuals, aiding in accurate diagnoses and treatment planning.

It holds the second-highest adoption rate at 30%, likely due to its ability to enhance diagnostic precision even in remote settings.

The integration of digital imaging improves treatment accuracy, reducing the need for repeated visits and ensuring better patient outcomes.

Mobile Health Apps

Mobile health applications provide essential dental education, appointment reminders, and basic consultations through smartphones and tablets.

These apps have a moderate adoption rate of 25%.

While they offer convenience, challenges such as digital literacy and limited smartphone access in rural areas may hinder their widespread use.

AI-Powered Diagnostics

AI-powered diagnostics utilize artificial intelligence to analyze dental data, including images and patient histories, to generate accurate diagnoses and predictive insights.

With an adoption rate of just 15%, it is the least utilized digital dental service in rural areas.

The lower percentage likely stems from factors such as higher costs, limited awareness, and insufficient infrastructure in remote regions.

Advancements in Digital Dentistry

Modern digital dentistry starts with intraoral scanners, which take accurate digital impressions of a patient's teeth and oral structures (Vaz & Kumar, 2021). These scans are then converted into 3D models that can be used with 3D printing technology. By using advanced materials like biocompatible resins, ceramics, and hybrid polymers, dental prosthetics can be created with exceptional precision and durability, often rivaling or surpassing the quality of traditional methods.

In addition to enhancing accuracy, 3D printing dramatically reduces production times while maintaining consistent, high-quality results. It also allows for the development of patient-specific solutions, making it easier to handle complex dental cases compared to conventional techniques. Dental professionals can utilize digital design software to refine prosthetic designs, optimizing both functionality and appearance to meet clinical and aesthetic standards (Zhu et al., 2016; Khorsandi et al., 2021).

Transforming Orthodontics

Orthodontics has also seen significant improvements with the incorporation of 3D printing. The production of clear aligners, retainers, and custom brackets has been transformed, offering more efficient and precise treatment options. Digital scans of a patient's teeth are turned into highly accurate 3D models, facilitating the creation of custom-fitted orthodontic appliances (Chu et al., 2020). This technology allows for quicker adjustments, shortening overall treatment time and enhancing patient comfort. By adopting these digital innovations, dentistry is becoming more accessible, efficient, and personalized, especially for patients in underserved rural areas.

Mass customization has become a reality, particularly for clear aligners. Previously, creating orthodontic devices involved physical molds, manual crafting, and lengthy production times. Now, with 3D printing, practitioners can design aligners tailored to each stage of tooth movement, increasing both efficiency and precision (Mallakpour et al., 2021). Furthermore, the digital workflow enables orthodontists to make real-time adjustments based on a patient's progress and print new aligners as necessary. This flexible approach enhances patient comfort, reduces the number of clinic visits, and speeds up treatment outcomes.

Enhancing Surgical Precision

In dental surgery, precision is crucial for achieving successful results. 3D-printed surgical guides, custom-made for each patient, have become essential tools for procedures like implant placement. These guides ensure accurate implant positioning, minimizing the risk of complications and improving long-term success rates (Arif et al., 2022; Lee et al., 2022). By integrating Cone Beam Computed Tomography (CBCT) with advanced planning software, dental professionals can generate detailed 3D images of a patient’s jaw. These high-resolution images allow for the design of surgical guides tailored to an individual’s anatomy, enabling even the most complex procedures to be performed with confidence and precision (Figure 2).

Figure 2. Implant's digital design.

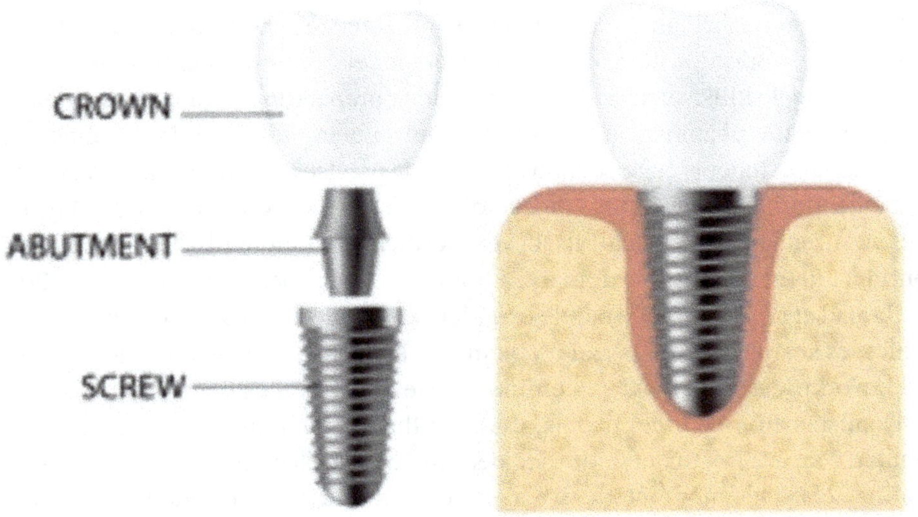

Beyond guides, 3D printing is revolutionizing implantology by facilitating the creation of custom implants and bone grafts. Patients with severe bone loss or structural irregularities benefit from implants designed specifically for their needs, leading to better integration, faster healing, and improved long-term outcomes (Wan et al., 2020).

Advancing Education and Diagnostics

3D printing has fundamentally transformed dental education and diagnostics by offering new ways to visualize, teach, and plan treatments. One of the most significant advancements is the ability to create highly detailed anatomical models of teeth, jaws, and other oral structures. These 3D-printed models are invaluable resources for treatment planning, patient education, and dental student training (Ashammakhi et al., 2018). Unlike traditional two-dimensional images or digital scans, physical models provide a three-dimensional perspective that enables a deeper understanding of the complex anatomy of the mouth. This tangible representation allows both dental professionals and students to explore oral structures from every angle, facilitating a more thorough comprehension of individual patient needs and the intricacies of various dental conditions.

For dental students, 3D-printed replicas offer a hands-on learning experience that is critical for bridging the gap between theoretical knowledge and real-world application. Working with realistic, physical models allows students to practice essential clinical skills, such as crown and bridge preparation, root canal treatments, and orthodontic planning, in a controlled and safe environment. By manipulating these models, students can better understand the precise anatomical details they will encounter during actual clinical procedures. This kind of experiential learning helps students to enhance their dexterity, develop critical thinking skills, and become more confident in their abilities before transitioning to live patients (Murphy et al., 2024; Al Hamad et al., 2022). The tactile experience provided by 3D-printed models also reinforces spatial awareness and problem-solving skills, both of which are essential when working in the complex, confined space of the oral cavity.

Dentists can rotate the models, examine them from multiple angles, and even simulate various treatment options to determine the best course of action (Abudula et al., 2022). This more interactive approach leads to more accurate, personalized treatment planning, as dentists can visualize the real-world application of different dental procedures in a way that traditional flat images cannot replicate.

In summary, 3D printing has revolutionized both dental education and diagnostics by providing highly detailed, three-dimensional models that enhance learning, diagnosis, and patient care. These models bridge the gap between theory and practice for dental students, offering them a hands-on learning experience that improves confidence and competence. In diagnostics, 3D-printed models offer a more precise and detailed understanding of oral conditions, helping dentists make more accurate treatment decisions. Furthermore, the use of physical models in patient education leads to better patient understanding, involvement, and trust in their treatment plans, which can contribute to improved outcomes.

The Role of 3D Printing in Rural Dentistry

While 3D printing is transforming dentistry around the globe, its effects are especially significant in rural areas. These regions often face challenges like limited access to specialized care, fewer resources, and financial constraints. 3D printing helps bridge these gaps by decentralizing production, lowering costs, and providing local clinics with advanced dental solutions.

Localized Manufacturing for Greater Accessibility

One of the primary benefits of 3D printing in rural dentistry is the ability to produce dental devices on-site. Instead of depending on distant laboratories, crowns, dentures, and aligners can be printed in-house within hours. This allows patients to receive their custom prosthetics on the same day, eliminating the need for multiple appointments and lengthy wait times (Li et al., 2016; Mallakpour et al., 2021).

In areas where dental specialists are scarce, general practitioners with 3D printing capabilities can offer a broader range of treatments. This helps to reduce geographic healthcare disparities, ensuring that more patients can access timely, high-quality care without needing to travel long distances.

By providing affordable, high-precision dental solutions directly to underserved areas, 3D printing is transforming access to oral healthcare, making it more efficient, inclusive, and centered around patient needs.

Enhancing Efficiency and Reducing Costs in Dental Prosthetics

Traditional dental prosthetic manufacturing involves multiple steps, specialized equipment, and substantial material waste. In contrast, 3D printing significantly reduces waste by utilizing only the required amount of material, which decreases costs and minimizes environmental impact. This efficiency makes advanced dental care more affordable, especially for economically disadvantaged populations in rural areas (Ramasamy et al., 2021).

Additionally, the lower production costs enable rural clinics to invest in state-of-the-art dental technology without significantly raising expenses for patients. As a result, high-quality dental care becomes more accessible and financially sustainable, leading to improved oral health outcomes in underserved communities.

Customization for Individual Patient Needs

Patients in rural areas often encounter unique oral health challenges due to factors such as diet, limited access to preventive care, and delays in treatment. 3D printing offers highly customized dental solutions, ensuring that each patient receives a prosthetic that fits comfortably and addresses their specific needs (Muthu et al., 2021). For instance, dentures and prosthetics can be tailored to accommodate patients with unusual oral structures, enhancing both comfort and functionality. By using advanced imaging and digital design tools, dental professionals can create personalized solutions that improve clinical effectiveness and aesthetic appeal.

Portability and Scalability: Expanding Access to Care

One of the most revolutionary aspects of 3D printing in dentistry is its portability. Compact and mobile 3D printers allow high-quality dental care to be brought directly to remote areas. Mobile dental units equipped with on-site 3D printing capabilities can deliver same-day prosthetics, crowns, and aligners, eliminating long wait times and reducing the need for patients to travel significant distances for treatment (Tappa et al., 2018; Vaz & Kumar, 2021).

This scalability is especially valuable for public health initiatives. Organizations focused on improving dental care in rural areas can deploy mobile clinics with 3D printing technology to efficiently meet the needs of multiple communities. As the cost of 3D printers continues to decrease, their adoption in rural dentistry is becoming increasingly feasible (Yang et al., 2022).

Transforming Rural Dentistry with On-Site Manufacturing

While 3D printing is revolutionizing dentistry globally, its impact on rural areas is particularly significant. These communities often face challenges such as limited access to specialized care, financial constraints, and shortages of trained professionals. By decentralizing production, lowering costs, and equipping local clinics with advanced technology, 3D printing offers practical solutions to these challenges (Jeong et al., 2023).

One of the key benefits of 3D printing is its ability to facilitate on-site production of dental devices. In rural clinics, this eliminates the need to send impressions to distant laboratories, which can lead to long waiting times. Instead, crowns, dentures, and aligners can be printed within hours, allowing patients to receive treatment the same day (Asanza et al., 2024).

By localizing production, rural clinics can make dental care more accessible, particularly for patients unable to travel long distances for treatment. Furthermore, in areas with a shortage of dental specialists, general practitioners equipped with 3D printers can fill the gap, offering a broader range of services and helping to reduce healthcare disparities (Gao et al., 2015).

Sustainability and Cost-Effectiveness in Dental Prosthetics

Traditional methods of producing dental prosthetics require multiple stages, specialized machinery, and a significant amount of raw material. 3D printing streamlines this process, utilizing only the required materials, thereby minimizing waste and lowering production costs. This cost-efficiency is particularly important for rural communities, where financial limitations often hinder access to advanced dental care (Kolesky et al., 2016).

The benefits extend beyond material savings. By reducing overall production costs, rural clinics can invest in 3D printing without burdening patients with high treatment expenses. This affordability enables clinics to deliver high-quality care at an accessible price point, significantly improving oral health outcomes in underserved regions.

Meeting the Unique Oral Health Needs of Rural Populations

Rural communities often experience distinct oral health issues due to dietary habits, lack of preventive care, and delayed treatment access. With 3D printing, dentists can develop customized treatment solutions that address these specific needs quickly and efficiently (Cui et al., 2020).

For example, patients with complex oral structures can receive dentures and prosthetics tailored for optimal comfort and function. The use of advanced imaging and digital modeling allows for the creation of precise, high-quality restorations that enhance both functionality and aesthetics.

Expanding Public Health Initiatives with 3D Printing

As 3D printing technology becomes more affordable, its integration into public health programs is increasingly viable. Mobile clinics equipped with 3D printers can effectively serve multiple rural communities, providing high-quality dental solutions in areas where traditional care might not be available (Liu et al., 2018).

Moreover, 3D printing is enhancing the field of implantology by facilitating the planning and production of surgical guides and prosthetic components for dental implants, which broadens treatment options in rural settings (Herschdorfer et al., 2020). The adoption of 3D printing in rural dentistry is transforming patient care through localized manufacturing, cost reduction, and the provision of customized treatment solutions. Its portability and scalability make it particularly beneficial for remote and underserved communities, ensuring that advanced dental care is both accessible and sustainable.

Modern intraoral scanning technology allows dental professionals to track changes in a patient's oral health over time. By comparing digital scans, they can identify issues such as wear, gum recession, or shifts in tooth positioning. This capability enables early intervention and personalized treatment adjustments, ultimately improving long-term patient outcomes.

The Future of Intraoral Scanning

As technology progresses, intraoral scanners are becoming more compact, faster, and increasingly affordable. The integration of artificial intelligence (AI) is enhancing their functionalities, allowing for the automatic detection of issues such as cavities, margin lines, and other critical dental features. Future developments will focus on improving accuracy, enabling cloud-based data management, and ensuring interoperability with other digital dentistry tools, solidifying the role of intraoral scanners as essential components of modern dental practices (Piedra Cascon et al., 2019).

CBCT (Cone Beam Computed Tomography): Advanced 3D Imaging

Cone Beam Computed Tomography (CBCT) represents an advanced imaging technique that provides detailed 3D images of a patient's dental structures, including bones and soft tissues. This technology enhances diagnostic capabilities, aiding in treatment planning for complex cases such as implants, extractions, and orthodontics. By offering high-resolution imaging, CBCT facilitates better decision-making and improved outcomes in dental care.For complex cases, such as dental implants or jaw surgeries, Cone Beam Computed Tomography (CBCT) generates detailed 3D images of the craniofacial anatomy. CBCT scans provide critical insights into bone density, nerve pathways, and other anatomical features, ensuring precise, safe, and functional treatment planning (Al Mortadi et al., 2015).

The process of 3D printing in dentistry involves several key steps. First, CAD software is used to refine digital impressions and create patient-specific designs, such as clear aligners, crowns, bridges, dentures, and virtual implants (Arifin et al., 2022; Osman et al., 2017). Next, the digital model is sliced into thin layers, and print settings such as layer thickness, speed, and material usage are adjusted to ensure precision and strength (de Andrade et al., 2019). Material selection is crucial for durability and biocompatibility, with options like photopolymer resins, metals (e.g., titanium), thermoplastics (e.g., PLA), and biocompatible materials tailored to specific dental applications (Ruschel et al., 2018; Teixeira et al., 2020). During 3D printing, techniques such as SLA, DLP, and SLS are used to fabricate the model layer by layer, offering high precision for detailed restorations and strong, durable objects (Sadowsky et al., 2021; Mosharraf et al., 2022). After printing, post-processing steps like curing, polishing, and sterilization ensure the final product meets quality and safety standards (Al-Qarni et al., 2022). Finally, quality assurance involves inspecting the printed object for accuracy and fit using advanced software tools and scanners, ensuring it meets the required specifications before use in clinical settings.

4. METHODOLOGY

This study examined the role of 3D printing in revolutionizing dental care in rural areas, highlighting its potential to enhance accessibility, reduce costs, and decentralize production. The methodology employed a comprehensive review of literature, case studies, and technical reports to examine the practical application of 3D printing in dentistry, particularly in underserved and rural settings. This systematic review was conducted following the PRISMA (Preferred Reporting Items for Systematic Reviews and Meta-Analyses) guidelines to ensure transparency, rigor, and reproducibility in the selection and analysis of sources. To support this objective, a literature search was conducted using major databases such as PubMed, Web of Science, and EMBASE (Figure 3).

Figure 3. PRISMA flow chart of the study's search strategy.

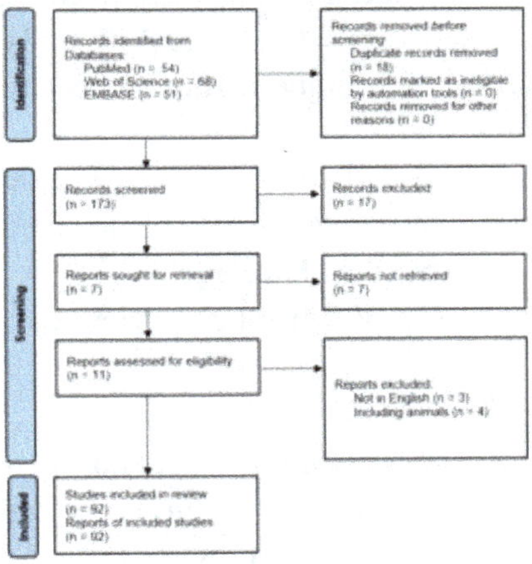

Inclusion Criteria:

From an initial pool of 173 articles, a total of 92 were selected for inclusion in the review based on the following criteria:

- Published in English;
- Dated between the years 2002 and 2025;
- Focused specifically on additive manufacturing methods, encompassing both clinical and laboratory (in vitro) studies in rural areas;

Offered valuable insights into fabrication techniques, clinical outcomes, or quality evaluations of 3D-printed dental restorations in rural areas.

Exclusion Criteria:

A total of 63 articles were excluded due to failure to meet the inclusion criteria or duplication of previously included content.

The selection process was carefully documented at each stage, ensuring transparency and reproducibility. The review focused on publications from January 1, 2002, to March 31, 2025, a period marked by a significant increase in the number of relevant clinical and in vitro studies. This systematic approach ensured that only high-quality, relevant literature was included in the final analysis.

Robustness Check

To ensure the rigor and reproducibility of this narrative review, a systematic and transparent selection process was employed, as illustrated in the PRISMA-style flow diagram.

A total of 173 studies were initially identified from three major databases—PubMed (n = 54), Web of Science (n = 68), and EMBASE (n = 51). Following the removal of 18 duplicate entries, 155 unique studies proceeded to the screening phase.

During screening:

- 6 articles were excluded based on irrelevance detected in the title,
- 5 were excluded after abstract evaluation,
- 7 articles were eliminated upon full-text review for not meeting inclusion criteria.

In addition, 7 articles were sought for retrieval, and 11 studies were assessed for eligibility, leading to the final inclusion of 92 studies in the review.

This comprehensive filtering process supports the robustness of the study in several ways:

- Multi-database sourcing reduced the likelihood of publication bias.
- Strict inclusion/exclusion criteria ensured thematic and methodological relevance.
- Documented rejections at every stage promote transparency and minimize selection bias.

The research was divided into the following components:

1. Data Collection

Survey Method: A survey was used to gather information on how digital dental services are being adopted in rural areas. It targeted dental professionals, healthcare providers, and rural residents who either use or are familiar with these services.

Target Population: The study focused on individuals and organizations in rural areas, including dental practitioners, local health clinics, and residents living in places with limited access to traditional dental care.

Types of Services: The survey looked at four key digital dental services:

Tele-Dentistry: This service enables remote consultations and evaluations, typically conducted via video calls or other digital platforms.

Digital Imaging: This involves using digital technology to capture dental images, like X-rays, for better diagnosis.

Mobile Health Apps: Apps that help individuals manage and track their dental health using their smartphones or tablets.

AI-Powered Diagnostics: Artificial intelligence tools that help analyze dental data and provide more accurate diagnoses.

Data Points: The survey measured the percentage of people or practices using each of these services, giving us a clear picture of adoption across rural areas.

2. Data Analysis

Descriptive Analysis: The data was summarized and displayed in a bar chart, showing the adoption rates for each digital dental service. The analysis provides a simple breakdown of how widely each service is being used in rural areas.

Visual Representation: The chart shows the percentage of adoption for each service. The vertical axis indicates the adoption rate (from 0% to 50%), and the horizontal axis lists the different types of services.

Key Findings:

Tele-Dentistry stands out as the most commonly adopted service, with 40% of respondents using it, likely due to its ability to overcome distance barriers.

Digital Imaging comes in second, with 30% adoption, showing it's a key tool for dental care.

Mobile Health Apps have a 25% adoption rate, still notable but lower than tele-dentistry and digital imaging.

AI-powered diagnostics had the lowest adoption rate at just 15%, possibly due to limited access or lower awareness of AI-based tools.

The data suggests that tele-dentistry is the most popular digital dental service in rural areas, likely because it makes dental care more accessible. Digital imaging and mobile health apps also have strong adoption rates, while AI-powered diagnostics have less traction, possibly due to limited availability or understanding of the technology.

3. **Case Studies Analysis**

Published reports from rural regions in India, Sub-Saharan Africa, and Southeast Asia were examined to evaluate the effectiveness and adaptability of 3D printing in producing custom dental devices. The study focused on key performance metrics, including:

- Treatment turnaround time
- Cost reduction
- Patient accessibility

Table 1 details the articles included in the review, highlighting those deemed highly relevant to the subject matter.

Table 1. Most esteemed articles included in our study.

Author's Name	Topic	Article Type	Year of Publication
Revilla-León, M.; et al.	Artificial intelligence models for fixed and removable prosthodontics	Systematic review	2023
Siqueira, R.; et al.	Intraoral scanning in fixed prosthodontics and implant dentistry	Systematic review	2021
Bernauer, S.A.; Zitzmann, N.U.; Joda, T.	Artificial intelligence in prosthodontics	Systematic review	2021
Ahmed, N.; et al.	Artificial intelligence techniques in dentistry	Systematic review	2021
Joda, T.; Zarone, F.; Ferrari, M.	The complete digital workflow in fixed prosthodontics	Systematic review	2017
Bernauer, S.A.; et al.	The complete digital workflow in fixed prosthodontics (updated)	Systematic review	2023
DeSimone, J.M.; et al.	Continuous Liquid Interphase Printing	US Patent	2015
Morsy, N.; El Kateb, M.	Intraoral scanners	Systematic review and meta-analysis	2022
Alghazzawi, T.F.	Advancements in CAD/CAM Technology	Literature review	2008
Joda, T.; Brägger, U.	Digital vs. conventional implant prosthetic workflows	Cost/time analysis	2015

Figure 4. Evaluation of Digital Dental Service Adoption in Rural Areas (based on the author's research data).

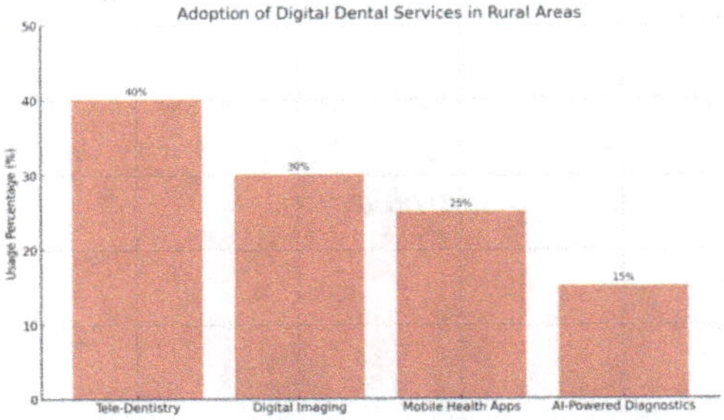

Figure 4 presents statistical insights into how digital dental services have been adopted in rural regions.

4. TECHNICAL EVALUATION

The study reviewed the layer-by-layer fabrication process, assessing the efficiency of Stereolithography (SLA), Digital Light Processing (DLP), and Fused Deposition Modeling (FDM) in creating accurate, durable, and cost-effective dental devices for rural settings. Each method was evaluated based on:

- Precision and durability of printed prosthetics
- Material efficiency and affordability
- Suitability for decentralized and mobile dental clinics

Addressing the Rural-Urban Disparity in Dental Care

Figure 5 highlights the significant shortage of dental specialists in rural areas compared to urban locations. This disparity limits access to specialized care, often leading to worse oral health outcomes in underserved communities.

To bridge this gap, potential strategies include:

- Tele-dentistry for remote diagnosis and treatment planning
- Incentives for dental specialists to work in rural settings
- Expansion of mobile dental services, integrating 3D printing for on-site prosthetic fabrication

By leveraging 3D printing technology, these initiatives can help ensure more equitable access to quality dental care, addressing the persistent healthcare challenges faced by rural populations.

Figure 5. Analysis of Dental Professional Availability Across Urban and Rural Regions (based on the author's research data).

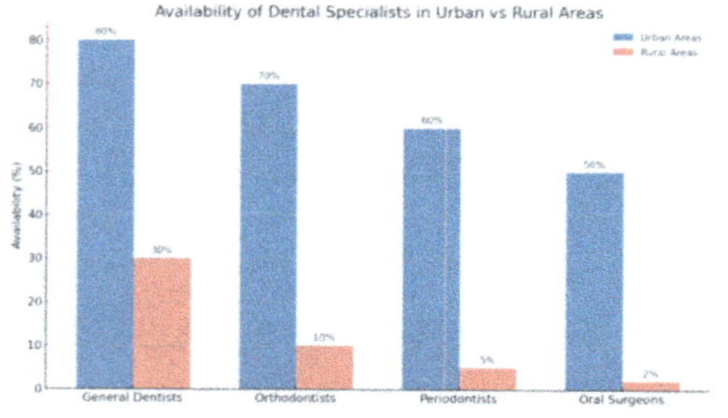

The figure clearly shows that urban areas have significantly more dental professionals available than rural areas, pointing to a disparity in access to dental care. This difference could be due to factors like population density, economic opportunities for practitioners, and the challenges of recruiting professionals to rural areas. The figure illustrates the gap in the availability of dental specialists between urban and rural areas, highlighting significant disparities across four key specializations:

1. General Dentists
    - Urban Areas: 80% availability
    - Rural Areas: 30% availability
    - Key Insight: General dental services are far more accessible in urban areas, leaving rural populations with limited options for routine and preventive care.
2. Orthodontists
    - Urban Areas: 70% availability
    - Rural Areas: 10% availability
    - Key Insight: The sharp contrast in orthodontist distribution highlights the scarcity of specialized orthodontic care in rural regions, leading to untreated misalignments and bite issues.
3. Periodontists
    - Urban Areas: 60% availability
    - Rural Areas: 5% availability

- Key Insight: While more balanced compared to other specialists, access to periodontal care remains significantly lower in rural areas, limiting treatment for gum disease and other oral health conditions.

4. Oral Surgeons
   - Urban Areas: 50% availability
   - Rural Areas: 2% availability
   - Key Insight: The stark difference in oral surgeon availability underscores the extreme lack of surgical dental services in rural areas, affecting patients who require extractions, implants, and other advanced procedures.

Economic and Infrastructure Feasibility

The economic feasibility of implementing 3D printing in rural dental clinics was evaluated through a comprehensive cost analysis. This included an examination of startup costs, such as the initial investment in 3D printers and associated training, as well as ongoing material expenses related to resins, metals, and thermoplastics. Additionally, production costs were analyzed to compare the efficiency and affordability of 3D printing versus traditional manufacturing methods.

In terms of infrastructure, the study assessed the specific challenges faced in low-resource environments. Critical factors included limited electricity access in remote areas, the need for reliable water supply and sanitation in dental laboratories, and the availability of technical expertise for maintaining and troubleshooting the equipment. To address these limitations, the study explored potential adaptations, including the use of solar-powered 3D printers and the deployment of mobile dental clinics, both of which could significantly enhance operational feasibility in rural contexts.

Survey of Training Needs

A review of existing training programs for rural dental professionals revealed significant knowledge gaps in digital dentistry and 3D printing technologies. The study evaluated the current levels of awareness and expertise among rural dental practitioners and investigated the feasibility of integrating 3D printing education into both undergraduate dental curricula and continuing professional development programs. Strategies were also considered to simplify and standardize the implementation of digital dental workflows in rural clinics, ensuring that new technologies could be adopted more uniformly and effectively.

Regulatory and Logistical Assessment

Several key barriers to the widespread adoption of 3D printing in rural dentistry were identified. One major concern was the limited availability of high-quality, biocompatible printing materials in remote regions. Regulatory compliance also posed a challenge, particularly with respect to meeting local health and safety standards for 3D-printed medical devices. Logistical difficulties, such as transporting and distributing 3D-printed dental products to geographically isolated areas, further complicated implementation efforts.

Data Synthesis

Data from the components as mentioned earlier were synthesized to identify best practices, challenges, and future opportunities for implementing 3D printing to enhance rural dental care. The findings provide insights into the role of 3D printing in decentralizing dental device production, addressing healthcare inequities, and improving oral health outcomes for underserved populations.

5. ISSUES, CONTROVERSIES, PROBLEMS

Challenges and Solutions in Implementing 3D Printing for Rural Dental Care

The integration of 3D printing in rural dental care has the potential to revolutionize accessibility, affordability, and efficiency. However, several barriers must be addressed before widespread adoption can be achieved. These challenges can be categorized into technological, economic, educational, ethical, and systemic issues (Fatima et al., 2021).

Technological Barriers

One of the key technological barriers is the limitation of available materials. High-quality dental devices require specialized biocompatible resins, metals, and thermoplastics, which are often either unavailable or prohibitively expensive in rural areas (Irfan et al., 2020; Bazli et al., 2020). Although cost-effective alternatives exist, they often lack the necessary durability and safety standards for clinical use. Equipment maintenance also poses a challenge, as 3D printers require regular calibration, repairs, and part replacements, necessitating technical expertise that is often scarce in rural regions (Haleem et al., 2020; Khan et al., 2021). Consequently, machine downtime can delay patient care due to the lack of immediate access to specialized repair services. Moreover, the infrastructure dependence of 3D printing systems further complicates implementation. These technologies rely on stable electricity, internet connectivity, and controlled environments (El-Mahdy et al., 2021; Arifin et al., 2022), all of which are unreliable or inconsistent in many rural regions.

Economic Barriers

Economic challenges also hinder the adoption of 3D printing in rural dentistry. The high initial costs associated with acquiring printers, software, and materials remain a significant barrier for clinics with limited funding (Bedarf et al., 2021). While cost-sharing models or government subsidies could alleviate this burden, recurring expenses continue to be problematic. Clinics must also manage ongoing costs such as material refills, maintenance, and software upgrades (Sumanasena et al., 2022), which may outweigh the long-term benefits, particularly for low-income communities. In addition, there is a growing inequity in accessibility. Urban dental institutions, with better infrastructure and funding, can adopt 3D printing more easily, while rural clinics lag behind. This technological divide risks exacerbating existing disparities in oral healthcare (Sun et al., 2022).

Educational and Training Barriers

The lack of training and awareness further inhibits the integration of 3D printing technologies in rural settings. Many rural dental professionals lack the necessary skills in CAD/CAM software, printer operation, and post-processing (Moelich et al., 2021). Resistance to change also plays a role, as some dentists and policymakers remain skeptical due to concerns over high costs, system complexity, and uncertain returns on investment. As a result, traditional dental techniques continue to dominate rural practices. Furthermore, limited awareness among dental professionals regarding the applications and benefits of 3D printing (Afshar et al., 2021) prevents widespread adoption. Addressing this gap through targeted workshops and awareness campaigns could significantly improve uptake.

Ethical Controversies

The ethical implications of 3D printing in rural dentistry are also significant. One concern is the potential compromise in patient safety due to cost-cutting measures, such as the use of substandard materials or accelerated production timelines (Sumanasena et al., 2022). Another issue involves the ownership of digital designs.

As custom dental devices rely on digital files, there are growing concerns around intellectual property rights, unauthorized use, and design security.

Systemic Barriers

Systemic challenges include sustainability concerns and fragmented implementation. Many of the materials used in 3D printing, such as resins and plastics, are non-biodegradable, posing serious waste management issues in rural areas (Australian Institute of Health and Welfare, 2021). Additionally, the uneven adoption of 3D printing technologies across rural regions results in inconsistencies in the availability and quality of dental care. While some communities benefit from localized production, others remain underserved.

Recommendations for Overcoming Challenges

To address these challenges, several recommendations are proposed. From a technological standpoint, there is a need to develop cost-effective, durable, and biocompatible materials suitable for rural use. The introduction of portable, solar-powered, or battery-operated 3D printers could also help reduce infrastructure dependence. Economically, governments and private stakeholders should provide subsidies, grants, or enter into public-private partnerships to reduce financial burdens. Cost-sharing models, where multiple clinics share 3D printing resources, could further ease implementation. Training and awareness should be prioritized through the establishment of regional training centers that offer hands-on workshops and certification programs. Awareness campaigns targeting rural healthcare providers and policymakers would also enhance engagement. In terms of policy and regulation, ethical guidelines are needed to ensure the safety and quality of 3D-printed dental devices.

Applications of 3D Printing in Dentistry

The integration of 3D printing technology into dentistry has revolutionized the field, offering a wide range of applications that improve accuracy, efficiency, and patient satisfaction. By leveraging the capabilities of additive manufacturing, dental professionals can create precise, cost-effective, and customized solutions tailored to individual patient needs. Below, the key applications of 3D printing in dentistry are expanded upon:

Table 2. Dental applications of 3D Printing (author's own research sources)

Application	Description	Benefits	Specific Examples
Prosthetics (Crowns, Bridges, Dentures)	3D printing is used to create custom crowns, bridges, and dentures directly at the point of care or in dental labs.	- Faster production times - Tailored fit - Reduced material waste - Lower costs	- Same-day restorations: Patients receive crowns or dentures in a single visit - SmileReach Program (India): Mobile dental units provide same-day dentures
Orthodontic Aligners	3D printing creates clear, custom aligners designed to straighten teeth.	- Precise fit - Faster treatment times - Enhanced comfort - Minimal adjustments required	- Invisalign: Custom aligners designed and printed using 3D technology for better treatment outcomes
Surgical Guides	Custom guides created with 3D printing for more accurate placement of implants and other surgical interventions.	- Improved accuracy - Reduced risk of complications - More efficient surgeries	- Implant surgeries: Guides help in precise placement of dental implants, minimizing risks and improving outcomes
Implants (Dental)	Customized dental implants are created using 3D printing to match the patient's anatomical needs.	- Better fit - Reduced surgery time - Increased success rates - Personalized treatment	- Titanium implants: 3D printing used to create patient-specific titanium dental implants
Temporary Restorations	Temporary crowns, bridges, or dentures can be 3D printed as a temporary solution while waiting for permanent prosthetics.	- Immediate restoration - Easy to customize - Quick production	- Temporary crowns: 3D printed as placeholders before final restoration
Dental Models for Diagnostics	3D printed models of patients' teeth and oral structures can be used for better diagnosis and treatment planning.	- Better visualization of patient anatomy - Helps in treatment planning - Can be shared with other specialists	- 3D printed anatomical models: Used to understand complex dental cases, improve diagnostics, and develop treatment strategies
Orthodontic Appliances	3D printing is used to create various orthodontic appliances, such as retainers, splints, and expanders.	- Custom fit - Enhanced comfort - Faster production - Reduced need for manual adjustments	- Nightguards and retainers: Printed based on 3D scans of the patient's teeth to provide a comfortable fit and faster delivery of the appliance
Bioprinting (Dental Tissues)	The development of 3D printed dental tissues, such as gums or even teeth, using biocompatible materials.	- Potential for tissue regeneration - Personalized treatment for severe oral health issues	- Bioprinted tissues: Experimental use of biocompatible materials for regenerating dental tissues (e.g., gums or pulp)

continued on following page

Table 2. Continued

Application	Description	Benefits	Specific Examples
Customized Abutments	3D printing is used to create customized abutments for dental implants, ensuring the implant fits precisely with the rest of the dental prosthetic.	- Improved fit - Reduces complications - Better aesthetic outcomes	- Custom abutments: Tailored to each patient's dental anatomy to ensure better integration of implants with crowns
Teeth Whitening Trays	Custom-fit teeth whitening trays are produced with 3D printing, ensuring a precise fit for the patient's dental structure.	- More comfortable - Improved treatment effectiveness - Faster production of custom trays	- Whitening trays: Custom-fit for patients who want personalized whitening solutions at home
Dentistry Education & Training	3D printed models are used for training dental students and professionals by providing realistic, hands-on practice.	- Realistic training - Reduces risk of errors in live procedures - Improves technical skills	- Dental schools: Using 3D printed tooth models to teach students about tooth anatomy, cavity preparation, and other dental procedures
Custom Dental Tools & Instruments	3D printing allows for the creation of custom dental tools or instruments needed for specific procedures.	- Tailored to specific needs - Cost-effective - Easier production of specialized tools	- Custom handpieces: Specially designed tools to accommodate unique patient needs, such as for difficult extractions or specific surgeries
Bridge & Retainer Designs	3D printing aids in the design and production of bridges and retainers with better accuracy, especially for complex cases or patients with unique dental needs.	- More accurate - Faster production times - Personalized fit	- 3D printed retainers: Custom-made to prevent teeth movement after orthodontic treatment
Maxillofacial Prosthetics	3D printing is used to produce custom prosthetics for patients who have suffered oral cancer or facial trauma.	- Precise fit - Better aesthetics - Enhanced comfort - Faster turnaround time	- Facial prosthetics: Used for reconstructing missing or damaged facial tissue after surgery
Personalized Mouthguards	Customized mouthguards for sports or medical purposes (e.g., for sleep apnea) can be 3D printed to fit an individual's unique oral anatomy.	- Custom fit - Improved comfort and protection - Faster delivery	- Sports mouthguards: Designed for comfort and better protection during sports, tailored for each athlete's teeth

This table summarizes how 3D printing is revolutionizing dentistry by providing faster, more affordable, and highly customized solutions for various dental applications. It emphasizes the significant benefits of speed, precision, cost reduction, and improved patient outcomes that come with adopting this technology.

1. Prosthetics

Crowns and Bridges: 3D printing ensures a precise fit using digital scans, cutting down the time needed for production and improving patient comfort (Figure 6).

Figure 6. 3D – Printed models.

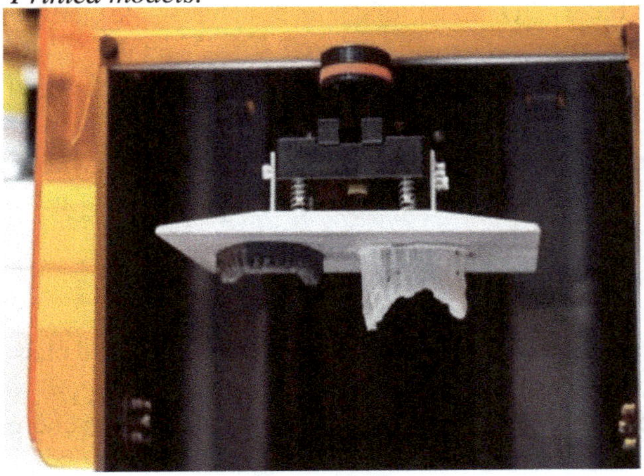

Removable Dentures: Custom-made dentures fit the patient's unique anatomy, speeding up the process and improving functionality.

Implant Components: Surgical precision is enhanced, and custom components are cost-effective, helping in the longevity and integration of dental implants.

2. Orthodontics

Clear Aligners: Digital customization results in a perfect fit and efficiency, with aligners printed in advance for faster treatment.

Retainers: Tailored retainers improve treatment outcomes by precisely matching the patient's dental contours.

Custom Brackets: Brackets are designed to fit each tooth individually, reducing discomfort and accelerating treatment progress.

3. Surgical Guides

Improved Accuracy: Surgical guides, based on CBCT scans, ensure precise implant placement, reducing risks and improving stability.

Time Efficiency: With minimal adjustments needed during surgery, procedures are faster, benefiting both the patient and the clinician.

Minimized Risks: By improving placement accuracy, the chances of surgical complications are significantly reduced.

4. Education and Diagnostics

Diagnostic Models: 3D models of dental structures help analyze complex cases and plan treatment approaches.

Patient Communication: Physical models improve patient understanding, setting realistic expectations, and enhancing confidence.

Training and Education: Dental students and specialists can practice and rehearse procedures on 3D-printed models, ensuring readiness for real-life scenarios.

5. Additional Applications

Restorative Models: 3D printing guides the preparation and placement of restorative treatments such as veneers, inlays, and onlays.

Occlusal Splints and Night Guards: Custom-made splints and guards alleviate bite issues like bruxism and TMJ disorders.

Orthognathic Surgery: Jaw surgeries benefit from accurate pre-surgical models, improving surgical planning.

Facial Prosthetics: Lifelike prosthetics for maxillofacial reconstruction restore both function and aesthetics.

Advantages of 3D Printing in Dentistry

Cost-Effectiveness: By reducing material waste and eliminating intermediaries, 3D printing lowers production costs, making dental treatments more affordable for patients.

Speed: The ability to produce dental devices and appliances in-house saves time compared to traditional off-site fabrication.

Customization: Personalization of dental products enhances comfort, fit, and outcomes, contributing to improved patient satisfaction.

The transformative nature of 3D printing in dentistry not only enhances the quality of care but also makes advanced treatments more accessible. The technology continues to grow, providing exciting opportunities for both practitioners and patients alike.Speed is another critical advantage of 3D printing. With the ability to produce dental devices in-house, clinics can accelerate turnaround times and, in many cases, provide same-day treatments. This rapid production process not only saves time for both patients and practitioners but also minimizes the logistical delays associated with traditional dental lab workflows.

Finally, the accessibility of 3D printing is revolutionizing dental care delivery, particularly in underserved areas. Portable and scalable 3D printing systems enable clinics to bring advanced treatments directly to remote or rural communities, bridging gaps in access and ensuring that patients receive high-quality care regardless of their location.

6. DISCUSSION

The integration of 3D printing into dentistry represents a significant milestone in the evolution of oral healthcare. Its capacity to produce highly accurate and customizable dental devices, lower costs, and enhance efficiency has transformed traditional practices. The discussion surrounding 3D printing becomes even more compelling when considering its implications for rural dentistry, where persistent challenges such as limited access to specialized care, inadequate infrastructure, and scarce resources pose significant barriers.

Public Health and Policy Trends

The adoption of 3D printing in dentistry must be examined within the broader framework of public health policies and government regulations. In many countries, the integration of new medical technologies into public health systems is influenced by regulatory bodies that oversee medical device approval, reimbursement policies, and healthcare infrastructure investments (Farah et al., 2016). Governments and international organizations can play a crucial role in subsidizing 3D printing initiatives, particularly in rural areas where economic constraints hinder technology adoption. Policy interventions should focus on training programs, funding models for clinics, and quality control measures to ensure safe and effective implementation of 3D-printed dental prosthetics.

Digital Trends and AI in 3D Printing

The role of artificial intelligence (AI) in digital dentistry is becoming increasingly significant, with applications in diagnosis, treatment planning, and automated design of dental prosthetics (Sun et al., 2022). AI-enhanced software can optimize the efficiency and accuracy of 3D-printed models, reducing manual errors and improving patient outcomes. Machine learning algorithms can also analyze patient data to predict treatment needs, enabling more personalized dental care in both urban and rural settings.

Another emerging trend is the integration of 3D printing with tele-dentistry services. Digital impressions from remote locations can be sent to centralized facilities where AI-powered design software refines the model before printing (Sumanasena et al., 2022). This approach reduces logistical challenges and ensures that even patients in isolated areas can access high-quality dental prosthetics. Future studies should explore how AI-driven automation can further streamline 3D printing workflows and improve accessibility.

Sustainability and Environmental Trends

As 3D printing gains traction in dentistry, sustainability concerns must be addressed. While additive manufacturing reduces material waste compared to traditional subtractive techniques, the environmental impact of resin-based printing materials and disposable components remains a challenge (Revilla-León & Özcan, 2017). The development of biodegradable and recyclable printing materials could mitigate some of these concerns and enhance the sustainability of 3D printing in healthcare settings.

In rural areas, where waste management infrastructure is often limited, strategies for responsible disposal and recycling of used materials must be considered (Prpić et al., 2020). Clinics should be encouraged to adopt eco-friendly materials and energy-efficient printing technologies. Additionally, research into sustainable production methods and lifecycle assessments of 3D-printed dental prosthetics could guide future innovations.

Patient Education and Literacy

An often overlooked aspect of 3D printing in dentistry is its potential to enhance patient education and literacy. By producing tangible 3D models of dental conditions and treatment plans, dentists can improve patient understanding and engagement (Al Jabbari et al., 2014). This is particularly valuable in rural areas, where health literacy levels may be lower, and patients may have limited exposure to advanced dental procedures.

Educational initiatives should incorporate interactive tools, such as virtual simulations and printed models, to help patients visualize their treatment options. Additionally, incorporating 3D printing into dental education curricula can equip future professionals with the skills needed to effectively communicate with and treat diverse patient populations (Tahayeri et al., 2018). Strengthening patient education efforts will not only improve treatment adherence but also foster greater acceptance of new dental technologies in rural communities.

7. SOLUTIONS AND RECOMMENDATIONS

Technological Solutions for 3D Printing in Rural Dentistry

One of the critical areas for technological advancement in rural dentistry is the development of affordable materials and equipment. Emphasis should be placed on creating cost-effective, biocompatible dental materials suitable for use in resource-constrained rural clinics. Manufacturers are encouraged to design portable and durable 3D printers optimized for low-resource environments. Open-source designs for both printers and materials could significantly reduce production costs and make these technologies more accessible, allowing for local customization and reducing dependency on proprietary equipment (Hegedus et al., 2022).

Equally important is the simplification of 3D printing systems. The design of user-friendly, intuitive machines that require minimal technical expertise would greatly benefit rural practitioners. These systems should be robust enough to withstand challenges such as fluctuating power supplies and harsh environmental conditions. Features like simplified interfaces and built-in troubleshooting guides can enhance usability for individuals with limited technical backgrounds (Vasamsetty et al., 2020).

In many rural regions, integrating renewable energy sources into 3D printing operations is essential. Solar-powered 3D printers, for instance, can provide a sustainable and consistent power supply, enabling uninterrupted services even in areas with frequent electricity outages (Daher et al., 2024).

Economic Strategies for Implementing 3D Printing in Rural Dentistry

To make 3D printing feasible in rural contexts, economic strategies must support its implementation. Public-private partnerships (PPPs) can play a pivotal role by providing subsidies, funding research and training, and facilitating local deployment of 3D printing technologies. Initiatives such as India's "Make in India" program exemplify how localized production can improve affordability and accessibility (Luu et al., 2024).

Another viable model involves the establishment of centralized 3D printing hubs that serve multiple rural clinics. This shared service approach allows clinics to pool resources, minimizing individual investments. For example, a regional health center could produce prosthetics and dental devices for neighboring communities, thereby streamlining logistics and costs (Palantza et al., 2024).

Micro-financing options, including low-interest loans or leasing plans, are also essential. Such financial mechanisms, supported by banks or microfinance institutions, can help clinics overcome initial capital barriers and adopt 3D printing technologies more easily.

Regulatory and Logistical Recommendations

Streamlining regulatory processes is essential for facilitating the adoption of 3D printing in rural dental care. Governments should develop simplified approval procedures for 3D-printed dental devices, particularly for rural applications. Regulatory bodies could adopt a "sandbox" model that enables the testing and fast-tracked approval of innovative products in controlled environments (Prakash et al., 2024).

Enhancing local supply chains is another priority. Establishing regional hubs for the production and distribution of 3D printing materials and spare parts can reduce reliance on imports and ensure a steady supply. Partnering with local manufacturers would further reinforce this effort.

In addition, setting global and regional standards for 3D-printed dental devices is crucial. These standards, potentially led by international bodies such as the International Organization for Standardization (ISO), would ensure safety, quality, and consistency across different regions.

Educational and Training Programs

Capacity building through targeted training programs is vital. These programs should cover essential skills, including CAD/CAM design, printer operation, and post-processing techniques. Short-term certification courses offered by universities and technical institutes could be tailored specifically to rural dental professionals (Aktas et al., 2024).

To support continuous learning and innovation, online platforms should be developed for knowledge sharing. These platforms can host open-source digital designs for dental devices, which rural practitioners can adapt to meet local needs. Platforms such as GitHub or dental-specific repositories could serve this purpose effectively.

Additionally, organizing hands-on workshops and outreach programs in rural communities can foster familiarity and confidence in using 3D printing technologies. Such initiatives allow practitioners to directly engage with the technology, thereby facilitating wider adoption (Arefin et al., 2021).

Ethical and Environmental Considerations

Ethical practices must guide the deployment of 3D printing in rural dentistry. Guidelines concerning intellectual property (IP) rights are necessary to protect the creators of digital designs while allowing rural practitioners to access and customize those resources. A fair licensing framework can help balance innovation with equitable access (Iftekar et al., 2023).

From an environmental standpoint, the use of biodegradable and recyclable materials should be prioritized. Local initiatives could also establish recycling and waste management programs to mitigate the environmental impact of 3D printing activities. Collaborating with environmental organizations will be key in developing sustainable systems (Mora et al., 2022).

Broader Systemic Recommendations

For long-term sustainability, 3D printing must be integrated into national health policies. Governments should formally recognize the role of this technology in reducing disparities in rural dental care. National health campaigns could emphasize the use of 3D printing to improve the availability and quality of dental treatments in underserved regions.

Incentives for innovation, such as grants, tax breaks, or awards, should be offered to encourage the development of 3D printing solutions tailored to rural healthcare. Innovation challenges could further stimulate creative approaches to making these technologies more accessible.

Finally, collaboration with NGOs and international organizations, including the World Health Organization (WHO), can help deploy 3D printing in rural areas globally. Joint projects can provide the necessary infrastructure, training, and support to bring this transformative technology to scale (Araujo et al., 2024).

Future Directions in 3D Printing for Rural Dentistry

Looking ahead, integrating artificial intelligence (AI) into 3D printing systems presents significant opportunities. AI can automate the design process, tailoring dental devices to individual patients and reducing the technical burden on rural practitioners. These intelligent systems can ensure high-quality outputs with minimal manual input (Kirby et al., 2024).

Additionally, combining 3D printing with telehealth platforms enables remote collaboration between rural clinics and urban dental specialists. In this model, specialists can design dental devices remotely and transmit the files to rural clinics for on-site printing, ensuring timely and expert-supported care (Caussin et al., 2024).

8. LIMITATIONS AND FUTURE RESEARCH

While this study provides valuable insights into the role of 3D printing in addressing the challenges of rural dentistry, several limitations should be acknowledged.

1. **Systematic Review Methodology:** This study is based on a systematic review of existing literature, which inherently limits the scope of data to the information available in published research. As such, any emerging technologies or advancements in the field that have not yet been documented may not be included in the findings. Moreover, the analysis relies on secondary data, which might not fully capture the complexities or nuances of real-world applications.
2. **Bias by Researchers:** As a systematic review without primary data collection, there is a potential for researcher bias. The selection of studies, data interpretation, and conclusions may reflect the researchers' perspectives or preferences, even when conducted with rigorous methodology. This bias may influence the overall findings and limit the generalizability of the conclusions drawn from this study.
3. **Lack of Respondent Input:** This study does not include input from practitioners, patients, or other stakeholders who may directly interact with or benefit from 3D printing technology in rural dentistry. The lack of firsthand experience or feedback from these groups means that certain practical challenges or benefits may not be fully understood.
4. **Financial Feasibility:** The financial feasibility of implementing mobile dental units with 3D printing technology in rural areas depends on several factors, including the initial cost of the equipment, maintenance expenses, and the ability to sustain operations long-term. While the upfront investment in portable 3D printers and the mobile units themselves can be substantial, the potential for cost savings in the long run is significant. Traditional dental treatments often require patients to travel long distances to urban clinics, which can be costly for both patients and the healthcare system.

5. **Regulatory Barriers:** The introduction of mobile dental units equipped with 3D printing technology will face several regulatory challenges. In many countries, medical devices, including dental materials and equipment, are subject to strict regulations to ensure their safety and effectiveness. These regulations can vary by region, making it necessary to navigate different legal frameworks when deploying 3D printing in rural areas.
6. **Infrastructure Limitations:** Infrastructure limitations are a significant challenge when implementing mobile dental units with 3D printers in rural areas. Many remote regions lack the basic infrastructure necessary for modern healthcare delivery, including reliable electricity, internet connectivity, and adequate roads for transportation. While mobile dental units powered by renewable energy sources like solar panels can help address the electricity challenges, logistical issues, such as transporting equipment to difficult-to-reach locations, must also be considered. Poor road conditions, lack of access to clean water, and inadequate waste disposal systems can make it difficult to maintain the hygiene standards required for dental procedures.
7. **Workforce Training Needs:** To maximize the effectiveness of mobile dental units, there is a critical need for comprehensive workforce training in rural areas. Dental professionals, including dentists, dental hygienists, and dental technicians, will need specialized training to operate 3D printing technology effectively. Although 3D printing can enhance dental procedures, it requires a different set of skills compared to traditional methods.

8. RECOMMENDATIONS FOR FUTURE STUDIES

1. **Incorporation of Primary Data:** Future research should include primary data collection through surveys, interviews, or questionnaires with dental practitioners, patients, and healthcare providers in rural areas. This would provide a more comprehensive understanding of the real-world challenges and successes associated with 3D printing in rural dentistry. Gathering qualitative data from respondents would offer valuable insights into user experiences, satisfaction, and practical barriers to implementation.
2. **Broader Scope of Studies:** Further studies should aim to include diverse rural settings across different geographical regions. Comparative studies can be conducted to evaluate the applicability of 3D printing in various economic, cultural, and infrastructural contexts, helping to identify region-specific challenges and solutions.

3. **Long-Term Impact Studies:** Longitudinal studies that assess the long-term impact of 3D printing adoption in rural dental practices should be conducted. These studies could measure improvements in patient outcomes, cost reductions, and the sustainability of 3D printing technologies over time.
4. **Focus on Education and Training:** Additional research is needed to evaluate the effectiveness of training programs, especially in resource-limited areas, to ensure that dental professionals can confidently operate 3D printing equipment. Investigating the potential for virtual training programs, mobile workshops, and other scalable educational initiatives can help bridge the skills gap in rural settings.

Development of Cost-Effective Solutions

To ensure that 3D printing technology becomes a viable option for rural dentistry, research efforts must focus on making dental-grade 3D printers and materials more affordable and accessible. This would enable rural clinics to adopt advanced dental technologies without being hindered by prohibitive costs. The priority should be the development of low-cost 3D printers capable of meeting the strict precision and durability requirements specific to dental applications. These printers need to be designed in a way that allows for accurate production of dental prosthetics, aligners, crowns, and other restorations, ensuring that the quality of care is not compromised. This could involve the use of more affordable manufacturing processes, local production models, and open-source technology that could drive down costs while still maintaining high standards for dental work.

Creation of Mobile 3D Printing Units

Mobile dental units equipped with lightweight, portable 3D printers present a transformative solution for overcoming the geographical and logistical barriers that often limit access to dental care in rural and remote areas. These mobile units can bring advanced dental technology directly to underserved communities, helping to bridge the gap where traditional dental clinics are few and far between. Research should focus on the design and engineering of 3D printers that are not only compact and portable but also energy-efficient, capable of functioning optimally with minimal power consumption.

To make these mobile units truly viable in rural environments, the 3D printers should be engineered for ease of transport and setup, ensuring they can be deployed quickly and efficiently. This includes making them lightweight without compromising on the accuracy and durability required for dental procedures. By focusing on developing energy-efficient printers, they can operate without placing heavy demands on the power sources available in these areas, which often struggle with unreliable electricity or limited access to grids.

Enhanced Training for Rural Practitioners

A significant barrier to adopting 3D printing technology in rural areas is the lack of skilled practitioners who are proficient in utilizing this advanced technology. As 3D printing continues to revolutionize dental care, it becomes increasingly important to ensure that dental professionals in rural settings are equipped with the necessary skills to operate and incorporate these tools into their practices effectively. Traditional dental education often lacks a strong emphasis on emerging technologies like 3D printing, and rural clinics may have fewer opportunities to access advanced training programs. Therefore, research should focus on developing and testing effective methods for training rural dentists and their staff in these technologies to make the process more accessible, cost-effective, and tailored to the unique needs of rural communities.

Infrastructure Solutions for Remote Areas

In regions where reliable internet and power infrastructure are lacking, research should focus on self-contained 3D printing systems that operate offline and feature backup power solutions. These systems would allow rural clinics to function independently from unreliable infrastructure, ensuring continuous service delivery despite power outages or poor internet connectivity.

Adapting Materials to Local Conditions

Research into the development of materials resistant to environmental challenges, such as temperature fluctuations, high humidity, and storage limitations, is essential. Developing durable materials for 3D-printed dental devices will ensure they remain stable and functional in rural clinics, improving the reliability of care in these regions.

Scaling Public Health Initiatives

Future research should also explore innovative ways to integrate 3D printing technology into public health campaigns aimed at improving oral health in underserved communities, particularly in rural and remote areas. Traditional public health efforts often focus on education, prevention, and basic care, but the inclusion of advanced technologies like 3D printing could significantly enhance these initiatives by making dental care more accessible and effective. Research should investigate how mobile 3D printing units or equipping local health centers with 3D printing technology could be used as part of broader public health strategies. This could involve exploring ways to provide essential dental treatments, such as custom-made dentures, crowns, and bridges, directly within underserved communities, reducing the need for patients to travel long distances to receive care.

The development of mobile 3D printing units could be particularly impactful for reaching remote areas where access to healthcare facilities is limited. These units could be designed to travel to various communities, bringing dental care to those who otherwise might not receive it. By outfitting these mobile units with state-of-the-art 3D printers, dental professionals could rapidly create customized dental prosthetics or other devices on-site, providing immediate relief to individuals in need.

Improving Patient Engagement and Trust

In rural populations, where advanced technology may be unfamiliar, research should focus on methods to effectively communicate the benefits of 3D-printed dental devices. Increasing patient trust and understanding is crucial for the successful adoption of these technologies. Using tangible 3D-printed models to explain procedures could significantly enhance patient education, fostering greater acceptance of new dental treatments.

9. CONCLUSION

3D printing holds significant potential for addressing the systemic challenges faced by rural dentistry, especially when analyzed through the lens of the Technology Acceptance Model (TAM) and digital intelligence frameworks. Case studies from regions such as India, Sub-Saharan Africa, and Southeast Asia demonstrate its transformative capacity to enhance localized, affordable, and efficient dental care in underserved communities.

According to TAM, the perceived usefulness and ease of use of 3D printing technology directly influence its acceptance among rural dental practitioners. The ability to overcome barriers such as long wait times, high costs, and logistical challenges positions 3D printing as a highly beneficial innovation. However, its perceived ease of use may be hindered by obstacles like high initial investment costs, regulatory complexities, and the need for specialized training. Addressing these barriers is crucial for broader adoption. Strategic approaches, including targeted training programs, public-private partnerships, and advancements in materials science, are essential for facilitating the acceptance and sustained use of 3D printing technology. Integrating artificial intelligence (AI) into the design process can further streamline operations by automating complex tasks, reducing human error, and improving efficiency. This convergence of AI with human intelligence enhances decision-making and optimizes patient outcomes, embodying the principles of digital intelligence.

Moreover, incorporating renewable energy solutions for off-grid operations and promoting sustainable practices for material recycling will ensure the technology's accessibility and environmental responsibility. These innovations align with the growing need for sustainable healthcare solutions in resource-limited rural settings. As 3D printing technology continues to evolve, collaborations among governments, private sectors, and non-governmental organizations (NGOs) will be instrumental in fostering widespread adoption. Such partnerships can facilitate knowledge sharing, provide financial support, and promote infrastructure development, enabling rural communities to benefit from advanced dental technologies.

In conclusion, by aligning 3D printing advancements with the variables of the TAM model and integrating digital intelligence, the global dental community can significantly advance toward universal access to quality dental care. Embracing these innovations will help bridge the gap between rural and urban dental services, ensuring equitable oral healthcare access regardless of geographical constraints.

ACKNOWLEDGMENT

This research received no specific grant from any funding agency in the public, commercial, or not-for-profit sectors.

REFERENCES

Afshar, A., & Mihut, D. (2020). Enhancing durability of 3D printed polymer structures by metallization. *Journal of Materials Science and Technology*, *53*, 185–191. DOI: 10.1016/j.jmst.2020.01.072

Al Hamad, K. Q., Al-Rashdan, B. A., Ayyad, J. Q., Al Omrani, L. M., Sharoh, A. M., Al Nimri, A. M., & Al-Kaff, F. T. (2022). Additive manufacturing of dental ceramics: A systematic review and meta-analysis. *Journal of Prosthodontics*, *31*(8), e67–e86. DOI: 10.1111/jopr.13553 PMID: 35675133

Al Mortadi, N., Jones, Q., Eggbeer, D., Lewis, J., & Williams, R. J. (2015). Fabrication of a resin appliance with alloy components using digital technology without an analog impression. *American Journal of Orthodontics and Dentofacial Orthopedics*, *148*(6), 862–867. DOI: 10.1016/j.ajodo.2015.06.014 PMID: 26522047

Al-Qarni, F. D. (2022). Customized post and cores fabricated with CAD/CAM technology: A literature review. *International Journal of General Medicine*, *15*, 4771–4779. DOI: 10.2147/IJGM.S365296 PMID: 35571288

Asanza, D. M. (2025). Emerging trends and future perspectives in digital dentistry for rural areas: An update. In Martínez Asanza, D. (Ed.), *Transforming dental health in rural communities: Digital dentistry* (pp. 1–20). IGI Global Scientific Publishing., DOI: 10.4018/979-8-3693-7165-7.ch001

Australian Institute of Health and Welfare. (2021). *Rural & Remote Health.* Retrieved from https://www.aihw.gov.au/reports/rural-remote-australians/rural-remote-health/contents/health-status-and-outcomes

Bedarf, P., Dutto, A., Zanini, M., & Dillenburger, B. (2021). Foam 3D printing for construction: A review of applications, materials, and processes. *Automation in Construction*, *130*, 103861. DOI: 10.1016/j.autcon.2021.103861

Campbell, S. D., Cooper, L., Craddock, H., Hyde, T. P., Nattress, B., Pavitt, S. H., & Seymour, D. W. (2017). Removable partial dentures: The clinical need for innovation. *The Journal of Prosthetic Dentistry*, *118*(3), 273–280. DOI: 10.1016/j.prosdent.2017.01.008 PMID: 28343666

Caviezel, C., Grünwald, R., Ehrenberg-Silies, S., Kind, S., Jetzke, T., & Bovenschulte, M. (2017). *Additive Fertigungsverfahren (3D-Druck)—Innovationsanalyse*. Berlin, Germany: TAB Arbeitsbereicht. Retrieved May 22, 2024, from https://www.google.com/scholar

Chen, J., Zhao, L., & Zhou, K. (2022). Multi-jet fusion 3D voxel printing of conductive elastomers. *Advanced Materials, 34*(47), e2205909. DOI: 10.1002/adma.202205909 PMID: 36125341

Chu, H., Yang, W., Sun, L., Cai, S., Yang, R., Liang, W., Yu, H., & Liu, L. (2020). 4D printing: A review on recent progresses. *Micromachines, 11*(796), 1–15. DOI: 10.3390/mi11090796 PMID: 32842588

Daher, R., Ardu, S., di Bella, E., Krejci, I., & Duc, O. (2024). Efficiency of 3D printed composite resin restorations compared with subtractive materials: Evaluation of fatigue behavior, cost, and time of production. *The Journal of Prosthetic Dentistry, 131*(5), 943–950. DOI: 10.1016/j.prosdent.2022.08.001 PMID: 36333176

Daher, R., Krejci, I., & Ardu, S. (2024). Time-and cost-effective 3-dimensional-printing workflow to rehabilitate worn dentitions: A clinical report. *The Journal of Prosthetic Dentistry, 131*(6), 996–999. DOI: 10.1016/j.prosdent.2023.02.013 PMID: 36959005

Daher, R., Krejci, I., & Ardu, S. (2024). Time-and cost-effective 3-dimensional-printing workflow to rehabilitate worn dentitions: A clinical report. *The Journal of Prosthetic Dentistry, 131*(6), 996–999. DOI: 10.1016/j.prosdent.2023.02.013 PMID: 36959005

Dawood, A., Marti, B., Sauret Jackson, V., & Darwood, A. (2015). 3D printing in dentistry. *British Dental Journal, 219*(11), 521–529. DOI: 10.1038/sj.bdj.2015.914 PMID: 26657435

Della Bona, A., Cantelli, V., Britto, V. T., Collares, K. F., & Stansbury, J. W. (2021). 3D printing restorative materials using a stereolithographic technique: A systematic review. *Dental Materials, 37*(2), 336–350. DOI: 10.1016/j.dental.2020.11.030 PMID: 33353734

Farah, S., Anderson, D. G., & Langer, R. (2016). Physical and mechanical properties of PLA, and their functions in widespread applications—A comprehensive review. *Advanced Drug Delivery Reviews, 107*, 367–392. DOI: 10.1016/j.addr.2016.06.012 PMID: 27356150

Fatima, S., Haleem, A., Bahl, S., Javaid, M., Mahla, S. K., & Singh, S. (2021). Exploring the significant applications of internet of things (IoT) with 3D printing using advanced materials in medical field. *Materials Today: Proceedings*, *45*(6), 4844–4851. DOI: 10.1016/j.matpr.2021.01.305

Galante, R., Figueiredo-Pina, C. G., & Serro, A. P. (2019). Additive manufacturing of ceramics for dental applications: A review. *Dental Materials*, *35*(6), 825–846. DOI: 10.1016/j.dental.2019.02.026 PMID: 30948230

Garcia, P. P., Wambier, L. M., de Geus, J. L., da Cunha, L. F., Correr, G. M., & Gonzaga, C. C. (2019). Do anterior and posterior teeth treated with post-and-core restorations have similar failure rates? A systematic review and meta-analysis. *The Journal of Prosthetic Dentistry*, *121*(6), 887–894.e4. DOI: 10.1016/j.prosdent.2018.08.004 PMID: 30617032

Goguta, L., Lungeanu, D., Negru, R., Birdeanu, M., Jivanescu, A., & Sinescu, C. (2021). Selective laser sintering versus selective laser melting and computer-aided design—Computer-aided manufacturing in double crowns retention. *Journal of Prosthodontic Research*, *65*(3), 371–378. DOI: 10.2186/jpr.JPOR_2019_556 PMID: 32981911

Hegedus, T., Kreuter, P., Kismarczi-Antalffy, A. A., Demeter, T., Banyai, D., Vegh, A., Geczi, Z., Hermann, P., Payer, M., Zsembery, A., Al-Hassiny, A., Mukaddam, K., Herber, V., Jakse, N., & Vegh, D. (2022). User experience and sustainability of 3D printing in dentistry. *International Journal of Environmental Research and Public Health*, *19*(4), 1921. DOI: 10.3390/ijerph19041921 PMID: 35206116

Herschdorfer, L., Negreiros, W., Gallucci, G., & Hamilton, A. (2020). Comparison of the accuracy of implants placed with CAD-CAM surgical templates manufactured with various 3D printers: An in vitro study. *The Journal of Prosthetic Dentistry*, *125*(6), 905–910. DOI: 10.1016/j.prosdent.2020.03.017 PMID: 32499166

Horn, T. J., & Harryson, O. L. A. (2012). Overview of current additive manufacturing technologies and selected applications. *Science Progress*, *95*(3), 255–282. DOI: 10.3184/003685012X13420984463047 PMID: 23094325

Jordan, R. A., & Micheelis, W. (2016). *Fünfte Deutsche Mundgesundheitsstudie (DMS V)*. Köln, Germany: Deutscher Zahnärzte Verlag. Retrieved December 10, 2020, from https://www.ncbi.nlm.nih.gov/pmc/

Kessler, A., Hickel, R., & Reymus, M. (2020). 3D printing in dentistry—State of the art. *Operative Dentistry*, *45*(1), 30–40. DOI: 10.2341/18-229-L PMID: 31172871

Khan, S. A., Koc, M., & Al-Ghamdi, S. G. (2021). Sustainability assessment, potentials and challenges of 3D printed concrete structures: A systematic review for built environmental applications. *Journal of Cleaner Production*, *303*, 127027. DOI: 10.1016/j.jclepro.2021.127027

Khorsandi, D., Fahimipour, A., Abasian, P., Saber, S. S., Seyedi, M., Ghanavati, S., Ahmad, A., De Stephanis, A. A., Taghavinezhaddilami, F., Leonova, A., Mohammadinejad, R., Shabani, M., Mazzolai, B., Mattoli, V., Tay, F. R., & Makvandi, P. (2021). 3D and 4D printing in dentistry and maxillofacial surgery: Printing techniques, materials, and applications. *Acta Biomaterialia*, *122*, 26–49. DOI: 10.1016/j.actbio.2020.12.044 PMID: 33359299

Kirby, S., Pesun, I., Nowakowski, A., & França, R. (2024). Effect of different post-curing methods on the degree of conversion of 3D-printed resin for models in dentistry. *Polymers*, *16*(4), 549. DOI: 10.3390/polym16040549 PMID: 38399926

Lalama, M., Rocha, M. G., O'Neill, E., & Zoidis, P. (2022). Polyetheretherketone (PEEK) post and core restorations: A 3D accuracy analysis between heat-pressed and CAD-CAM fabrication methods. *Journal of Prosthodontics*, *31*(5), 537–542. DOI: 10.1111/jopr.13452 PMID: 34755428

Lee, Y. C., Zheng, J., Kuo, J., Acosta-Vélez, G. F., Linsley, C. S., & Wu, B. M. (2022). Binder jetting of custom silicone powder for direct three-dimensional printing of maxillofacial prostheses. *3D Printing and Additive Manufacturing, 9,* 520-534. https://doi.org/DOI: 10.1089/3dp.2021.0099

Liu, F., Vyas, C., Poologasundarampillai, G., Pape, I., Hinduja, S., Mirihanage, W., & Bartolo, P. (2018). Structural evolution of PCL during melt extrusion 3D printing. *Macromolecular Materials and Engineering*, *303*(2), 1700494. DOI: 10.1002/mame.201700494

Μαλχανγι, Γ., Πατανο, Α., Μορολλα, Ρ., Δε Σαντισ, Μ., Πιρασ, Φ., Σετταννι, ς., Μανχινι, Α., Δι ςενερε, Δ., Ινχηινγολο, Φ., Ινχηινγολο, Α. Δ., Διπαλμα, Γ., & Ινχηινγολο, Α. Μ. (2023). Αναλψσισ οφ δενταλ εναμελ ρεμινεραλιζατιον: Α σψστεματιχ ρεϖιεω οφ τεχηνιθυε χομπαρισονσ. *Βιοενγινεερινγ (Βασελ, Σωιτζερλανδ)*, 10(4), 472. ηττπσ:// ωωω .μδπι .χομ/ 2306 – 5354/ 10/ 4/ 472. ΔΟΙ: ΠΜΙΔ: 37106659DOI: 10.3390/βιοενγινεερινγ10040472

Μανσκι, Ρ. ϑ., & Μεψερηοεφερ, Χ. Δ. (2017). Προφεχτινγ τηε δεμανδ φορ δενταλ χαρε ιν 2040. *ϑουρναλ οφ Δενταλ Εδυχατιον*, 81(8), eS133–eS145. https:// onlinelibrary .wiley .com/ doi/ abs/ . DOI: PMID: 28765465DOI: 10.21815/JDE.017.020

Mallakpour, S., Tabesh, F., & Hussain, C. M. (2021). 3D and 4D printing: From innovation to evolution. *Advances in Colloid and Interface Science*, *294*, 102482. DOI: 10.1016/j.cis.2021.102482 PMID: 34274721

Manyika, J. (2021). The Future of Think Tanks: Trends and Transformations. *The Future of Think Tanks and Policy Advice in the United States*, 139–143. https:// link .springer .com/ chapter/ _21DOI: 10.1007/978-3-030-60386-1

Palantza, E., Sykaras, N., Zoidis, P., & Kourtis, S. (2024). *In vitro* comparison of accuracy between conventional and digital impression using elastomeric materials and two intraoral scanning devices. *Journal of Esthetic and Restorative Dentistry*, *36*(8), 1179–1198. DOI: 10.1111/jerd.13227 PMID: 38534043

Phuangsuwan, P., Siripipatthanakul, S., Limna, P., & Pariwongkhuntorn, N. (2024). The Impact of Google Maps Application on the Digital Economy. *Phuangsuwan, P., Siripipatthanakul, S., Limna, P., & Pariwongkhuntorn*, 192-203. https://papers .ssrn.com/sol3/papers.cfm?abstract_id=4785205

Piedra Cascon, W., Parra Nunez, A., Charlen Diez, I., & Revilla León, M. (2019). Laboratory workflow to obtain long-term injected resin composite interim restorations from an additive manufactured esthetic diagnostic template. *Journal of Esthetic and Restorative Dentistry*, *31*(1), 13–19. DOI: 10.1111/jerd.12419 PMID: 30367695

Prakash, J., Shenoy, M., Alhasmi, A., Al Saleh, A. A., Shivakumar, G. C., & Shivakumar, S. (2024). Biocompatibility of 3D-printed dental resins: A systematic review. *Cureus*, *16*, e51721. DOI: 10.7759/cureus.51721 PMID: 38318586

Rathee, M., Alam, M., Divakar, S., & Malik, S. (2022). Resin-bonded bridge as a simplified approach to restore missing teeth in esthetic zone by conventional and digital techniques. *Dental Research Journal (Isfahan)*, *19*(1), 92. DOI: 10.4103/1735-3327.361341 PMID: 36605148

Ruschel, G. H., Gomes, É. A., Silva-Sousa, Y. T., Pinelli, R. G. P., Sousa-Neto, M. D., Pereira, G. K. R., & Spazzin, A. O. (2018). Mechanical properties and superficial characterization of a milled CAD-CAM glass fiber post. *Journal of the Mechanical Behavior of Biomedical Materials*, *82*, 187–192. DOI: 10.1016/j.jmbbm.2018.03.035 PMID: 29609139

Sadowsky, S. J. (2021). Comments regarding: Batista V. E. S., Bitencourt S. B., Bastos N. A., Pellizzer E. P., Goiato M. C., Dos Santos D. M. Influence of the ferrule effect on the failure of fiber-reinforced composite post-and-core restorations: A systematic review and meta-analysis. *The Journal of Prosthetic Dentistry*, *125*(5), 554. DOI: 10.1016/j.prosdent.2020.02.036 PMID: 32807404

Schweiger, J., Edelhoff, D., & Güth, J. F. (2020). Update digitale Zahnheilkunde 2020—Aktuelle Möglichkeiten und Limitationen. *Bayerisches Zahnärzte Blatt, 57*, 42–52. Retrieved May 12, 2024, from https://www.google.com/scholar

Schweiger, J., & Güth, J. F. (2020). Neue Entwicklungen in der additiven und subtraktiven Fertigung. *Teamwork Journal of Continuing Dental Education, 23*, 82–90. Retrieved December 10, 2020, from https://www.google.com/scholar

Simpson, D. D. (2011). A framework for implementing sustainable oral health promotion interventions. *Journal of Public Health Dentistry, 71*(s1), S84–S94. DOI: 10.1111/j.1752-7325.2011.00234.x PMID: 21499507

Sumanasena, V., Rajabipour, A., Bazli, M., Kutay, C., & Guo, D. (2022). Strength and erosion resistance of mudbrick as an alternative local material for Australia's Northern Territory remote housing. *Case Studies in Construction Materials, 16*, e01023. DOI: 10.1016/j.cscm.2022.e01023

Sumanasena, V., Rajabipour, A., Bazli, M., Kutay, C., & Guo, D. (2022). Strength and erosion resistance of mudbrick as an alternative local material for Australia's Northern Territory remote housing. *Case Studies in Construction Materials, 16*, e01023. Advance online publication. DOI: 10.1016/j.cscm.2022.e01023

Sun, X., Zhou, J., Wang, Q., Shi, J., & Wang, H. (2022). PVA fibre reinforced high-strength cementitious composite for 3D printing: Mechanical properties and durability. *Additive Manufacturing, 49*, 102500. Advance online publication. DOI: 10.1016/j.addma.2021.102500

Τανγ, Ω. Λ., Χηαο, Ξ. Ψ., Ψε, Ζ., Λιυ, Μ. Ω., & ϑιανγ, Η. (2024). Τηε υσε οφ δψναμιχ ναϖιγατιον σψστεμσ ασ α χομπονεντ οφ διγιταλ δεντιστρψ. *ϑουρναλ οφ Δενταλ Ρεσεαρχη*, 103(2), 119–128. https:// journals .sagepub .com/ doi/ abs/ . DOI: PMID: 38098369DOI: 10.1177/00220345231212811

Tahayeri, A., Morgan, M., Fugolin, A. P., Bompolaki, D., Athirasala, A., Pfeifer, C. S., Ferracane, J. L., & Bertassoni, L. E. (2018). 3D printed versus conventionally cured provisional crown and bridge dental materials. *Dental Materials, 34*(2), 192–200. DOI: 10.1016/j.dental.2017.10.003 PMID: 29110921

Takeuchi, Y., Koizumi, H., Furuchi, M., Sato, Y., Ohkubo, C., & Matsumura, H. (2018). Use of digital impression systems with intraoral scanners for fabricating restorations and fixed dental prostheses. *Journal of Oral Science, 60*(1), 1–7. DOI: 10.2334/josnusd.17-0444 PMID: 29576569

Teixeira, K. N., Duque, T. M., Maia, H. P., & Gonçalves, T. (2020). Fracture resistance and failure mode of custom-made post-and-cores of polyetheretherketone and nano-ceramic composite. *Operative Dentistry*, *45*(5), 506–515. DOI: 10.2341/19-080-L PMID: 32101501

Thurzo, A., Strunga, M., Urban, R., Surovková, J., & Afrashtehfar, K. I. (2023). *Impact of artificial intelligence on dental education: A review and guide for curricυλυμ υπδατε. Εδυχατιον Σχιευχεσ, 13(2), 150. ηττπσ:// ωωω. μδπι. χομ/ 2227 – 7102/ 13/ 2/ 150.* ΔOI., DOI: 10.3390/εδυχσχι13020150

Tian, Y., Chen, C., Xu, X., Wang, J., Hou, X., Li, K., Lu, X., Shi, H., Lee, E., & Jiang, H. (2021). A review of 3D printing in dentistry: Technologies, affecting factors, and applications. *Scanning*, *9950131*, 1–19. Advance online publication. DOI: 10.1155/2021/9950131 PMID: 34367410

Uctasli, S., Boz, Y., Sungur, S., Vallittu, P. K., Garoushi, S., & Lassila, L. (2021). Influence of post-core and crown type on the fracture resistance of incisors submitted to quasistatic loading. *Polymers*, *13*(7), 1130. DOI: 10.3390/polym13071130 PMID: 33918203

Valenti, C., Isabella Federici, M., Masciotti, F., Marinucci, L., Xhimitiku, I., Cianetti, S., & Pagano, S. (2022). Mechanical properties of 3D-printed prosthetic materials compared with milled and conventional processing. *The Journal of Prosthetic Dentistry*. Advance online publication. DOI: 10.1016/j.prosdent.2022.05.004 PMID: 35934576

Van Noort, R. (2012). The future of dental devices is digital. *Dental Materials*, *28*(1), 3–12. DOI: 10.1016/j.dental.2011.10.014 PMID: 22119539

van Noort, R. (2012). The future of dental devices is digital. *Dental Materials*, *28*(1), 3–12. DOI: 10.1016/j.dental.2011.10.014 PMID: 22119539

Vasamsetty, P., Pss, T., Kukkala, D., Singamshetty, M., & Gajula, S. (2020). 3D printing in dentistry—Exploring the new horizons. *Materials Today: Proceedings*, *26*, 838–841. DOI: 10.1016/j.matpr.2020.01.049

Verband Deutscher Zahntechniker-Innungen (VDZI). (2024). Betriebe—Beschäftigte—Auszubildende im Zahntechniker-Handwerk. Retrieved May 20, 2024, from https://www.vdzi.de/statistik.html

Wesemann, C., Spies, B. C., Sterzenbach, G., Beuer, F., Kohal, R., Wemken, G., Krügel, M., & Pieralli, S. (2021). Polymers for conventional, subtractive, and additive manufacturing of occlusal devices differ in hardness and flexural properties but not in wear resistance. *Dental Materials*, *37*(3), 432–442. DOI: 10.1016/j.dental.2020.11.020 PMID: 33288324

Wong, B. K. M., Vengusamy, S., & Bastrygina, T. (2024). Healthcare digital transformation through the adoption of artificial intelligence. In *Artificial Intelligence, big data, blockchain, and 5G for the digital transformation of the healthcare industry* (pp. 87–110). Academic Press., DOI: 10.1016/B978-0-443-21598-8.00014-2

Wuersching, S. N., Hickel, R., Edelhoff, D., & Kollmuss, M. (2022). Initial biocompatibility of novel resins for 3D-printed fixed dental prostheses. *Dental Materials*, *38*(10), 1587–1597. DOI: 10.1016/j.dental.2022.08.001 PMID: 36008188

Yang, J., Li, H., Xu, L., & Wang, Y. (2022). Selective laser sintering versus conventional lost-wax casting for single metal copings: A systematic review and meta-analysis. *The Journal of Prosthetic Dentistry*, *128*(5), 897–904. DOI: 10.1016/j.prosdent.2021.02.011 PMID: 33789799

Zhu, W., Ma, X., Gou, M., Mei, D., Zhang, K., & Chen, S. (2016). 3D printing of functional biomaterials for tissue engineering. *Current Opinion in Biotechnology*, *40*, 103–112. DOI: 10.1016/j.copbio.2016.03.014 PMID: 27043763

KEY TERMS AND DEFINITIONS

AI-Powered Diagnostics: The application of artificial intelligence to analyze dental data for accurate diagnoses and predictive insights, enabling more efficient and expert-level care.

Digital Dental Services: Technology-driven solutions, such as tele-dentistry, digital imaging, mobile health apps, and AI-powered diagnostics, are designed to enhance accessibility, precision, and efficiency in dental care.

Digital Imaging: The use of advanced imaging technologies to capture detailed visuals for accurate dental diagnosis and treatment planning.

Mobile Health Apps: Smartphone-based tools providing dental education, reminders, and basic consultations, with a 25% adoption rate, though limited by digital literacy and smartphone access.

Tele-Dentistry: The use of digital technology to provide dental care, consultation, and education remotely, overcoming geographical barriers and improving access, especially in rural areas.

3D Printing: A manufacturing process that creates three-dimensional objects layer by layer using digital designs, offering customizable, cost-effective, and efficient solutions for producing dental devices and prosthetics.

Chapter 9
Ethical Considerations in Using Technology for Medical Education: Ethics in Medical Education

Ioannis Adamopoulos
https://orcid.org/0000-0002-4942-7123
School of Public Health, University of West Attica, Greece

Pramila Thapa
https://orcid.org/0000-0003-4950-9855
Life Skills Education, Nepal

Niki Syrou
https://orcid.org/0000-0002-0849-7272
University of Thessaly, Greece

ABSTRACT

Background: Medical education is integrating technology, including artificial intelligence, but ethical concerns remain. Objective: This study aims to enhance the role of ethics in medicine, focusing on the integration of human intelligence, particularly social and emotional intelligence, for ethical decision-making in medical education. Methods: The study uses a scoping review design to examine and explore key approaches to ethical considerations in using technology for medical education. Results: The data synthesis process identifies themes concerning behavior changes, technology acceptance, digital distraction, and AI mobile learning. Technology integration in medical education has led to significant advancements in assessment, learning, and professional development. Conclusions: Using Technology for Medical Education has enhanced learning outcomes, provided creative teaching methods,

DOI: 10.4018/979-8-3373-1519-5.ch009

and increased resource access. The digitalization of medical education has led to the development of clinical skills and increased access to resources.

1. INTRODUCTION

The integration of technology into educational settings is becoming increasingly prevalent, offering innovative approaches to assessment, learning, and professional development (Nissen & Andersen, 2021; Austin & Kent-Wilkinson, 2023; Dickens et al., 2024; Puras, 2022; Okhrimenko et al., 2023; Lombardi et al., 2022; Goulah-Pabst, 2023). In medical education, emerging technologies hold vast potential, but it is crucial to explore the ethical and professional implications that accompany these advancements (Cherkowski et al., 2020; Duchac & Duchac, 2023; Wu, 2022; Zhou et al., 2024; Al-kfairy et al., 2024). The primary objective of Medical Education Technology (MET) is to train competent healthcare professionals. However, ethical considerations play a pivotal role in ensuring that this goal is achieved responsibly.

As technology reshapes medical training, it is essential to consider how it affects the physical, psychological, and social well-being of students, educators, and patients. Medical students are expected to develop professionalism, encompassing knowledge, attitudes, and behaviors that align with these values as they transition into their careers in medicine (Sallam, 2023; Koelen & Van den Ban, 2023; Varkey, 2021; Kaplan, 2020). This chapter aims to explore the ethical challenges and opportunities posed by MET, focusing specifically on how these technologies impact human intelligence, emotional aspects of learning, and the overall learning experience.

1.1. Overview of MET

Medical education is continuously evolving, integrating modern tools and methodologies into the curriculum to enhance teaching and learning outcomes (Chiu & Chai, 2020; Su & Zhong, 2022). Digital platforms such as virtual and augmented reality simulations, recorded lectures, question banks (Chiu et al., 2021; Xu & Babaian, 2021; Yang, 2022; Southworth et al., 2023), and flashcard applications are increasingly used to improve students' learning experiences. Mobile applications play a key role in helping students grasp new medical content more effectively (Huang, 2021). Moreover, artificial intelligence (AI) and machine learning are being integrated into health professional education for both student-facing and educator-facing purposes (Chiu, 2021; Fitria, 2021).

These technologies support educational technology purposes, such as personalized learning experiences, and facilitate the management of learning objectives and resources. A prominent application of AI in medical education is the use of electronic health records (EHRs), which assist in shaping learning objectives, determining curricula, and optimizing resource allocation (Chen et al., 2020).

1.2 Proposed Future Research

The theoretical framework of this study can be enhanced through a cross-sectional study, factor analysis, and both exploratory and confirmatory factor analyses (EFA & CFA). Additionally, a mixed-methods approach and a proposal for further development of this research are outlined.

The research hypotheses proposed by the authors are illustrated in Figure 1.

Figure 1. Research model and hypotheses of this study, proposed model by authors Adamopoulos et al., (2025).

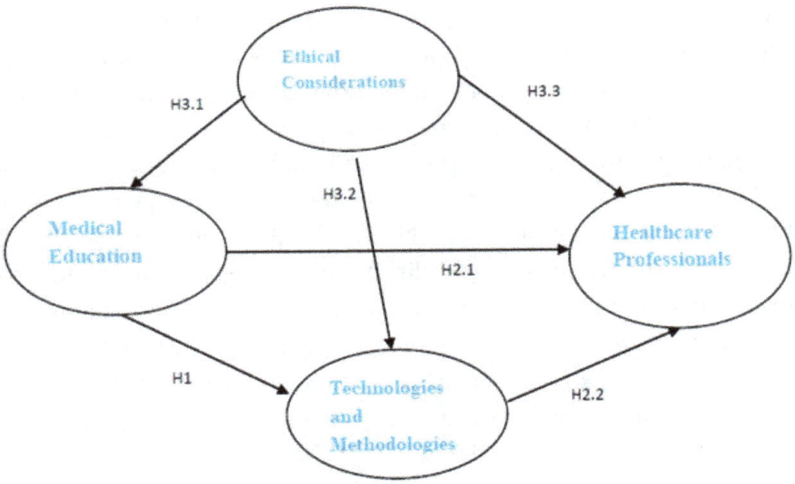

2. LITERATURE REVIEW

2.1 Benefits of MET

Advances in technology have profoundly enhanced medical education, leading to improvements in both teaching and learning outcomes (Goh & Sandars, 2020; Baniasadi et al., 2020; Al-Balas et al., 2020). Key benefits include engaging students through innovative and interactive teaching methodologies (Lee, 2024; Shah et al.,

2020; Barteit et al., 2021; Jumreornvong et al., 2020). These methodologies focus on developing clinical skills, annotating digital models, and correlating computed tomography images with clinical findings (Sahi et al., 2020; Senbekov et al., 2020; Alowais et al., 2023; Bărbuceanu, 2020).

Furthermore, technology facilitates interactive learning processes and provides a wealth of educational resources, including didactic materials and self-assessment tools (Reddy et al., 2020; Tran et al., 2020; Evans & Robertson, 2020; Reid et al., 2023). Increased access to educational content and enhanced collaboration within institutions and globally via online platforms have further enriched the learning experience (Emosda & Annisa, 2020; Öncül, 2021; Kirovska-Simjanoska, 2021; Rubach & Lazarides, 2021).

2.2. Enhanced Accessibility

Technology has significantly improved the accessibility of education, particularly through the expansion of large-scale open online courses, which have democratized learning on a global scale (Bozkurt, 2021; Rodríguez et al., 2021; Samuel et al., 2021; Meaney, 2021). This democratization helps address equity disadvantages in publishing, reduces costs for both students and institutions, and provides learners with the flexibility to access educational materials from anywhere (Berlivet & Löwy, 2020; Spencer & Temple, 2021; Norris, 2023; Kirchgasler & Choi, 2024).

Technology also offers greater flexibility by enabling learners to create and engage with course materials at their own pace (Chisadza et al., 2021; Thai et al., 2020; Stevens et al., 2021), which can lead to more engaging and personalized learning experiences. However, early-career or new educators may face challenges due to unfamiliarity or apprehension with online educational technologies (Bergeler & Read, 2021; Nennig et al., 2020; Pollock, 2022; Beatty et al., 2022). Overall, MET contributes to a more inclusive and accessible learning environment for a diverse range of students (Enoch et al., 2022; Mullen, 2020).

3. METHODOLOGY

3.1. Methods-Design

This book chapter utilizes a methodical scoping review design, guided by the PRISMA 2020 guidelines (Page et al., 2021), to examine the current state of the proposed topic. It presents an innovative review study, grounded in scientific methodology and guidelines, which serves as a foundation for future research and proposals to be developed by the authors at later stages. The aim of this study is to highlight and improve the crucial role of ethics in medicine, with a particular focus on the significant ethical considerations involved in the use of Medical Education Technology (MET).

The review includes studies published between 2010 and 2023, providing a comprehensive overview of recent advancements in MET. To ensure rigor and relevance, the following databases were searched: PubMed, Scopus, Web of Science, and Google Scholar. Inclusion criteria encompassed peer-reviewed articles, conference papers, and reports related to MET in medical education, focusing on ethical concerns such as privacy, bias, and transparency. Studies were excluded if they were not available in English or did not focus on educational settings within healthcare.

3.2. Research-Strategy

The purpose of this review is to explore the use of Medical Education Technology (MET) through mobile learning, digital distraction, and artificial intelligence (AI). To ensure the relevance and quality of the studies included, the selection process was guided by clearly defined inclusion and exclusion criteria.

3.3. Synthesis-Data-Findings

The data synthesis process involves summarizing key findings from selected research to examine evidence-based methodologies and best practices. The goal is to provide actionable insights and recommendations for stakeholders in Ethical Considerations in Using MET, including policymakers, educators, technology developers, and students, on improving healthcare services and educational outcomes through mobile learning.

Figure 2 illustrates the PRISMA flow diagram of the literature review conducted for this book chapter.

Figure 2. Research methods of Book Chapter study, PRISMA flow Diagram.

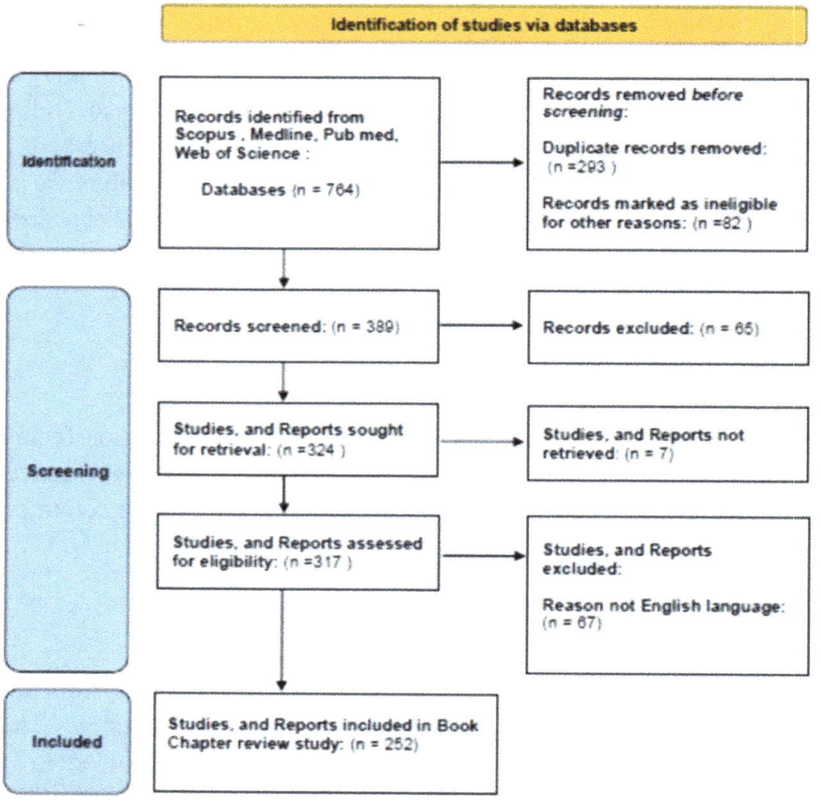

4. RESULTS

4.1. Theoretical Perspectives and Challenges of MET

The integration of Medical Education Technology (MET) has significantly transformed teaching and learning in the 21st century (Hayat et al., 2021; Rajab et al., 2020; Baniasadi et al., 2020; Gaur et al., 2020; Papapanou et al., 2022; Dedeilia et al., 2020). Medical educators are transitioning from traditional methods to technology-enhanced learning, which presents numerous opportunities to advance medical education (Regmi & Jones, 2020; Sharma & Bhaskar, 2020; Zalat et al., 2021; Goh & Sandars, 2020; Tabatabai, 2020; Wilcha, 2020). However, challenges remain, including the need for a balanced educational system and careful consideration of how technology is applied in educational settings (Khan et al., 2023; Sallam, 2023; Katz & Nandi, 2021; Cecilio-Fernandes et al., 2020). Online learning, which supports the continuum of care from patient diagnosis to skill development (Jumreornvong et al., 2020; Vallée et al., 2020; Binks et al., 2021; Gordon et al., 2020), often uses a case-based format with well-regulated content and blended learning approaches (Daniel et al., 2021; Wilcha, 2020; Hilburg et al., 2020). However, this method requires systematic coordination between faculty members and robust academic evaluations (Sahi et al., 2020; Kaul et al., 2021; Teele et al., 2021). Medical educators must engage faculty in all educational activities and offer solutions that contribute to academic growth and development (Rose, 2020; Papapanou et al., 2022).

4.2. Privacy and Data Security Concerns

The use of technology in medical education raises significant concerns about the privacy and protection of sensitive personal information. Participants in training programs may share various types of data, exposing them to risks such as data loss, exposure, or ransomware attacks (Alam, 2023; Huang, 2023; Amo et al., 2021; Alier et al., 2021; Jones et al., 2020; Tzimas & Demetriadis, 2021; Malone, 2020). This can result in unauthorized access to personal data, including transcripts, registration details, learning activities, grades, communication logs, and login credentials (Mutimukwe et al., 2022; Braunack-Mayer et al., 2020; Gudmundsdottir & Hatlevik, 2020). Furthermore, educational data mining practices can lead to the creation of detailed student profiles linked to personal identities (Clifford, 2024; Rubinstein & Margulies, 2022). Instructors have an ethical responsibility to ensure the safety and security of their students' personal information, and the use of Learning Management Systems (LMS) introduces additional ethical concerns (Di Fede et al., 2023). Medical professionals may also be hesitant to engage with eLearning platforms due to concerns about convenience and efficiency. University directors must guarantee the responsible and ethical use of records and data (Schünemann & Windwehr, 2021; Sun, 2023).

4.3 Real-world Applications and Exemplary Models in MET

Medical education seeks to integrate innovation with traditional methods, and learner-centered pedagogy is particularly well-suited to the nontraditional approaches enabled by technology (Winter et al., 2021; Kohnke et al., 2023; Oyedotun, 2020; Chan, 2023; Alamri et al., 2021). This study aims to highlight examples of technology use in medical education (Cardullo et al., 2021; Syauqi et al., 2020; Guan et al., 2020; Yates et al., 2021; Haleem et al., 2022), demonstrate the investment made by programs and faculty in these approaches, and show that the effective use of technology is driven by pedagogical goals (Papapanou et al., 2022; Goh & Sandars, 2020; Mbakwe et al., 2023). MET innovations are designed to achieve specific objectives, such as improving effectiveness before investing in new curricular materials (McKenney & Reeves, 2021; Binks et al., 2021; Sahi et al., 2020). Effective use of MET shares similarities with outcomes management projects, quality initiatives, and research efforts. Lessons learned from these projects can provide valuable guidance for educators in developing their own materials using similar approaches (Krishnamurthy et al., 2022; Baniasadi et al., 2020; Sapci & Sapci, 2020).

4.3.1. Virtual Reality Simulations

Virtual reality (VR) simulations are a valuable tool in MET, offering immersive learning experiences that generate greater interest compared to traditional classroom-based activities (Lee et al., 2020; Shorey et al., 2020; Liaw et al., 2020; Shorey & Ng, 2021; Jiang et al., 2022). VR enables students to practice patient communication and manage realistic clinical scenarios in a safe, controlled environment, allowing them to acquire clinical skills more quickly than through traditional instruction (Bagacean et al., 2020; Van et al., 2022; Coyne et al., 2021; Almousa et al., 2021). Additionally, VR has potential benefits in enhancing simulation-based critical thinking and decision-making skills. However, challenges remain, including high costs, the need for specialized skills for VR training (Mergen et al., 2024; Maqsoom et al., 2023; Baniasadi et al., 2020), extensive faculty development, and limited access to the necessary internet infrastructure and hardware (Badamasi et al., 2022; Sarkar et al., 2021; Almousa et al., 2021; Regmi & Jones, 2020). Despite these limitations, it is essential for educators to consider the technical and ethical implications associated with implementing VR technology (Kulkov et al., 2023; Oke & Arowoiya, 2022).

5. ETHICAL PRINCIPLES IN MET

Integrating technology into medical education requires adherence to ethical principles such as beneficence, non-malfeasance, and the promotion of a healthy educational environment (Langenfeld, 2020; Adams et al., 2023). Technology should enhance the educational journey without causing disruption; educators must remain mindful of potential distractions and actively work to minimize them (Qizi et al., 2024). Justice and fairness must be upheld in the use of technology for instruction (Krupiy, 2020). MET spans a wide range of technologies, from traditional blackboards to holographic augmented reality (AR), all of which require careful ethical consideration (Legg, 2021; Coghlan et al., 2021). As technology continues to evolve, educators must prioritize the avoidance of harm and the safeguarding of student engagement (Liu et al., 2022). Medical educators should continually refine their ethical frameworks and practices to remain responsive to the dynamic nature of technological advancements (Solomonides et al., 2022; Chan, 2023).

5.1. Autonomy and Informed Consent

MET places significant emphasis on informed consent and autonomy, recognizing individuals as rational agents capable of making informed choices (Sallam et al., 2023; Pokhrel et al., 2020; Xu et al., 2020). Educators should support students in making informed decisions by ensuring that they fully understand the program and its data. They must also respect students' autonomy by allowing them to opt out of digital tools when necessary (Harries et al., 2021; Glaser et al., 2020; Abd-Alrazaq et al., 2023; Kim et al., 2020; Alowais et al., 2023). The ethical principle of respecting learners' autonomy and ensuring voluntary participation must guide the use of technological innovations in medical education (Emanuel, 2020; Eysenbach, 2023; Rawas, 2024). The focus should be on the lived experiences of students with the technology, ensuring transparency and honesty in the presentation of educational opportunities (Jumreornvong et al., 2020; Hwang & Chien, 2022). This approach will enhance the student experience and positively influence educational outcomes, encouraging more technologically adept students to engage in patient care-oriented research and practice (Yan et al., 2024; Nimavat et al., 2021; Tang et al., 2022).

6. DISCUSSION

6.1. Challenges of the reviews and the ethical principles inherent in MET

The integration of technology in medical education has emerged as a significant area of research (Safranek et al., 2023; Al-kfairy et al., 2024; Haltaufderheide & Ranisch, 2024), accompanied by a growing recognition of the ethical implications it entails (Raman et al., 2024; Akkila et al., 2024; Fawns et al., 2020; Syed & ES, 2024; Osasona et al., 2024). The use of artificial intelligence (AI) (Goisauf & Cano Abadía, 2022; Brand et al., 2021) and computer-based learning systems has raised concerns regarding potential biases and moral challenges (Marinucci et al., 2023; Cheng et al., 2021; Nishant et al., 2024). These discussions are vital to ensuring that future medical professionals are equipped with a comprehensive understanding of the ethical responsibilities associated with these innovations (Ray, 2023; Koçak et al., 2024; Schwartz et al., 2022; Williams, 2024). Khan et al. emphasized the need for a humanistic approach in medical education, advocating for a curriculum that promotes human connection and collaboration among learners (Khan et al., 2021; Ashok et al., 2022; Akram, 2024; D'Souza et al., 2024; Franco et al., 2024). Naeem et al. conducted a scoping review identifying key components of technology-enhanced learning (TEL) environments in medical education, revealing nine essential thematic elements for effective learning (Li, 2023; Williams, 2022; Naeem et al., 2023; Fatima et al., 2024). They also highlighted the importance of robust pedagogical frameworks that incorporate ethical dimensions and learner characteristics (D'Souza & Rebello, 2021; Cortes-Briones et al., 2022; Sanchez et al., 2024). D'Souza et al. addressed ethical concerns arising from AI implementation in medical education, focusing on its transformative potential in personalizing learning and improving teaching methodologies (Shetty et al., 2022; Kabongo et al., 2021; Rapanta et al., 2021; Irasuti & Bachtiar, 2024). However, they cautioned about the ethical dilemmas associated with AI, such as privacy concerns, algorithmic biases (Greenhow & Galvin, 2020; Petraki & Khat, 2022; Carrillo & Flores, 2020; Yang, 2022; VanTassel-Baska & Wood, 2023; Yeung & Ng, 2024), and the potential erosion of human judgment in educational settings (Han & Kim, 2024; Tiwari et al., 2023; Yamashiro & de Riese, 2021; Froese et al., 2023; Sermonesi et al., 2024; LoPresti & Igarashi, 2024). The study "Understanding the Functional Components of Technology-Enhanced Learning Environments in MET" (Manzer et al., 2024; Fariani et al., 2023; Liu et al., 2024) provides a comprehensive overview of TEL in undergraduate medical education, identifying nine critical themes essential for establishing effective TEL environments (Newman et al., 2021; Kooli, 2023; Nassar & Kamal, 2021; Paul et al., 2023; Prakash et al., 2023; Baskara, 2023; Hensen et al., 2021; Elbanna & Armstrong, 2024). These themes include cognitive enhancement, content curation, digital capability, technological usability, pedagogical practices, learner characteristics, learning facilitators, social representations, and institutional support (Fu et al., 2020; Grant et al., 2020; Saini et al., 2020; Wang et al., 2020). However, the article could benefit from a deeper exploration of ethical issues, such as equity, accessibility, and the ethical responsibilities of educational institutions (Cui et al., 2021; Juan et al., 2020; Chen et al., 2022; Morawska & Milton, 2020). Additionally, ethical concerns related to indoor air quality in educational institutions, as well as socio-demographic factors correlated with risk factors like nomophobia and digital distractions in classrooms, should be considered (Adamopoulos et al., 2025; Thapa et al., 2025; Mahajan et al., 2025).

6.2. Humans judgment in the face of AI advancements

The article Twelve Tips for Addressing Ethical Concerns in the Implementation of Artificial Intelligence in Medical Education by Franco D'Souza et al. explores the ethical implications of AI integration into MET (Franco D'Souza et al., 2024;

Grunhut et al., 2022; van der Niet & Bleakley, 2021). While AI offers significant potential to enhance medical training through personalized learning, improved diagnostic capabilities, and more efficient administrative processes, it also presents profound ethical challenges (Lee, 2024; Abulibdeh et al., 2024; Ahuja et al., 2023; Katznelson & Gerke, 2021; Masters, 2023; McLennan et al., 2022; Jiang et al., 2021; Pillai, 2021). Medical educators must understand the ethical dimensions of AI deployment in educational settings, as AI's ability to personalize learning experiences may unintentionally perpetuate existing biases (Quinn & Coghlan, 2021; Alrashed et al., 2024; Pregowska & Perkins, 2023; Almansour & Alfhaid, 2024; Nur et al., 2024). Transparency in AI systems used in MET is essential, as a lack of clarity in AI-driven decisions can erode trust among students and educators (Memarian & Doleck, 2023; Karabacak et al., 2023; Amann et al., 2020; Akinrinola et al., 2024; Lee, 2024). During the COVID-19 pandemic, it was crucial to address these ethical concerns, mitigate burnout, improve job satisfaction, and reduce occupational risks in medical and public health services (Adamopoulos et al., 2024; Thapa et al., 2024; Adamopoulos et al., 2023; Hegedűs et al., 2024; Adamopoulos et al., 2022; Adamopoulos, 2023). Ethical considerations in MET also include reducing the emotional influence of healthcare providers on the cognitive development of preschoolers (Sharma et al., 2025; Adamopoulos et al., 2025). Furthermore, predicting public health hazards through AI-driven analysis, particularly in the context of climate change, requires proper ethical approval (Adamopoulos et al., 2025). Additionally, the use of graph theory algorithms to model and analyze COVID-19 infection dynamics, taking into account digital distractions and mobile phone use in classrooms among medical students, should be prioritized (Thapa et al., 2025).

Limitations and Recommendations Challenges

The adoption of technology in medical education requires comprehensive digital literacy training for both educators and students, emphasizing the development of human-centered skills, ethical decision-making, and patient care. It is essential to establish clear ethical guidelines and foster collaboration between developers and educators. Additionally, ongoing monitoring of the impact of technology on student well-being is crucial to ensure that it enhances, rather than hinders, the learning experience.

Future Directions and Opportunities

Medical institutions are increasingly adopting AI technologies to enhance patient care. However, it is critical that ethical standards are maintained to ensure the fair use of these technologies, particularly in low-resource settings. This ensures that AI development adheres to principles of equity and supports ethical decision-making processes throughout the development and implementation stages.

Applications and Benefits

This chapter emphasizes the significance of using current citations to enhance the organization and flow of a manuscript, while also highlighting the strengths and weaknesses of current practices.

7. CONCLUSION

The integration of MET has raised important ethical concerns, underscoring the need for a humanistic approach that balances technological advancements with ethical considerations. The literature highlights the importance of a curriculum that fosters human connection and collaboration, while advocating for continued research to ethically incorporate technology-enhanced learning environments. The proposed research model in this study strengthens the hypotheses, particularly concerning the negative effects of ethical considerations on healthcare professionals, medical practice, and medical education. While MET technologies and approaches enhance training quality and meet the professional development needs of healthcare providers, full integration into medical education is hindered by ethical constraints. The study underscores the transformative potential of AI in MET but also cautions about the risks related to privacy concerns and algorithmic biases. It stresses the importance for educators to develop a comprehensive understanding of AI ethics to ensure its equitable and responsible use in MET.

Funding information state: This research received no specific grant from any funding agency in the public, commercial, or not-for-profit sectors.

REFERENCES

Abd-Alrazaq, A., AlSaad, R., Alhuwail, D., Ahmed, A., Healy, P. M., Latifi, S., Aziz, S., Damseh, R., Alabed Alrazak, S., & Sheikh, J. (2023). Large language models in medical education: Opportunities, challenges, and future directions. *JMIR Medical Education, 9*(1), e48291. DOI: 10.2196/48291 PMID: 37261894

Abulibdeh, A., Zaidan, E., & Abulibdeh, R. (2024). Navigating the confluence of artificial intelligence and education for sustainable development in the era of industry 4.0: Challenges, opportunities, and ethical. *Journal of Cleaner Production, 437*, 140527. DOI: 10.1016/j.jclepro.2023.140527

Adamopoulos, I., Frantzana, A., & Syrou, N. (2024e). Climate crises associated with epidemiological, environmental, and ecosystem effects of a storm: Flooding, landslides, and damage to urban and rural areas. *Med-Sci-Forum, 25*(1), 7.

Adamopoulos, I., Lamnisos, D., Syrou, N., & Boustras, G. (2022). Public health and work safety pilot study: Inspection of job risks, burn out syndrome and job satisfaction of public health inspectors in Greece. *Safety Science, 147*, 105592. DOI: 10.1016/j.ssci.2021.105592

Adamopoulos, I., Lamnisos, D., Syrou, N., & Boustras, G. (2022a, October). Training needs and quality of public health inspectors in Greece during the COVID-19 pandemic. *European Journal of Public Health, 32*(Suppl_3), ckac131.373, 1.

Adamopoulos, I., Syrou, N., Lamnisos, D., & Boustras, G. (2023b, February). Cross-sectional nationwide study in occupational safety & health: Inspection of job risks context, burn out syndrome and job satisfaction of public health inspectors in the period of the COVID-19 pandemic in Greece. *Safety Science, 158*, 105960. DOI: 10.1016/j.ssci.2022.105960

Adamopoulos, I., Syrou, N., Lamnisos, D., & Dounias, G. (2024d). Public health inspectors classification and assessment of environmental, psychosocial, organizational risks and workplace hazards in the context of the global climate crisis. *Preprints*, 2024120639.

Adamopoulos, I., Valamontes, A., Syrou, N., Adamopoulou, J., & Bardavouras, A. (2025a). Utilizing graph theory algorithms for the modeling and analysis of COVID-19 infection dynamics. *Mesopotamian Journal of Artificial Intelligence in Healthcare, 2025*, 1–11. DOI: 10.58496/MJAIH/2025/001

Adamopoulos, I., Valamontes, A., Tsirkas, P., & Dounias, G. (2025c). Predicting workplace hazard, stress and burnout among public health inspectors: An AI-driven analysis in the context of climate change. *European Journal of Investigation in Health, Psychology and Education, 15*(5), 65. DOI: 10.3390/ejihpe15050065 PMID: 40422294

Adamopoulos, I. P. (2022b). Job satisfaction in public health care sector, measures scales and theoretical background. *European Journal of Environment and Public Health, 6*(2), em0116. Advance online publication. DOI: 10.21601/ejeph/12187

Adamopoulos, I. P., Frantzana, A. A., & Syrou, N. F. (2024a). Medical educational study burnout and job satisfaction among general practitioners and occupational physicians during the COVID-19 epidemic. *Electronic Journal of Medical Education and Technology, 17*(1), em2402.

Adamopoulos, I. P., Frantzana, A. A., & Syrou, N. F. (2024c). General practitioners, health inspectors, and occupational physicians' burnout syndrome during COVID-19 pandemic and job satisfaction: A systematic review. *European Journal of Environment and Public Health, 8*(3), em0160. DOI: 10.29333/ejeph/14997

Adamopoulos, I. P., Syrou, N. F., & Adamopoulou, J. P. (2024b). Greece's current water and wastewater regulations and the risks they pose to environmental hygiene and public health, as recommended by the European Union Commission. *European Journal of Sustainable Development Research, 8*(2), em0251. DOI: 10.29333/ejosdr/14301

Adamopoulos, I. P., Syrou, N. F., Mijwil, M., Thapa, P., Ali, G., & Dávid, L. D. (2025b). Quality of indoor air in educational institutions and adverse public health in Europe: A scoping review. *Electronic Journal of General Medicine, 22*(2), em632. DOI: 10.29333/ejgm/15962

Adamopoulou, J. P., Frantzana, A. A., & Adamopoulos, I. P. (2023). Addressing water resource management challenges in the context of climate change and human influence. *European Journal of Sustainable Development Research, 7*(3), em0223. DOI: 10.29333/ejosdr/13297

Adams, C., Pente, P., Lemermeyer, G., & Rockwell, G. (2023). Ethical principles for artificial intelligence in K-12 education. *Computers and Education: Artificial Intelligence, 4*, 100131. DOI: 10.1016/j.caeai.2023.100131

Ahuja, A. S., Polascik, B. W., Doddapaneni, D., Byrnes, E. S., & Sridhar, J. (2023). The digital metaverse: Applications in artificial intelligence, medical education, and integrative health. *Integrative Medicine Research, 12*(1), 100917. DOI: 10.1016/j.imr.2022.100917 PMID: 36691642

Akhtar, N., Aslam, N., Hussain, S. Q., & Memon, A. (2021). *Qualitative analysis of diffusing ERE cycle in teaching at higher education: Experiential learning practices in Pakistan*. Ilkogretim Online.

Akinrinola, O., et al. (2024). Navigating and reviewing ethical dilemmas in AI development: Strategies for transparency, fairness, and accountability. *GSC Advanced Research and Reviews, 18*(3), 050–058.

Akkila, A. N., et al. (2024). Navigating the ethical landscape of artificial intelligence: Challenges and solutions.

Akram, M.. (2024). Enhancing secondary education: Diagnosing, developing, and assessing a novel educational management model. *Remittances Review*, *9*(2), 4306–4337.

Al-Balas, M., Al-Balas, H. I., Jaber, H. M., Obeidat, K., Al-Balas, H., Aborajooh, E. A., Al-Taher, R., & Al-Balas, B. (2020). Distance learning in clinical medical education amid COVID-19 pandemic in Jordan: Current situation, challenges, and perspectives. *BMC Medical Education*, *20*, 1–7.

Al-kfairy, M., Mustafa, D., Kshetri, N., Insiew, M., & Alfandi, O. (2024). Ethical challenges and solutions of generative AI: An interdisciplinary perspective.

Alamri, H. A., Watson, S., & Watson, W. (2021). Learning technology models that support personalization within blended learning environments in higher education.

Alier, M., Casañ Guerrero, M. J., Amo, D., Severance, C., & Fonseca, D. (2021). Privacy and e-learning: A pending task. *Sustainability (Basel)*, *13*(16), 9206. DOI: 10.3390/su13169206

Almansour, M., & Alfhaid, F. M. (n.d.). Generative artificial intelligence and the personalization of health professional education: A narrative review.

Almousa, O., Zhang, R., Dimma, M., Yao, J., Allen, A., Chen, L., Heidari, P., & Qayumi, K. (2021). Virtual reality technology and remote digital application for tele-simulation and global medical education: An innovative hybrid system for clinical training. *Simulation & Gaming*, *52*(5), 614–634. DOI: 10.1177/10468781211008258

Alowais, S. A., Alghamdi, S. S., Alsuhebany, N., Alqahtani, T., Alshaya, A. I., Almohareb, S. N., Aldairem, A., Alrashed, M., Bin Saleh, K., Badreldin, H. A., Al Yami, M. S., Al Harbi, S., & Albekairy, A. M. (2023). Revolutionizing healthcare: The role of artificial intelligence in clinical practice. *BMC Medical Education*, *23*(1), 689. DOI: 10.1186/s12909-023-04698-z PMID: 37740191

Alrashed, F. A., Ahmad, T., Almurdi, M., Alderaa, A., Alhammad, S., Serajuddin, M., & Alsubiheen, A. (2024). Incorporating technology adoption in medical education: A qualitative study of medical students' perspectives. *Advances in Medical Education and Practice, 15*, 615–625. DOI: 10.2147/AMEP.S464555 PMID: 38975614

Amann, J., Blasimme, A., Vayena, E., Frey, D., & Madai, V. I. (2020). Explainability for artificial intelligence in healthcare: A multidisciplinary perspective. *BMC Medical Informatics and Decision Making, 20*(1), 1–9. DOI: 10.1186/s12911-020-01332-6 PMID: 33256715

Amo Filvá, D., Prinsloo, P., Alier Forment, M., Fonseca Escudero, D., Torres Kompen, R., Canaleta Llampallas, X., & Herrero Martín, J. (2021). Local technology to enhance data privacy and security in educational technology. *International Journal of Interactive Multimedia and Artificial Intelligence, 7*(2), 262–273. DOI: 10.9781/ijimai.2021.11.006

Ashok, M., Madan, R., Joha, A., & Sivarajah, U. (2022). Ethical framework for artificial intelligence and digital technologies. *International Journal of Information Management, 62*, 102433. DOI: 10.1016/j.ijinfomgt.2021.102433

Austin, W., & Kent-Wilkinson, A. (2023). *Legal and ethical aspects of practice*. Psychiatric & Mental Health Nursing for Canadian Practice.

Badamasi, A. A., Aryal, K. R., Makarfi, U. U., & Dodo, M. (2022). Drivers and barriers of virtual reality adoption in UK AEC industry. *Engineering, Construction, and Architectural Management, 29*(3), 1307–1318.

Baniasadi, T., Ayyoubzadeh, S. M., & Mohammadzadeh, N. (2020). Challenges and practical considerations in applying virtual reality in medical education and treatment. *Oman Medical Journal, 35*(3), e125. DOI: 10.5001/omj.2020.43 PMID: 32489677

Bărbuceanu, C. D. (2020). Teaching the digital natives. *Revista de Stiinte Politice*, (65), 136–145.

Barteit, S., Lanfermann, L., Bärnighausen, T., Neuhann, F., & Beiersmann, C. (2021). Augmented, mixed, and virtual reality-based head-mounted devices for medical education: Systematic review. *JMIR Serious Games, 9*(3), e29080. DOI: 10.2196/29080 PMID: 34255668

Baskara, R., & Mukarto, M. (2023). Exploring the implications of ChatGPT for language learning in higher education. *Indonesian Journal of English Language Teaching and Applied Linguistics, 7*(2), 343–358. DOI: 10.21093/ijeltal.v7i2.1387

Beatty, A. E., Esco, A., Curtiss, A. B., & Ballen, C. J. (2022). Students who prefer face-to-face tests outperform their online peers in organic chemistry. *Chemistry Education Research and Practice*, *23*(2), 464–474. DOI: 10.1039/D1RP00324K

Bergeler, E., & Read, M. F. (2021). Comparing learning outcomes and satisfaction of an online algebra-based physics course with a face-to-face course. *Journal of Science Education and Technology*, *30*(1), 97–111. DOI: 10.1007/s10956-020-09878-w

Berlivet, L., & Löwy, I. (2020). Hydroxychloroquine controversies: Clinical trials, epistemology, and the democratization of science. *Medical Anthropology Quarterly*, *34*(4), 525–541. DOI: 10.1111/maq.12622 PMID: 33210338

Binks, A. P., LeClair, R. J., Willey, J. M., Brenner, J. M., Pickering, J. D., Moore, J. S., Huggett, K. N., Everling, K. M., Arnott, J. A., Croniger, C. M., Zehle, C. H., Kranea, N. K., & Schwartzstein, R. M. (2021). Changing medical education, overnight: The curricular response to COVID-19 of nine medical schools. *Teaching and Learning in Medicine*, *33*(3), 334–342. DOI: 10.1080/10401334.2021.1891543 PMID: 33706632

Bozkurt, A. (2021). *Surfing on three waves of MOOCs: An examination and snapshot of research in Massive Open Online Courses*. Open Praxis.

Brand, G., Sheers, C., Wise, S., Seubert, L., Clifford, R., Griffiths, P., & Etherton-Beer, C. (2021). A research approach for co-designing education with healthcare consumers. *Medical Education*, *55*(5), 574–581. DOI: 10.1111/medu.14411 PMID: 33155301

Braunack-Mayer, A. J., Street, J. M., Tooher, R., Feng, X., & Scharling-Gamba, K. (2020). Student and staff perspectives on the use of big data in the tertiary education sector: A scoping review and reflection on the ethical issues. *Review of Educational Research*, *90*(6), 788–823. DOI: 10.3102/0034654320960213

Breton, M., Sullivan, E. E., & Deville-Stoetzel, N. (2021). *Telehealth challenges during COVID-19 as reported by primary healthcare physicians in Quebec and Massachusetts*. BMC Family. DOI: 10.1186/s12875-021-01543-4

Cardullo, V., Wang, C. H., Burton, M., & Dong, J. (2021). K-12 teachers' remote teaching self-efficacy during the pandemic. *Journal of Research in Innovative Teaching & Learning*, *14*(1), 32–45. DOI: 10.1108/JRIT-10-2020-0055

Carrillo, C., & Flores, M. A. (2020). COVID-19 and teacher education: A literature review of online teaching and learning practices. *European Journal of Teacher Education*, *43*(4), 466–487. DOI: 10.1080/02619768.2020.1821184

Cecilio-Fernandes, D., Parisi, M. C. R., Santos, T. M., & Sandars, J. (2020). The COVID-19 pandemic and the challenge of using technology for medical education in low and middle income countries.

Chan, C. K. Y. (2023). A comprehensive AI policy education framework for university teaching and learning. *International Journal of Educational Technology in Higher Education*, *20*(1), 38. DOI: 10.1186/s41239-023-00408-3

Chen, H., Gomez, C., Huang, C. M., & Unberath, M. (2022). Explainable medical imaging AI needs human-centered design: Guidelines and evidence from a systematic review. *NPJ Digital Medicine*, *5*(1), 156. DOI: 10.1038/s41746-022-00699-2 PMID: 36261476

Cheng, L., Varshney, K. R., & Liu, H. (2021). Socially responsible AI algorithms: Issues, purposes, and challenges. *Journal of Artificial Intelligence Research*, *71*, 1137–1181. DOI: 10.1613/jair.1.12814

Cherkowski, S., Kutsyuruba, B., & Walker, K. (2020). Positive leadership: Animating purpose, presence, passion and play for flourishing in schools. *Journal of Educational Administration*, *58*(4), 401–415. DOI: 10.1108/JEA-04-2019-0076

Chisadza, C., Clance, M., Mthembu, T., Nicholls, N., & Yitbarek, E. (2021). Online and face-to-face learning: Evidence from students' performance during the COVID-19 pandemic. *African Development Review*, *33*(S1), S114–S125. DOI: 10.1111/1467-8268.12520 PMID: 38607902

Chiu, T. K., Meng, H., Chai, C. S., King, I., Wong, S., & Yam, Y. (2021). Creation and evaluation of a pretertiary artificial intelligence (AI) curriculum. *IEEE Transactions on Education*, *65*(1), 30–39. DOI: 10.1109/TE.2021.3085878

Coghlan, S., Miller, T., & Paterson, J. (2021). Good proctor or "big brother"? Ethics of online exam supervision technologies. *Philosophy & Technology*, *34*(4), 1581–1606. DOI: 10.1007/s13347-021-00476-1 PMID: 34485025

Cortes-Briones, J. A., Tapia-Rivas, N. I., D'Souza, D. C., & Estevez, P. A. (2022). Going deep into schizophrenia with artificial intelligence. *Schizophrenia Research*, *245*, 122–140. DOI: 10.1016/j.schres.2021.05.018 PMID: 34103242

Coyne, E., Calleja, P., Forster, E., & Lin, F. (2021). A review of virtual-simulation for assessing healthcare students' clinical competency. *Nurse Education Today*, *96*, 104623. DOI: 10.1016/j.nedt.2020.104623 PMID: 33125979

Cui, X., Zhao, Z., Zhang, T., Guo, W., Guo, W., Zheng, J., Zhang, J., Dong, C., Na, R., Zheng, L., Li, W., Liu, Z., Ma, J., Wang, J., He, S., Xu, Y., Si, P., Shen, Y., & Cai, C. (2021). A systematic review and meta-analysis of children with coronavirus disease 2019 (COVID-19). *Journal of Medical Virology*, *93*(2), 1057–1069. DOI: 10.1002/jmv.26398 PMID: 32761898

Daniel, M., Gordon, M., Patricio, M., Hider, A., Pawlik, C., Bhagdev, R., Ahmad, S., Alston, S., Park, S., Pawlikowska, T., Rees, E., Doyle, A. J., Pammi, M., Thammasitboon, S., Haas, M., Peterson, W., Lew, M., Khamees, D., Spadafore, M., & Stojan, J. (2021). An update on developments in medical education in response to the COVID-19 pandemic: A BEME scoping review: BEME Guide No. 64. *Medical Teacher*, *43*(3), 253–271. DOI: 10.1080/0142159X.2020.1864310 PMID: 33496628

Dedeilia, A., Sotiropoulos, M. G., Hanrahan, J. G., Janga, D., Dedeilias, P., & Sideris, M. (2020). Medical and surgical education challenges and innovations in the COVID-19 era: A systematic review. *In Vivo (Athens, Greece)*, *34*(3, Suppl), 1603–1611. DOI: 10.21873/invivo.11950 PMID: 32503818

Di Fede, O., La Mantia, G., Cimino, M. G. C. A., & Campisi, G. (2023). Protection of patient data in digital oral and general health care: A scoping review with respect to the current regulations.

Dickens, G. L., Watson, F., Schoultz, M., Kemp, C., Ion, R., Hallett, N., & Al Maqbali, M. (2024). Mental health risk assessment and safety planning during UK Covid-19 pandemic lockdown: Mixed methods survey and interview study. *Issues in Mental Health Nursing*, *45*(10), 1111–1119. DOI: 10.1080/01612840.2024.2415468 PMID: 39447076

Duchac, J. N., & Duchac, N. E. (2023). A servant leadership model of social awareness development in a higher education non-profit setting. *Emotional Intelligence in Organizational Leadership*, *13*(1), 67.

Elbanna, S., & Armstrong, L. (2024). Exploring the integration of ChatGPT in education: Adapting for the future. *Management & Sustainability: An Arab Review*, *3*(1), 16–29. DOI: 10.1108/MSAR-03-2023-0016

Emosda, E., & Annisa, V. (2020, May). Digital literacy skills on the generation of digital immigrants. In *Proceeding of International Conference on Social Sciences* (pp. 81–88).

Enoch, L. C., Abraham, R. M., & Singaram, V. S. (2022). A comparative analysis of the impact of online, blended, and face-to-face learning on medical students' clinical competency in the affective, cognitive, and. *BMC Medical Education*, *22*(1), 753. DOI: 10.1186/s12909-022-03777-x PMID: 36320031

Evans, C., & Robertson, W. (2020). The four phases of the digital natives debate. *Human Behavior and Emerging Technologies*, *2*(3), 269–277. DOI: 10.1002/hbe2.196

Eysenbach, G. (2023). The role of ChatGPT, generative language models, and artificial intelligence in medical education: A conversation with ChatGPT and a call for papers. *JMIR Medical Education*, *9*, e46885. DOI: 10.2196/46885 PMID: 36863937

Fariani, R. I., Junus, K., & Santoso, H. B. (n.d.). A systematic literature review on personalised learning in the higher education context. *Technology*.

Fatima, N.. (2024). The role of feedback in enhancing creative writing skills in ELT contexts. *Remittances Review*, *9*(3), 350–368.

Fawns, T., Jones, D., & Aitken, G. (2020). Challenging assumptions about "moving online" in response to COVID-19, and some practical advice. *MedEdPublish*.

Fitria, T. N. (2021). *Artificial intelligence (AI) in education: Using AI tools for teaching and learning process*. Prosiding Seminar Nasional & Call for Paper STIE AAS.

Franco D'Souza, R., Mathew, M., Mishra, V., & Mohan Surapaneni, K. (2024). Twelve tips for addressing ethical concerns in the implementation of artificial intelligence in medical education.

Froese, T., Richter, M., Hofmann, F., & Lüdeke-Freund, F. (2023). Degrowth-oriented organisational value creation: A systematic literature review of case studies. *Ecological Economics*, *207*, 107765. DOI: 10.1016/j.ecolecon.2023.107765

Fu, L., Wang, B., Yuan, T., Chen, X., Ao, Y., Fitzpatrick, T., Li, P., Zhou, Y., Lin, Y., Duan, Q., Luo, G., Fan, S., Lu, Y., Feng, A., Zhan, Y., Liang, B., Cai, W., Zhang, L., Du, X., & Zou, H. (2020). Clinical characteristics of coronavirus disease 2019 (COVID-19) in China: A systematic review and meta-analysis. *The Journal of Infection*, *80*(6), 656–665. DOI: 10.1016/j.jinf.2020.03.041 PMID: 32283155

Gaur, U., Majumder, M. A. A., Sa, B., Sarkar, S., Williams, A., & Singh, K. (2020). Challenges and opportunities of preclinical medical education: COVID-19 crisis and beyond. *SN Comprehensive Clinical Medicine*, *2*(11), 1992–1997. DOI: 10.1007/s42399-020-00528-1 PMID: 32984766

Goh, P. S., & Sandars, J. (2020). A vision of the use of technology in medical education after the COVID-19 pandemic. *MedEdPublish*. Advance online publication. DOI: 10.15694/mep.2020.000049.1 PMID: 38058893

Goisauf, M., & Cano Abadía, M. (2022). Ethics of AI in radiology: A review of ethical and societal implications. *Frontiers in Big Data*, *5*, 850383. DOI: 10.3389/fdata.2022.850383 PMID: 35910490

Goulah-Pabst, D. M. (2023). Suicide loss survivors: Navigating social stigma and threats to social bonds. *Omega*, *87*(3), 769–792. DOI: 10.1177/00302228211026513 PMID: 34218692

Grant, M. C., Geoghegan, L., Arbyn, M., Mohammed, Z., McGuinness, L., Clarke, E. L., & Wade, R. G. (2020). The prevalence of symptoms in 24,410 adults infected by the novel coronavirus (SARS-CoV-2; COVID-19): A systematic review and meta-analysis of 148 studies from 9 countries. *PLoS One*, *15*(6), e0234765. DOI: 10.1371/journal.pone.0234765 PMID: 32574165

Greenhow, C., & Galvin, S. (2020). Teaching with social media: Evidence-based strategies for making remote higher education less remote. *Information and Learning Science*, *121*(7/8), 513–524. DOI: 10.1108/ILS-04-2020-0138

Grunhut, J., Marques, O., & Wyatt, A. T. M. (2022). Needs, challenges, and applications of artificial intelligence in medical education curriculum. *JMIR Medical Education*, *8*(2), e35587. DOI: 10.2196/35587 PMID: 35671077

Guan, C., Mou, J., & Jiang, Z. (2020). Artificial intelligence innovation in education: A twenty-year data-driven historical analysis. *International Journal of Innovation Studies*.

Gudmundsdottir, G. B., & Hatlevik, O. E. (2020). "I just Google it"–Developing professional digital competence and preparing student teachers to exercise responsible ICT use. [NJCIE]. *Nordic Journal of Comparative and International Education*, *4*(3), 39–55. DOI: 10.7577/njcie.3752

Haleem, A., Javaid, M., Qadri, M. A., & Suman, R. (2022). Understanding the role of digital technologies in education: A review. *Sustainable Operations and Computers*, *3*, 275–285. DOI: 10.1016/j.susoc.2022.05.004

Haltaufderheide, J., & Ranisch, R. (2024). The ethics of ChatGPT in medicine and healthcare: A systematic review on large language models (LLMs). *NPJ Digital Medicine*, *7*(1), 183. DOI: 10.1038/s41746-024-01157-x PMID: 38977771

Harries, A. J., Lee, C., Jones, L., Rodriguez, R. M., Davis, J. A., Boysen-Osborn, M., & Langsfeld, J. M. (2021). Effects of the COVID-19 pandemic on medical students: A multicenter quantitative study. *BMC Medical Education*, *21*(1), 1–8. DOI: 10.1186/s12909-020-02462-1 PMID: 33407422

Hayat, A. A., Keshavarzi, M. H., Zare, S., Bazrafcan, L., Rezaee, R., Faghihi, S. A., Amini, M., & Kojuri, J. (2021). Challenges and opportunities from the COVID-19 pandemic in medical education: A qualitative study. *BMC Medical Education*, *21*(1), 247. DOI: 10.1186/s12909-021-02682-z PMID: 33926439

Hegedűs, M., Szivós, E., Adamopoulus, I., & Dávid, L. D. (2024). Hospital integration to improve the chances of recovery for decubitus (pressure ulcer) patients through centralised procurement procedures. *Journal of Infrastructure. Policy and Development*, *8*(10), 7273.

Hendricks, S., & Mwapwele, S. D. (2024). A systematic literature review on the factors influencing e-commerce adoption in developing countries. *Data and Information Management*, *8*(1), 100045. DOI: 10.1016/j.dim.2023.100045

Hensen, B., Mackworth-Young, C. R. S., Simwinga, M., Abdelmagid, N., Banda, J., Mavodza, C., Doyle, A. M., Bonell, C., & Weiss, H. A. (2021). Remote data collection for public health research in a COVID-19 era: Ethical implications, challenges and opportunities. *Health Policy and Planning*, *36*(3), 360–368. DOI: 10.1093/heapol/czaa158 PMID: 33881138

Hilburg, R., Patel, N., Ambruso, S., Biewald, M. A., & Farouk, S. S. (2020). Medical education during the coronavirus disease-2019 pandemic: Learning from a distance. *Advances in Chronic Kidney Disease*, *27*(5), 412–417. DOI: 10.1053/j.ackd.2020.05.017 PMID: 33308507

Huang, L. (2023). *Ethics of artificial intelligence in education: Student privacy and data protection*. Science Insights Education Frontiers.

Hwang, G. J., & Chien, S. Y. (2022). Definition, roles, and potential research issues of the metaverse in education: An artificial intelligence perspective. *Computers and Education: Artificial Intelligence*.

Ide, T., Bruch, C., Carius, A., Conca, K., Dabelko, G. D., Matthew, R., & Weinthal, E. (2021). The past and future (s) of environmental peacebuilding. *International Affairs*, *97*(1), 1–16. DOI: 10.1093/ia/iiaa177

Irasuti, I., & Bachtiar, B. (2024). Empowering Indonesian EFL teachers: The transformative impact of visual literacy training on teaching materials. *International Journal of Learning. Teaching and Educational Research*, *23*(8), 116–136.

Javaid, M., Haleem, A., Singh, R. P., Suman, R., & Gonzalez, E. S. (2022). Understanding the adoption of Industry 4.0 technologies in improving environmental sustainability. *Sustainable Operations and Computers*, *3*, 203–217. DOI: 10.1016/j.susoc.2022.01.008

Jiang, L., et al. (2021). Opportunities and challenges of artificial intelligence in the medical field: Current application, emerging problems, and problem-solving strategies. *Journal of International Medical Research, 49*(3), 030.

Jones, K. M., Asher, A., Goben, A., Perry, M. R., Salo, D., Briney, K. A., & Robertshaw, M. B. (2020). "We're being tracked at all times": Student perspectives of their privacy in relation to learning analytics in higher education. *Journal of the Association for Information Science and Technology*, *71*(9), 1044–1059. DOI: 10.1002/asi.24358

Juan, J., Gil, M. M., Rong, Z., Zhang, Y., Yang, H., & Poon, L. C. (2020). Effect of coronavirus disease 2019 (COVID-19) on maternal, perinatal and neonatal outcome: Systematic review. *Ultrasound in Obstetrics & Gynecology*, *56*(1), 15–27. DOI: 10.1002/uog.22088 PMID: 32430957

Jumreornvong, O., Yang, E., Race, J., & Appel, J. (2020). Telemedicine and medical education in the age of COVID-19. *Academic Medicine*.

Kabongo, S., D'Souza, J., & Auer, S. (2021). Automated mining of leaderboards for empirical AI research. In *Towards Open and Trustworthy Digital Societies:23rd International Conference on Asia-Pacific Digital Libraries, ICADL 2021*. Springer International Publishing. DOI: 10.1007/978-3-030-91669-5_35

Kaplan, B. (2020). Revisiting health information technology ethical, legal, and social issues and evaluation: Telehealth/telemedicine and COVID-19. *International Journal of Medical Informatics*.

Karabacak, M., Ozkara, B. B., Margetis, K., Wintermark, M., & Bisdas, S. (2023). The advent of generative language models in medical education. *JMIR Medical Education*, *9*, e48163. DOI: 10.2196/48163 PMID: 37279048

Katz, M., & Nandi, N. (2021). Social media and medical education in the context of the COVID-19 pandemic: Scoping review. *JMIR Medical Education*, *7*(2), e25892. DOI: 10.2196/25892 PMID: 33755578

Katznelson, G., & Gerke, S. (2021). The need for health AI ethics in medical school education. *Advances in Health Sciences Education : Theory and Practice*, *26*(4), 1447–1458. DOI: 10.1007/s10459-021-10040-3 PMID: 33655433

Kaul, V., de Moraes, A. G., Khateeb, D., Greenstein, Y., Winter, G., Chae, J., & Dangayach, N. S. (2021). Medical education during the COVID-19 pandemic. *Chest*, *159*(5), 1949–1960. DOI: 10.1016/j.chest.2020.12.026 PMID: 33385380

Khan, N. U., Wei, H., Yue, G., Nazir, N., & Zainol, N. R. (2021). Exploring themes of sustainable practices in manufacturing industry: Using thematic networks approach. *Sustainability (Basel)*, *13*(18), 10288. DOI: 10.3390/su131810288

Khan, R. A., Jawaid, M., Khan, A. R., & Sajjad, M. (2023). ChatGPT—Reshaping medical education and clinical management. *Pakistan Journal of Medical Sciences*, *39*(2), 605. DOI: 10.12669/pjms.39.2.7653 PMID: 36950398

Kim, J. W., Myung, S. J., Yoon, H. B., Moon, S. H., Ryu, H., & Yim, J. J. (2020). How medical education survives and evolves during [Our experience and future direction.]. *COVID*, •••, 19. PMID: 33338045

Kirchgasler, C., & Choi, S. (2024). Performing a global learning crisis: Citizen-led assessments, social accountability, and directing democracy. *Compare: A Journal of Comparative Education*, •••, 1–18. DOI: 10.1080/03057925.2024.2314015

Kirovska-Simjanoska, D. (2021). Designing an ESP course for the 21st century students: The clash of the digital immigrants and natives. *Journal of Teaching English for Specific and Academic Purposes*, 17–30.

Koçak, B.. (2024). *Bias in artificial intelligence for medical imaging: Fundamentals, detection, avoidance, mitigation, challenges, ethics, and prospects*. Diagnostic and Interventional Radiology.

Kohnke, L., Moorhouse, B. L., & Zou, D. (2023). ChatGPT for language teaching and learning. *RELC Journal*, *54*(2), 537–550. DOI: 10.1177/00336882231162868

Kulkov, I., Tsvetkova, A., & Ivanova-Gongne, M. (2023). Identifying institutional barriers when implementing new technologies in the healthcare industry. *European Journal of Innovation Management*, *26*(4), 909–932. DOI: 10.1108/EJIM-02-2021-0093

Langenfeld, T. (2020). Internet-based proctored assessment: Security and fairness issues. *Educational Measurement: Issues and Practice*, *39*(3), 24–27. DOI: 10.1111/emip.12359

Lee, J., Kim, H., Kim, K. H., Jung, D., Jowsey, T., & Webster, C. S. (2020). Effective virtual patient simulators for medical communication training: A systematic review. *Medical Education*, *54*(9), 786–795. DOI: 10.1111/medu.14152 PMID: 32162355

Legg, M. (2021). The COVID-19 pandemic, the courts and online hearings: Maintaining open justice, procedural fairness and impartiality. *Federal Law Review*.

Li, N. (2023). Ethical considerations in artificial intelligence: A comprehensive discussion from the perspective of computer vision. *SHS Web of Conferences*.

Liaw, S. Y., Tan, J. Z., Lim, S., Zhou, W., Yap, J., Ratan, R., Ooi, S. L., Wong, S. J., Seah, B., & Chua, W. L. (2023). Artificial intelligence in virtual reality simulation for interprofessional communication training: Mixed method study. *Nurse Education Today, 122*, 105718. DOI: 10.1016/j.nedt.2023.105718 PMID: 36669304

Liu, Y., Wang, D., Wu, S., Liu, X., & Xiao, C. (2024). Literature review of the clinical features of sulfasalazine-induced drug reaction with eosinophilia and systemic symptoms/drug-induced hypersensitivity syndrome. *Frontiers in Pharmacology, 15*, 1488483. DOI: 10.3389/fphar.2024.1488483 PMID: 39687296

Lombardi, B. M., Zerden, L. D. S., & Thyberg, C. (2022). Social work answers the (video) call: Tele-behavioral health use during COVID-19. *Journal of the Society for Social Work and Research, 13*(1), 67–87. DOI: 10.1086/715621

LoPresti, M., & Igarashi, A. (2024). A pragmatic review of cost-effectiveness evaluations of reimbursed medical devices conducted for Japan. *Journal of Medical Economics, 27*(1), 1456–1471. DOI: 10.1080/13696998.2024.2420542 PMID: 39436025

Mahajan, S., Thapa, P., Sharma, P., Tsirkas, P., Ali, G., & Adamopoulos, I. (2025). Prevalence and risk factors of nomophobia among students studying in private colleges. *Preprints*.

Malone, D. M. (2020). Ethics education in teacher preparation: A case for stakeholder responsibility. *Ethics and Education, 15*(1), 77–97. DOI: 10.1080/17449642.2019.1700447

Manzer, J. L., Carrillo-Perez, A., Tingey, L., Ouellette, L., Hogan, C., Atkins, N., Carmichael, K., Ramirez, G. G., Magee, M. M., Miller, M. A., Nwankwo, C., Reid, S., Strelevitz, T., Taylor, V., Waddell, W., Wong, M., Yuksel, B., & Blum, J. (2024). Client perspectives on contraceptive care: A systematic review. *American Journal of Preventive Medicine, 67*(6), S22–S31. DOI: 10.1016/j.amepre.2024.07.019 PMID: 39570202

Maqsoom, A., Zulqarnain, M., Irfan, M., Ullah, F., Alqahtani, F. K., & Khan, K. I. A. (2023). Drivers of, and barriers to, the adoption of mixed reality in the construction industry of developing countries. *Buildings (Basel, Switzerland), 13*(4), 872. DOI: 10.3390/buildings13040872

Marinucci, L., Mazzuca, C., & Gangemi, A. (2023). Exposing implicit biases and stereotypes in human and artificial intelligence: State of the art and challenges with a focus on gender. *AI & Society, 38*(2), 747–761. DOI: 10.1007/s00146-022-01474-3

Masters, K. (2023). Ethical use of artificial intelligence in health professions education: AMEE Guide No. 158. *Medical Teacher, 45*(6), 574–584. DOI: 10.1080/0142159X.2023.2186203 PMID: 36912253

Mbakwe, A. B., Lourentzou, I., Celi, L. A., Mechanic, O. J., & Dagan, A. (2023). ChatGPT passing USMLE shines a spotlight on the flaws of medical education. *PLOS Digital Health, 2*(2), e0000205. DOI: 10.1371/journal.pdig.0000205 PMID: 36812618

McKenney, S., & Reeves, T. C. (2021). Educational design research: Portraying, conducting, and enhancing productive scholarship. *Medical Education, 55*(1), 82–92. DOI: 10.1111/medu.14280 PMID: 32564385

McLennan, S., Fiske, A., Tigard, D., Müller, R., Haddadin, S., & Buyx, A. (2022). Embedded ethics: A proposal for integrating ethics into the development of medical AI. *BMC Medical Ethics, 23*(1), 6. DOI: 10.1186/s12910-022-00746-3 PMID: 35081955

Meaney, M. (2021). Essays on the design of inclusive learning in Massive Open Online Courses, and implications for educational futures.

Memarian, B., & Doleck, T. (2023). Fairness, accountability, transparency, and ethics (FATE) in artificial intelligence (AI), and higher education: A systematic review. *Computers and Education: Artificial Intelligence.*

Mergen, M., Graf, N., & Meyerheim, M. (2024). Reviewing the current state of virtual reality integration in medical education—A scoping review. *BMC Medical Education, 24*(1), 788. DOI: 10.1186/s12909-024-05777-5 PMID: 39044186

Morawska, L., & Milton, D. K. (2020). It is time to address airborne transmission of COVID-19. *Clinical Infectious Diseases: An Official Publication of the Infectious Diseases Society of America.*

Mullen, C. A. (2020). Does modality matter? A comparison of aspiring leaders' learning online and face-to-face. *Journal of Further and Higher Education, 44*(5), 670–688. DOI: 10.1080/0309877X.2019.1576859

Mutimukwe, C., Viberg, O., Oberg, L. M., & Cerratto-Pargman, T. (2022). Students' privacy concerns in learning analytics: Model development. *British Journal of Educational Technology, 53*(4), 932–951. DOI: 10.1111/bjet.13234

Naeem, N. K., Hadie, S. N. H., Ismail, I. M., Ullah, S., & Yusoff, M. S. B. (2024). Buzz or fuss: Gauging the online learning environments in undergraduate medical education—A mixed-method study. *Education in Medicine Journal, 16*(2), 63–83. DOI: 10.21315/eimj2024.16.2.5

Naik, N., Hameed, B. Z., Shetty, D. K., Swain, D., Shah, M., Paul, R., Aggarwal, K., Ibrahim, S., Patil, V., Smriti, K., Shetty, S., Rai, B. P., Chlosta, P., & Somani, B. K. (2022). Legal and ethical consideration in artificial intelligence in healthcare: Who takes responsibility? *Frontiers in Surgery*, *9*, 862322. DOI: 10.3389/fsurg.2022.862322 PMID: 35360424

Nassar, A., & Kamal, M. (2021). Ethical dilemmas in AI-powered decision-making: A deep dive into big data-driven ethical considerations. *International Journal of Responsible Artificial Intelligence*, *11*(8).

Nennig, H. T., Idárraga, K. L., Salzer, L. D., Bleske-Rechek, A., & Theisen, R. M. (2020). Comparison of student attitudes and performance in an online and a face-to-face inorganic chemistry course. *Chemistry Education Research and Practice*, *21*(1), 168–177. DOI: 10.1039/C9RP00112C

Newman, P. A., Guta, A., & Black, T. (2021). Ethical considerations for qualitative research methods during the COVID-19 pandemic and other emergency situations: Navigating the virtual field. *International Journal of Qualitative Methods*, *20*, 16094069211047823. DOI: 10.1177/16094069211047823

Nguyen, A., Ngo, H. N., Hong, Y., Dang, B., & Nguyen, B.-P. T. (2023). Ethical principles for artificial intelligence in education. *Education and Information Technologies*, *28*(4), 4221–4241. DOI: 10.1007/s10639-022-11316-w PMID: 36254344

Nishant, R., Schneckenberg, D., & Ravishankar, M. N. (2024). The formal rationality of artificial intelligence-based algorithms and the problem of bias. *Journal of Information Technology*, *39*(1), 19–40. DOI: 10.1177/02683962231176842

Nissen, R. D., & Andersen, A. H. (2021). Addressing religion in secular healthcare: Existential communication and the post-secular negotiation. *Religions*, *13*(1), 34. DOI: 10.3390/rel13010034

Norris, T. (2023). Educational futures after [Big tech and pandemic profiteering versus education for democracy. *Policy Futures in Education*.]. *COVID*, •••, 19.

Oke, A. E., & Arowoiya, V. A. (2022). Critical barriers to augmented reality technology adoption in developing countries: A case study of Nigeria. *Journal of Engineering. Defence Technology*, *20*(5), 1320–1333.

Öncül, G. (2021). Defining the need: Digital literacy skills for first-year university students. *Journal of Applied Research in Higher Education*.

Osasona, F.. (2024). Reviewing the ethical implications of AI in decision-making processes. *International Journal of Management & Entrepreneurship Research*, *6*(2), 322–335. DOI: 10.51594/ijmer.v6i2.773

Oyedotun, T. D. (2020). *Sudden change of pedagogy in education driven by COVID-19: Perspectives and evaluation from a developing country*. Research in Globalization.

Page, M. J., McKenzie, J. E., Bossuyt, P. M., Boutron, I., Hoffmann, T. C., Mulrow, C. D., Shamseer, L., Tetzlaff, J. M., Akl, E. A., Brennan, S. E., Chou, R., Glanville, J., Grimshaw, J. M., Hróbjartsson, A., Lalu, M. M., Li, T., Loder, E. W., Mayo-Wilson, E., McDonald, S., & Moher, D. (2021). The PRISMA 2020 statement: An updated guideline for reporting systematic reviews. *BMJ (Clinical Research Ed.), 372*(71), n71. Advance online publication. DOI: 10.1136/bmj.n71 PMID: 33782057

Papapanou, M., Routsi, E., Tsamakis, K., Fotis, L., Marinos, G., Lidoriki, I., Karamanou, M., Papaioannou, T. G., Tsiptsios, D., Smyrnis, N., Rizos, E., & Schizas, D. (2022). Medical education challenges and innovations during COVID-19 pandemic. *Postgraduate Medical Journal, 98*(1159), 321–327. DOI: 10.1136/postgradmedj-2021-140032 PMID: 33782202

Parmentola, A., Petrillo, A., Tutore, I., & De Felice, F. (2022). Is blockchain able to enhance environmental sustainability? A systematic review and research agenda from the perspective of Sustainable Development Goals (SDGs). *Business Strategy and the Environment, 31*(1), 194–217. DOI: 10.1002/bse.2882

Paul, J., Ueno, A., & Dennis, C. (2023). ChatGPT and consumers: Benefits, pitfalls and future research agenda. *International Journal of Consumer Studies, 47*(4), 1213–1225. DOI: 10.1111/ijcs.12928

Petraki, E., & Khat, K. (2022). Challenges and constraints in the design of an ESP course in Cambodia: Implications for higher education institutions. *Asia Pacific Journal of Education, 42*(2), 260–275. DOI: 10.1080/02188791.2020.1798738

Pillai, A. S. (2021). Utilizing deep learning in medical image analysis for enhanced diagnostic accuracy and patient care: Challenges, opportunities, and ethical implications. *Journal of Deep Learning in Genomic Data Analysis*.

Pokhrel, N. B., Khadayat, R., & Tulachan, P. (2020). Depression, anxiety, and burnout among medical students and residents of a medical school in Nepal: A cross-sectional study. *BMC Psychiatry, 20*(1), 298. DOI: 10.1186/s12888-020-02645-6 PMID: 32539732

Pregowska, A., & Perkins, M. (2023). Artificial Intelligence in medical education: Technology and ethical risk. *Available at SSRN* 4643763. DOI: 10.2139/ssrn.4643763

Puras, D. (2022). *Report of the Special Rapporteur on the right of everyone to the enjoyment of the highest attainable standard of physical and mental health*. Phil. LJ.

Qizi, R. S. S., Shukhratovna, T. S., & Karamatovna, M. A. (2024). Implementation of education and protection of children's rights in the age of technology.

Quinn, T. P., & Coghlan, S. (2021). Readying medical students for medical AI: The need to embed AI ethics education. *arXiv preprint arXiv:2109.02866*.

Rajab, M. H., Gazal, A. M., & Alkattan, K. (2020). Challenges to online medical education during the COVID-19 pandemic.

Raman, R., Pattnaik, D., Hughes, L., & Nedungadi, P. (2024). Unveiling the dynamics of AI applications: A review of reviews using scientometrics and BERTopic modeling. *Journal of Innovation & Knowledge*, *9*(3), 100517. DOI: 10.1016/j.jik.2024.100517

Rapanta, C., Botturi, L., Goodyear, P., Guàrdia, L., & Koole, M. (2021). Balancing technology, pedagogy and the new normal: Post-pandemic challenges for higher education. *Postdigital Science and Education*, *3*(3), 715–742. DOI: 10.1007/s42438-021-00249-1

Rawas, S. (2024). ChatGPT: Empowering lifelong learning in the digital age of higher education. *Education and Information Technologies*, *29*(6), 6895–6908. DOI: 10.1007/s10639-023-12114-8

Ray, P. P. (2023). ChatGPT: A comprehensive review on background, applications, key challenges, bias, ethics, limitations and future scope. *Internet of Things and Cyber-Physical Systems*, *3*, 121–154. DOI: 10.1016/j.iotcps.2023.04.003

Reddy, P., Chaudhary, K., Sharma, B., & Chand, R. (2020, December). Digital literacy: A catalyst for the 21st-century education. In *2020 IEEE Asia-Pacific Conference on Computer Science and Data Engineering (CSDE)* (pp. 1–6).

Regmi, K., & Jones, L. (2020). A systematic review of the factors–enablers and barriers–affecting e-learning in health sciences education. *BMC Medical Education*, *20*(1), 91. DOI: 10.1186/s12909-020-02007-6 PMID: 32228560

Reid, L., Button, D., & Brommeyer, M. (2023). Challenging the myth of the digital native: A narrative review. *Nursing Reports*, *13*(2), 573–600. DOI: 10.3390/nursrep13020052 PMID: 37092480

Rubach, C., & Lazarides, R. (2021). Addressing 21st-century digital skills in schools–Development and validation of an instrument to measure teachers' basic ICT competence beliefs. *Computers in Human Behavior*, *118*, 106636. DOI: 10.1016/j.chb.2020.106636

Rubinstein, I., & Margulies, P. (2022). *Risk and rights in transatlantic data transfers: EU privacy law, US surveillance, and the search for common ground*. L. Rev.

Safranek, C. W., Sidamon-Eristoff, A. E., Gilson, A., & Chartash, D. (2023). The role of large language models in medical education: Applications and implications. *JMIR Medical Education*, *9*, e50945. DOI: 10.2196/50945 PMID: 37578830

Sahi, P. K., Mishra, D., & Singh, T. (2020). Medical education amid the COVID-19 pandemic. *Indian Pediatrics*, *57*(7), 652–657. DOI: 10.1007/s13312-020-1894-7 PMID: 32412913

Saini, K. S., Tagliamento, M., Lambertini, M., McNally, R., Romano, M., Leone, M., Curigliano, G., & de Azambuja, E. (2020). Mortality in patients with cancer and coronavirus disease 2019: A systematic review and pooled analysis of 52 studies. *European Journal of Cancer*, *139*, 43–50. DOI: 10.1016/j.ejca.2020.08.011 PMID: 32971510

Sallam, M., Salim, N. A., Barakat, M., & Ala'a, B. (2023). ChatGPT applications in medical, dental, pharmacy, and public health education: A descriptive study highlighting the advantages and limitations. *Narra J*, *3*(1), e103. DOI: 10.52225/narra.v3i1.103 PMID: 38450035

Samuel, J., Brennan-Tonetta, M., Samuel, Y., Subedi, P., & Smith, J. (2021). Strategies for democratization of supercomputing: Availability, accessibility and usability of high performance computing for education and practice of big data analytics. *arXiv preprint arXiv:2104.09091*.

Sanchez, T. W., Brenman, M., & Ye, X. (2024). The ethical concerns of artificial intelligence in urban planning. *Journal of the American Planning Association*, •••, 1–14.

Sapci, A. H., & Sapci, H. A. (2020). Artificial intelligence education and tools for medical and health informatics students: Systematic review. *JMIR Medical Education*, *6*(1), e19285. DOI: 10.2196/19285 PMID: 32602844

Sarkar, U., Lee, J. E., Nguyen, K. H., Lisker, S., & Lyles, C. R. (2021). Barriers and facilitators to the implementation of virtual reality as a pain management modality in academic, community, and safety-net settings: Qualitative analysis. *Journal of Medical Internet Research*, *23*(9), e26623. DOI: 10.2196/26623 PMID: 34550074

Schünemann, W. J., & Windwehr, J. (2021). Towards a 'gold standard for the world'? The European General Data Protection Regulation between supranational and national norm entrepreneurship. *Journal of European Integration*, *43*(7), 859–874. DOI: 10.1080/07036337.2020.1846032

Schwartz, R.. (2022). *Towards a standard for identifying and managing bias in artificial intelligence* (Vol. 3). U.S. Department of Commerce, National Institute of Standards and Technology. DOI: 10.6028/NIST.SP.1270

Sermonesi, G., Bertelli, R., Pieracci, F. M., Balogh, Z. J., Coimbra, R., Galante, J. M., Hecker, A., Weber, D., Bauman, Z. M., Kartiko, S., Patel, B., Whitbeck, S. A. S., White, T. W., Harrell, K. N., Perrina, D., Rampini, A., Tian, B., Amico, F., Beka, S. G., & Catena, F. (2024). Surgical stabilization of rib fractures (SSRF): The WSES and CWIS position paper. *World Journal of Emergency Surgery; WJES, 19*(1), 33. DOI: 10.1186/s13017-024-00559-2 PMID: 39425134

Shah, S., Diwan, S., Kohan, L., Rosenblum, D., Gharibo, C., Soin, A., Sulindro, A., Quinn, N., & Provenzano, D. A. (2020). The technological impact of COVID-19 on the future of education and health care delivery. *Pain Physician, 23*(23, 4S), S367–S380. DOI: 10.36076/ppj.2020/23/S367 PMID: 32942794

Shamsuzzoha, A., Nieminen, J., Piya, S., & Rutledge, K. (2021). *Smart city for sustainable environment: A comparison ofparticipatory strategiesfrom Helsinki*. Cities.

Sharma, P., Adamopoulos, I. P., Syrou, N. F., Budhathoki, C. B., & Thapa, P. P. (2025). The impact of health-caregivers emotional nurturance on cognitive development in preschoolers: A nationwide public health cross-sectional study. *EJGM, 22*(3), em643. DOI: 10.29333/ejgm/16184

Shetty, A., Shetty, A. D., Pai, R. Y., Rao, R. R., Bhandary, R., Shetty, J., Nayak, S., Keerthi Dinesh, T., & Dsouza, K. J. (2022). Blockchain application in insurance services: A systematic review of the evidence. *SAGE Open, 12*(1), 21. DOI: 10.1177/21582440221079877

Shorey, S., & Ng, E. D. (2021). The use of virtual reality simulation among nursing students and registered nurses: A systematic review. *Nurse Education Today, 98*, 104662. DOI: 10.1016/j.nedt.2020.104662 PMID: 33203545

Solomonides, A. E., Koski, E., Atabaki, S. M., Weinberg, C., & Lehmann, C. U. (2022). Defining AMIA's artificial intelligence principles. *Journal of the American Medical Informatics Association : JAMIA, 29*(4), 585–591. DOI: 10.1093/jamia/ocac006 PMID: 35190824

Southworth, J., Migliaccio, K., Glover, J., Reed, D., McCarty, C., Brendemuhl, J., & Thomas, A. (2023). Developing a model for AI across the curriculum: Transforming the higher education landscape via innovation in AI literacy. *Artificial Intelligence, 4*, 100127.

Souza, A. D., & Vaswani, V. (2020). Diversity in approach to teaching and assessing ethics education for medical undergraduates: A scoping review. *Annals of Medicine and Surgery (London), 56*, 178–185. DOI: 10.1016/j.amsu.2020.06.028 PMID: 32642060

Spencer, D., & Temple, T. (2021). Examining students' online course perceptions and comparing student performance outcomes in online and face-to-face classrooms.

Stahl, B. C., & Eke, D. (2024). The ethics of ChatGPT–Exploring the ethical issues of an emerging technology. *International Journal of Information Management, 74*, 102700. DOI: 10.1016/j.ijinfomgt.2023.102700

Stevens, G. J., Bienz, T., Wali, N., Condie, J., & Schismenos, S. (2021). Online university education is the new normal: But is face-to-face better? *Interactive Technology and Smart Education, 18*(3), 278–297. DOI: 10.1108/ITSE-08-2020-0181

Sun, J. C. (2023). Gaps, guesswork, and ghosts lurking in technology integration: Laws and policies applicable to student privacy. *British Journal of Educational Technology, 54*(6), 1604–1618. DOI: 10.1111/bjet.13379

Syauqi, K., Munadi, S., & Triyono, M. B. (2020). Students' perceptions toward vocational education on online learning during the COVID-19 pandemic. *International Journal of Evaluation and Research in Education, 9*(4), 881–886. DOI: 10.11591/ijere.v9i4.20766

Syed, F. M., & ES, F. K. (2024). AI-powered security for Internet of Medical Things (IoMT) devices. *Revista de Inteligencia Artificial en Medicina.*

Tabatabai, S. (2020). COVID-19 impact and virtual medical education. *Journal of Advances in Medical Education & Professionalism, 8*(3), 140. PMID: 32802908

Tang, Y. M., Chau, K. Y., Kwok, A. P. K., Zhu, T., & Ma, X. (2022). A systematic review of immersive technology applications for medical practice and education–trends, application areas, recipients, teaching contents, evaluation methods, and performance. *Educational Research Review, 35*, 100429. DOI: 10.1016/j.edurev.2021.100429

Teele, S. A., Sindelar, A., Brown, D., Kane, D. A., Thatte, N., Williams, R. J., Gueverra, J., & Wolbrink, T. A. (2021). Online education in a hurry: Delivering pediatric graduate medical education during COVID-19. *Progress in Pediatric Cardiology, 60*, 101320. DOI: 10.1016/j.ppedcard.2020.101320 PMID: 33169056

Temsah, O., Khan, S. A., Chaiah, Y., Senjab, A., Alhasan, K., Jamal, A., Aljamaan, F., Malki, K. H., Halwani, R., Al-Tawfiq, J. A., Temsah, M.-H., & Al-Eyadhy, A. (2023). Overview of early ChatGPT's presence in medical literature: Insights from a hybrid literature review by ChatGPT and human experts. *Cureus, 15*(4). Advance online publication. DOI: 10.7759/cureus.37281 PMID: 37038381

Thai, N. T. T., De Wever, B., & Valcke, M. (2020). Face-to-face, blended, flipped, or online learning environment? Impact on learning performance and student cognitions. *Journal of Computer Assisted Learning, 36*(3), 397–411. DOI: 10.1111/jcal.12423

Thapa, P., Adamopoulos, I. P., Sharma, P., & Lordkipanidze, R. (2024). Public hygiene and the awareness of beauty parlor: A study of consumer perspective. *European Journal of Environment and Public Health, 8*(2), em0157. DOI: 10.29333/ejeph/14738

Thapa, P., Rijal, A., Sharma, P., Tsirkas, P., Valamontes, A., & Adamopoulos, I. (2025). Impact of mobile phone use on distracted driving and the moderating role of self-regulatory skills. *Preprints.*

Thapa, P., Sharma, P., Goundar, S., Tsirkas, P., Valamontes, A., & Adamopoulos, I. (2025). Digital distractions in the classroom among students: A cross-sectional study. *Preprints*. DOI: 10.20944/preprints202502.1931.v1

Tiwari, A., Kumar, A., Jain, S., Dhull, K. S., Sajjanar, A., Puthenkandathil, R., Paiwal, K., & Singh, R. (2023). Implications of ChatGPT in public health dentistry: A systematic review. *Cureus, 15*(6). Advance online publication. DOI: 10.7759/cureus.40367 PMID: 37456464

Tran, T., Ho, M. T., Pham, T. H., Nguyen, M. H., Nguyen, K. L. P., Vuong, T. T., Nguyen, T. H. T., Nguyen, T. D., Nguyen, T. L., Khuc, Q., La, V. P., & Vuong, Q.-H. (2020). How digital natives learn and thrive in the digital age: Evidence from an emerging economy. *Sustainability (Basel), 12*(9), 3819. DOI: 10.3390/su12093819

Tzimas, D., & Demetriadis, S. (2021). Ethical issues in learning analytics: A review of the field. *Educational Technology Research and Development, 69*(2), 1101–1133. DOI: 10.1007/s11423-021-09977-4

Vallée, A., Blacher, J., Cariou, A., & Sorbets, E. (2020). Blended learning compared to traditional learning in medical education: Systematic review and meta-analysis. *Journal of Medical Internet Research, 22*(8), e16504. DOI: 10.2196/16504 PMID: 32773378

Valverde-Berrocoso, J., Garrido-Arroyo, M. C., Burgos-Videla, C., & Morales-Cevallos, M. B. (2020). Trends in educational research about e-learning: A systematic literature review. *Sustainability (Basel)*, *12*(12), 5153. DOI: 10.3390/su12125153

van der Kruk, S. R., Zielinski, R., MacDougall, H., Hughes-Barton, D., & Gunn, K. M. (2022). Virtual reality as a patient education tool in healthcare: A scoping review. *Patient Education and Counseling*, *105*(7), 1928–1942. DOI: 10.1016/j.pec.2022.02.005 PMID: 35168856

van der Niet, A. G., & Bleakley, A. (2021). Where medical education meets artificial intelligence: "Does technology care?". *Medical Education*, *55*(1), 30–36. DOI: 10.1111/medu.14131 PMID: 32078175

VanTassel-Baska, J., & Wood, S. M. (2023). The integrated curriculum model. In *Systems and models for developing programs for the gifted and talented* (pp. 655–691). Routledge. DOI: 10.4324/9781003419426-24

Varkey, B. (2021). Principles of clinical ethics and their application to practice. *Medical Principles and Practice : International Journal of the Kuwait University, Health Science Centre*, *30*(1), 17–28. DOI: 10.1159/000509119 PMID: 32498071

Wang, Y., Kala, M. P., & Jafar, T. H. (2020). Psychological distress during the coronavirus disease 2019 (COVID-19) pandemic on the predominantly general population: A systematic review and meta-analysis. *PLOS ONE.*

Wilcha, R. J. (2020). Effectiveness of virtual medical teaching during the COVID-19 crisis: Systematic review. *JMIR Medical Education*, *6*(2), e20963. DOI: 10.2196/20963 PMID: 33106227

Williams, D. P. (2024). Disabling AI: Biases and values embedded in artificial intelligence. In *Handbook on the ethics of artificial intelligence.*

Winter, E., Costello, A., O'Brien, M., & Hickey, G. (2021). Teachers' use of technology and the impact of Covid-19. *Irish Educational Studies*, *40*(2), 235–246. DOI: 10.1080/03323315.2021.1916559

Wu, K. (2022). First Generation Asian Americans obstacles to seeking mental health services.

Xu, A., Baysari, M. T., Stocker, S. L., Leow, L. J., Day, R. O., & Carland, J. E. (2020). Researchers' views on, and experiences with, the requirement to obtain informed consent in research involving human participants: A qualitative study. *BMC Medical Ethics*, *21*(1), 1–11. DOI: 10.1186/s12910-020-00538-7 PMID: 33008387

Xu, T., Weng, H., Liu, F., Yang, L., Luo, Y., Ding, Z., & Wang, Q. (2024). Current status of ChatGPT use in medical education: Potentials, challenges, and strategies. *Journal of Medical Internet Research, 26*, e57896. DOI: 10.2196/57896 PMID: 39196640

Yamashiro, J. R., & de Riese, W. T. W. (2021). Any correlation between prostate volume and incidence of prostate cancer: A review of reported data for the last thirty years. *Research and Reports in Urology, 13*, 749–757. DOI: 10.2147/RRU.S331506 PMID: 34676178

Yan, L., Sha, L., Zhao, L., Li, Y., Martinez-Maldonado, R., Chen, G., Li, X., Jin, Y., & Gašević, D. (2024). Practical and ethical challenges of large language models in education: A systematic scoping review. *British Journal of Educational Technology, 55*(1), 90–112. DOI: 10.1111/bjet.13370

Yang, W. (2022). Artificial Intelligence education for young children: Why, what, and how in curriculum design and implementation. *Computers and Education: Artificial Intelligence.*

Yates, A., Starkey, L., Egerton, B., & Flueggen, F. (2021). High school students' experience of online learning during Covid-19: The influence of technology and pedagogy. *Technology, Pedagogy and Education, 30*(1), 59–73. DOI: 10.1080/1475939X.2020.1854337

Yeung, W.-L., & Ng, O.-L. (2024). Using empathy maps to support design-thinking enhanced transdisciplinary STEM innovation in K-12 setting. *International Journal of Technology and Design Education, 34*(4), 1325–1350. DOI: 10.1007/s10798-023-09861-7

Zalat, M. M., Hamed, M. S., & Bolbol, S. A. (2021). The experiences, challenges, and acceptance of e-learning as a tool for teaching during the COVID-19 pandemic among university medical staff.

Zhong, W., Schröder, T., & Bekkering, J. (2022). Biophilic design in architecture and its contributions to health, well-being, and sustainability: A critical review. *Frontiers of Architectural Research, 11*(1), 114–141. DOI: 10.1016/j.foar.2021.07.006

Zhou, J., Müller, H., Holzinger, A., & Chen, F. (2024). Ethical ChatGPT: Concerns, challenges, and commandments. *Electronics (Basel).*

Compilation of References

Abd-Alrazaq, A., AlSaad, R., Alhuwail, D., Ahmed, A., Healy, P. M., Latifi, S., Aziz, S., Damseh, R., Alabed Alrazak, S., & Sheikh, J. (2023). Large language models in medical education: Opportunities, challenges, and future directions. *JMIR Medical Education, 9*(1), e48291. DOI: 10.2196/48291 PMID: 37261894

Abubakari, M. S., Shafik, W., & Hidayatullah, A. F. (2024). Evaluating the potential of artificial intelligence in Islamic religious education: A SWOT analysis overview. In *AI-Enhanced Teaching Methods* (pp. 216–239). IGI Global., DOI: 10.4018/979-8-3693-2728-9.ch010

Abulibdeh, A., Zaidan, E., & Abulibdeh, R. (2024). Navigating the confluence of artificial intelligence and education for sustainable development in the era of industry 4.0: Challenges, opportunities, and ethical. *Journal of Cleaner Production, 437*, 140527. DOI: 10.1016/j.jclepro.2023.140527

Acharya, V., Padhan, P., Bahinipati, J., Mishra, S., Aggarwal, K., Jhajharia, S., Parida, P., Sahu, D., & Pradhan, T. (2023). Artificial Intelligence in Medical Education. *The Journal of International Medical Research, 1*(3), 87–91. DOI: 10.4103/jimr.jimr_17_23

Acut, D. P., Gamusa, E. V., Pernaa, J., Yuenyong, C., Pantaleon, A. T., Espina, R. C., Sim, M. J. C., & Garcia, M. B. (2025). AI Shaming Among Teacher Education Students: A Reflection on Acceptance and Identity in the Age of Generative Tools. In *Pitfalls of AI Integration in Education: Skill Obsolescence, Misuse, and Bias*. IGI Global., DOI: 10.4018/979-8-3373-0122-8.ch005

Acut, D. P., Malabago, N. K., Malicoban, E. V., Galamiton, N. S., & Garcia, M. B. (2024). "ChatGPT 4.0 Ghosted Us While Conducting Literature Search:" Modeling the Chatbot's Generated Non-Existent References Using Regression Analysis. *Internet Reference Services Quarterly, 29*(1), 27–54. DOI: 10.1080/10875301.2024.2426793

Adamopoulos, I. P., Frantzana, A. A., & Syrou, N. F. (2024a). Medical educational study burnout and job satisfaction among general practitioners and occupational physicians during the COVID-19 epidemic. *Electronic Journal of Medical Education and Technology, 17*(1), em2402.

Adamopoulos, I., Lamnisos, D., Syrou, N., & Boustras, G. (2022a, October). Training needs and quality of public health inspectors in Greece during the COVID-19 pandemic. *European Journal of Public Health, 32*(Suppl_3), ckac131.373, 1.

Adamopoulos, I. P. (2022b). Job satisfaction in public health care sector, measures scales and theoretical background. *European Journal of Environment and Public Health*, *6*(2), em0116. Advance online publication. DOI: 10.21601/ejeph/12187

Adamopoulos, I. P., Frantzana, A. A., & Syrou, N. F. (2024c). General practitioners, health inspectors, and occupational physicians' burnout syndrome during COVID-19 pandemic and job satisfaction: A systematic review. *European Journal of Environment and Public Health*, *8*(3), em0160. DOI: 10.29333/ejeph/14997

Adamopoulos, I. P., Syrou, N. F., & Adamopoulou, J. P. (2024b). Greece's current water and wastewater regulations and the risks they pose to environmental hygiene and public health, as recommended by the European Union Commission. *European Journal of Sustainable Development Research*, *8*(2), em0251. DOI: 10.29333/ejosdr/14301

Adamopoulos, I. P., Syrou, N. F., Mijwil, M., Thapa, P., Ali, G., & Dávid, L. D. (2025b). Quality of indoor air in educational institutions and adverse public health in Europe: A scoping review. *Electronic Journal of General Medicine*, *22*(2), em632. DOI: 10.29333/ejgm/15962

Adamopoulos, I., Frantzana, A., & Syrou, N. (2024e). Climate crises associated with epidemiological, environmental, and ecosystem effects of a storm: Flooding, landslides, and damage to urban and rural areas. *Med-Sci-Forum*, *25*(1), 7.

Adamopoulos, I., Lamnisos, D., Syrou, N., & Boustras, G. (2022). Public health and work safety pilot study: Inspection of job risks, burn out syndrome and job satisfaction of public health inspectors in Greece. *Safety Science*, *147*, 105592. DOI: 10.1016/j.ssci.2021.105592

Adamopoulos, I., Syrou, N., Lamnisos, D., & Boustras, G. (2023b, February). Cross-sectional nationwide study in occupational safety & health: Inspection of job risks context, burn out syndrome and job satisfaction of public health inspectors in the period of the COVID-19 pandemic in Greece. *Safety Science*, *158*, 105960. DOI: 10.1016/j.ssci.2022.105960

Adamopoulos, I., Syrou, N., Lamnisos, D., & Dounias, G. (2024d). Public health inspectors classification and assessment of environmental, psychosocial, organizational risks and workplace hazards in the context of the global climate crisis. *Preprints*, 2024120639.

Adamopoulos, I., Valamontes, A., Syrou, N., Adamopoulou, J., & Bardavouras, A. (2025a). Utilizing graph theory algorithms for the modeling and analysis of COVID-19 infection dynamics. *Mesopotamian Journal of Artificial Intelligence in Healthcare, 2025*, 1–11. DOI: 10.58496/MJAIH/2025/001

Adamopoulos, I., Valamontes, A., Tsirkas, P., & Dounias, G. (2025c). Predicting workplace hazard, stress and burnout among public health inspectors: An AI-driven analysis in the context of climate change. *European Journal of Investigation in Health, Psychology and Education, 15*(5), 65. DOI: 10.3390/ejihpe15050065 PMID: 40422294

Adamopoulou, J. P., Frantzana, A. A., & Adamopoulos, I. P. (2023). Addressing water resource management challenges in the context of climate change and human influence. *European Journal of Sustainable Development Research, 7*(3), em0223. DOI: 10.29333/ejosdr/13297

Adams, C., Pente, P., Lemermeyer, G., & Rockwell, G. (2023). Ethical principles for artificial intelligence in K-12 education. *Computers and Education: Artificial Intelligence, 4*, 100131. DOI: 10.1016/j.caeai.2023.100131

Afshar, A., & Mihut, D. (2020). Enhancing durability of 3D printed polymer structures by metallization. *Journal of Materials Science and Technology, 53*, 185–191. DOI: 10.1016/j.jmst.2020.01.072

Ahmady, S., Khajeali, N., Kohan, N., Zarei, A., Biswas, B., Barzegar, M., & Moghaddam, A. K. (2024). Medical students' perception of mobile learning during COVID-19 in Iran: A national study. *PLoS One, 19*(10), e0308248. DOI: 10.1371/journal.pone.0308248 PMID: 39423220

Ahmed, A., Kerr, E., & O'Malley, A. (2025). Quality assurance and validity of AI-generated single best answer questions [Article]. *BMC Medical Education, 25*(1), 300. Advance online publication. DOI: 10.1186/s12909-025-06881-w PMID: 40001164

Ahuja, A. S., Polascik, B. W., Doddapaneni, D., Byrnes, E. S., & Sridhar, J. (2023). The digital metaverse: Applications in artificial intelligence, medical education, and integrative health. *Integrative Medicine Research, 12*(1), 100917. DOI: 10.1016/j.imr.2022.100917 PMID: 36691642

Akhtar, N., Aslam, N., Hussain, S. Q., & Memon, A. (2021). *Qualitative analysis of diffusing ERE cycle in teaching at higher education: Experiential learning practices in Pakistan*. Ilkogretim Online.

Akinrinola, O., et al. (2024). Navigating and reviewing ethical dilemmas in AI development: Strategies for transparency, fairness, and accountability. *GSC Advanced Research and Reviews, 18*(3), 050–058.

Akkila, A. N., et al. (2024). Navigating the ethical landscape of artificial intelligence: Challenges and solutions.

Akour, I., Alshurideh, M., Al Kurdi, B., Al Ali, A., & Salloum, S. (2021). Using machine learning algorithms to predict people's intention to use mobile learning platforms during the COVID-19 pandemic: Machine learning approach. *JMIR Medical Education, 7*(1), e24032. DOI: 10.2196/24032 PMID: 33444154

Akram, M.. (2024). Enhancing secondary education: Diagnosing, developing, and assessing a novel educational management model. *Remittances Review, 9*(2), 4306–4337.

Al Hamad, K. Q., Al-Rashdan, B. A., Ayyad, J. Q., Al Omrani, L. M., Sharoh, A. M., Al Nimri, A. M., & Al-Kaff, F. T. (2022). Additive manufacturing of dental ceramics: A systematic review and meta-analysis. *Journal of Prosthodontics, 31*(8), e67–e86. DOI: 10.1111/jopr.13553 PMID: 35675133

Al Kuwaiti, A., Nazer, K., Al-Reedy, A., Al-Shehri, S., Al-Muhanna, A., Subbarayalu, A. V., Al Muhanna, D., & Al-Muhanna, F. A. (2023). A Review of the Role of Artificial Intelligence in Healthcare. *Journal of Personalized Medicine, 13*(6), 951. DOI: 10.3390/jpm13060951 PMID: 37373940

Al Mortadi, N., Jones, Q., Eggbeer, D., Lewis, J., & Williams, R. J. (2015). Fabrication of a resin appliance with alloy components using digital technology without an analog impression. *American Journal of Orthodontics and Dentofacial Orthopedics, 148*(6), 862–867. DOI: 10.1016/j.ajodo.2015.06.014 PMID: 26522047

Alamri, H. A., Watson, S., & Watson, W. (2021). Learning technology models that support personalization within blended learning environments in higher education.

Alawneh, Y. J. J., Sleema, H., Salman, F. N., Alshammat, M. F., & Oteer, R. S., & ALrashidi, N. K. N. (2024). Adaptive Learning Systems: Revolutionizing Higher Education through AI-Driven Curricula. *2024 International Conference on Knowledge Engineering and Communication Systems (ICKECS), 1*, 1-5. https://doi.org/ DOI: 10.1109/ICKECS61492.2024.10616675

Al-Balas, M., Al-Balas, H. I., Jaber, H. M., Obeidat, K., Al-Balas, H., Aborajooh, E. A., Al-Taher, R., & Al-Balas, B. (2020). Distance learning in clinical medical education amid COVID-19 pandemic in Jordan: Current situation, challenges, and perspectives. *BMC Medical Education*, *20*(1), 1–7. DOI: 10.1186/s12909-020-02257-4 PMID: 33008392

Al-Emran, M., Arpaci, I., & Salloum, S. A. (2020). An empirical examination of continuous intention to use m-learning: An integrated model. *Education and Information Technologies*, *25*(4), 2899–2918. DOI: 10.1007/s10639-019-10094-2

Alfallaj, H. A., Afrashtehfar, K. I., Asiri, A. K., Almasoud, F. S., Alnaqa, G. H., & Al-Angari, N. S. (2023). The Status of Digital Dental Technology Implementation in the Saudi Dental Schools' Curriculum: A National Cross-Sectional Survey for Healthcare Digitization. *International Journal of Environmental Research and Public Health*, *20*(1), 321. DOI: 10.3390/ijerph20010321 PMID: 36612639

AlGerafi, M. A. M., Zhou, Y., Oubibi, M., & Wijaya, T. T. (2023). Unlocking the Potential: A Comprehensive Evaluation of Augmented Reality and Virtual Reality in Education. *Electronics (Basel)*, *12*(18), 3953. DOI: 10.3390/electronics12183953

Alghazi, S. S., Kamsin, A., Almaiah, M. A., Wong, S. Y., & Shuib, L. (2021). For sustainable application of mobile learning: An extended UTAUT model to examine the effect of technical factors on the usage of mobile devices as a learning tool. *Sustainability (Basel)*, *13*(4), 1856. DOI: 10.3390/su13041856

Ali, A. S. M., Ali, S., Ziaullah, K., Joo, M.-I., & Kim, H.-C. (2025). *IoMT and blockchain synergy: A novel approach to health data validation and storage*. IEEE., DOI: 10.1109/ACCESS.2025.3555289

Alier, M., Casañ Guerrero, M. J., Amo, D., Severance, C., & Fonseca, D. (2021). Privacy and e-learning: A pending task. *Sustainability (Basel)*, *13*(16), 9206. DOI: 10.3390/su13169206

Ali, R., Afzal, A., Shakil, S., Sultan, A., Babar, S., Rehman, J., Malik, M. G. R., Qadir, M. S., Khan, S., & Saeed, S. (2025). Transforming Education: Case-Based Integrated Learning Development and Implementation – A Mixed Methods Study at a Private Medical College [Article]. *Journal of Advances in Medical Education & Professionalism*, *13*(1), 49–58. DOI: 10.30476/jamp.2024.104285.2048 PMID: 39906080

Al-kfairy, M., Mustafa, D., Kshetri, N., Insiew, M., & Alfandi, O. (2024). Ethical challenges and solutions of generative AI: An interdisciplinary perspective.

Almansour, M., & Alfhaid, F. M. (n.d.). Generative artificial intelligence and the personalization of health professional education: A narrative review.

Almeida, R. S. d. (2023). Redefining Health Education in the Post-Pandemic World: How to Integrate Digital Technologies into the Curricula? In *Handbook of Research on Instructional Technologies in Health Education and Allied Disciplines*. IGI Global., DOI: 10.4018/978-1-6684-7164-7.ch001

Almousa, O., Zhang, R., Dimma, M., Yao, J., Allen, A., Chen, L., Heidari, P., & Qayumi, K. (2021). Virtual reality technology and remote digital application for tele-simulation and global medical education: An innovative hybrid system for clinical training. *Simulation & Gaming*, *52*(5), 614–634. DOI: 10.1177/10468781211008258

Alowais, S. A., Alghamdi, S. S., Alsuhebany, N., Alqahtani, T., Alshaya, A. I., Almohareb, S. N., Aldairem, A., Alrashed, M., Bin Saleh, K., Badreldin, H. A., Al Yami, M. S., Al Harbi, S., & Albekairy, A. M. (2023). Revolutionizing healthcare: The role of artificial intelligence in clinical practice. *BMC Medical Education*, *23*(1), 689. DOI: 10.1186/s12909-023-04698-z PMID: 37740191

Alqahtani, S. A. H. (2024). Enhancing dental practice. Cutting-edge digital innovations. *Brazilian Journal of Oral Sciences*, *23*, e0244785. https://dpi.org/10.20396/bjos.v23i00.8674785. DOI: 10.20396/bjos.v23i00.8674785

Al-Qarni, F. D. (2022). Customized post and cores fabricated with CAD/CAM technology: A literature review. *International Journal of General Medicine*, *15*, 4771–4779. DOI: 10.2147/IJGM.S365296 PMID: 35571288

Alqutaibi, A. Y., Hamadallah, H. H., Oqbi, H. F., Almuzaini, S. A., & Borzangy, S. (2024). Current applications and future perspective of virtual reality in dental education and practice in Saudi Arabia: A scoping review. *The Saudi Dental Journal*, *36*(11), 1406–1416. DOI: 10.1016/j.sdentj.2024.09.007 PMID: 39619710

Alrashed, F. A., Ahmad, T., Almurdi, M., Alderaa, A., Alhammad, S., Serajuddin, M., & Alsubiheen, A. (2024). Incorporating technology adoption in medical education: A qualitative study of medical students' perspectives. *Advances in Medical Education and Practice*, *15*, 615–625. DOI: 10.2147/AMEP.S464555 PMID: 38975614

Al-Shamsi, A., Al-Mekhlafi, A. M., Al Busaidi, S., & Hilal, M. M. (2020). The effects of mobile learning on listening comprehension skills and attitudes of Omani EFL adult learners. *International Journal of Learning. Teaching and Educational Research*, *19*(8), 16–39. DOI: 10.26803/ijlter.19.8.2

Alsharif, M. A., Bahbah, A. A., Ghonaim, M. M., Omran, J. A., Rihan, M. M., Zayed, M. A., Tabour, M. S., Alwardany, M. H., & Aboshady, O. A. (2024). Usage and attitude of medical students towards mobile medical applications during and after COVID-19 lockdown: Repeated cross-sectional study. *BMC Medical Education*, *24*(1), 233. DOI: 10.1186/s12909-024-05216-5 PMID: 38438883

Alshurideh, M., Al Kurdi, B., Salloum, S. A., Arpaci, I., & Al-Emran, M. (2023). Predicting the actual use of m-learning systems: A comparative approach using PLS-SEM and machine learning algorithms. *Interactive Learning Environments*, *31*(3), 1214–1228. DOI: 10.1080/10494820.2020.1826982

Alsoufi, A., Alsuyihili, A., Msherghi, A., Elhadi, A., Atiyah, H., Ashini, A., Ashwieb, A., Ghula, M., Ben Hasan, H., Abudabuos, S., Alameen, H., Abokhdhir, T., Anaiba, M., Nagib, T., Shuwayyah, A., Benothman, R., Arrefae, G., Alkhwayildi, A., Alhadi, A., & Elhadi, M. (2020). Impact of the COVID-19 pandemic on medical education: Medical students' knowledge, attitudes, and practices regarding electronic learning. *PLoS One*, *15*(11), e0242905. DOI: 10.1371/journal.pone.0242905 PMID: 33237962

Altintas, L., & Sahiner, M. (2024). Transforming medical education: The impact of innovations in technology and medical devices. *Expert Review of Medical Devices*, *21*(9), 797–809. DOI: 10.1080/17434440.2024.2400153 PMID: 39235206

Amann, J., Blasimme, A., Vayena, E., Frey, D., & Madai, V. I. (2020). Explainability for artificial intelligence in healthcare: A multidisciplinary perspective. *BMC Medical Informatics and Decision Making*, *20*(1), 1–9. DOI: 10.1186/s12911-020-01332-6 PMID: 33256715

Amo Filvá, D., Prinsloo, P., Alier Forment, M., Fonseca Escudero, D., Torres Kompen, R., Canaleta Llampallas, X., & Herrero Martín, J. (2021). Local technology to enhance data privacy and security in educational technology. *International Journal of Interactive Multimedia and Artificial Intelligence*, *7*(2), 262–273. DOI: 10.9781/ijimai.2021.11.006

Annamma, L. M., Varma, S. R., Abuttayem, H., Prasad, P., Azim, S. A., Odah, R., George, B. T., Nair, C., & Karobari, M. I. (2024). Current challenges in dental education- a scoping review. *BMC Medical Education*, *24*(1), 1523. DOI: 10.1186/s12909-024-06545-1 PMID: 39716191

Aquino, Y. S. J., Carter, S. M., Houssami, N., Braunack-Mayer, A., Win, K. T., Degeling, C., Wang, L., & Rogers, W. A. (2023). Practical, epistemic and normative implications of algorithmic bias in healthcare artificial intelligence: A qualitative study of multidisciplinary expert perspectives [Article]. *Journal of Medical Ethics*, jme-2022-108850. Advance online publication. DOI: 10.1136/jme-2022-108850 PMID: 36823101

Araujo, A. A. C., Gardim, L., Salma, J., Stephen, T., Santos, S. S. D., Silva, Í. R., Godoy, S., & Mendes, I. A. C. (2024). Advancing nursing education through wearable electronic devices: A scoping review. *Nurse Education in Practice*, *79*, 104075. DOI: 10.1016/j.nepr.2024.104075 PMID: 39068061

Arch Virtual. (2018, August 21). Virtual reality medical simulation: 7 ways VR is revolutionizing healthcare training. *Arch Virtual*. https://archvirtual.com/2018/08/21/vr-medical-simulation-7-ways/

Arivu, S. A., Amutha, R., Muthumeenakshi, K., & Edna, E. N. (2018). Design of smart vest to monitor physical activities of children. In *2018 Fourth International Conference on Advances in Electrical, Electronics, Information, Communication and Bio-Informatics (AEEICB)* (pp. 1–4). IEEE. DOI: 10.1109/AEEICB.2018.8480993

Arslan, B., Lehman, B., Tenison, C., Sparks, J. R., López, A. A., Gu, L., & Zapata-Rivera, D. (2024). 2024-October-07). Opportunities and challenges of using generative AI to personalize educational assessment [Perspective]. *Frontiers in Artificial Intelligence*, *7*, 1460651. Advance online publication. DOI: 10.3389/frai.2024.1460651 PMID: 39434872

Artaza, O., Santacruz, J., Girard, J. E., Alvarez, D., Barria, S., Tetelboin, C., Tomasina, F., & Medina, A. (2020). Formación de recursos humanos para la salud universal: Acciones estratégicas desde las instituciones académicas. *Revista Panamericana de Salud Pública = Pan American Journal of Public Health*, *44*(e83), 1. Advance online publication. DOI: 10.26633/RPSP.2020.83 PMID: 32733545

As'ad, M. (2024). Intelligent Tutoring Systems, Generative Artificial Intelligence (AI), and Healthcare Agents: A Proof of Concept and Dual-Layer Approach. *Cureus*. Advance online publication. DOI: 10.7759/cureus.69710 PMID: 39308847

Ashok, M., Madan, R., Joha, A., & Sivarajah, U. (2022). Ethical framework for artificial intelligence and digital technologies. *International Journal of Information Management*, *62*, 102433. DOI: 10.1016/j.ijinfomgt.2021.102433

Aslam, M. S., & Nisar, S. (2023). *Artificial intelligence applications using ChatGPT in education: Case studies and practices* [Book]. IGI Global., DOI: 10.4018/978-1-6684-9300-7

Aster, A., Laupichler, M. C., Rockwell-Kollmann, T., Masala, G., Bala, E., & Raupach, T. (2024). ChatGPT and Other Large Language Models in Medical Education — Scoping Literature Review. *Medical Science Educator, 35*(1), 1–13. DOI: 10.1007/s40670-024-02206-6 PMID: 40144083

Atkinson, C. J., Seth, I., Xie, Y., Ross, R. J., Hunter-Smith, D. J., Rozen, W. M., & Cuomo, R. (2024). Artificial Intelligence Language Model Performance for Rapid Intraoperative Queries in Plastic Surgery: ChatGPT and the Deep Inferior Epigastric Perforator Flap [Article]. *Journal of Clinical Medicine, 13*(3), 900. Advance online publication. DOI: 10.3390/jcm13030900 PMID: 38337594

Atuhurra, J., & Kaffenberger, M. (2022). Measuring education system coherence: Alignment of curriculum standards, examinations, and teacher instruction in Tanzania and Uganda. *International Journal of Educational Development, 92*, 102598. DOI: 10.1016/j.ijedudev.2022.102598

Austin, W., & Kent-Wilkinson, A. (2023). *Legal and ethical aspects of practice.* Psychiatric & Mental Health Nursing for Canadian Practice.

Australian Institute of Health and Welfare. (2021). *Rural & Remote Health.* Retrieved from https://www.aihw.gov.au/reports/rural-remote-australians/rural-remote-health/contents/health-status-and-outcomes

Awadallah Alkouk, W., & Khlaif, Z. N. (2024). AI-resistant assessments in higher education: Practical insights from faculty training workshops. *Frontiers in Education, 9*, 1499495. DOI: 10.3389/feduc.2024.1499495

Babu, M., Lautman, Z., Lin, X., Sobota, M. H. B., & Snyder, M. P. (2024). Wearable devices: Implications for precision medicine and the future of health care. *Annual Review of Medicine, 75*(1), 401–415. DOI: 10.1146/annurev-med-052422-020437 PMID: 37983384

Badamasi, A. A., Aryal, K. R., Makarfi, U. U., & Dodo, M. (2022). Drivers and barriers of virtual reality adoption in UK AEC industry. *Engineering, Construction, and Architectural Management, 29*(3), 1307–1318.

Baethge, C., Goldbeck-Wood, S., & Mertens, S. (2019). SANRA—A scale for the quality assessment of narrative review articles. *Research Integrity and Peer Review, 4*(1), 5. DOI: 10.1186/s41073-019-0064-8 PMID: 30962953

Bahroun, Z., Anane, C., Ahmed, V., & Zacca, A. (2023). Transforming education: A comprehensive review of generative artificial intelligence in educational settings through bibliometric and content analysis. *Sustainability (Basel), 15*(17), 12983. DOI: 10.3390/su151712983

Bajwa, J., Munir, U., Nori, A., & Williams, B. (2021). Artificial intelligence in healthcare: Transforming the practice of medicine. *Future Healthcare Journal*, *8*(2), e188–e194. DOI: 10.7861/fhj.2021-0095 PMID: 34286183

Baker, L. R., Phelan, S., Woods, N. N., Boyd, V. A., Rowland, P., & Ng, S. L. (2021). Re-envisioning paradigms of education: Towards awareness, alignment, and pluralism. *Advances in Health Sciences Education : Theory and Practice*, *26*(3), 1045–1058. DOI: 10.1007/s10459-021-10036-z PMID: 33742339

Baniasadi, T., Ayyoubzadeh, S. M., & Mohammadzadeh, N. (2020). Challenges and practical considerations in applying virtual reality in medical education and treatment. *Oman Medical Journal*, *35*(3), e125. DOI: 10.5001/omj.2020.43 PMID: 32489677

Bărbuceanu, C. D. (2020). Teaching the digital natives. *Revista de Stiinte Politice*, (65), 136–145.

Barteit, S., Lanfermann, L., Bärnighausen, T., Neuhann, F., & Beiersmann, C. (2021). Augmented, mixed, and virtual reality-based head-mounted devices for medical education: Systematic review. *JMIR Serious Games*, *9*(3), e29080. DOI: 10.2196/29080 PMID: 34255668

Barton, G., & Lennon, S. (2020). Literacy. In *Teaching Middle Years* (pp. 115–132). Routledge. DOI: 10.4324/9781003117780-9

Barwise, A. K., Curtis, S., Diedrich, D. A., & Pickering, B. W. (2024). Using Artificial Intelligence to Promote Equitable Care for Inpatients With Language Barriers and Complex Medical Needs: Clinical Stakeholder Perspectives. *Journal of the American Medical Informatics Association : JAMIA*, *31*(3), 611–621. DOI: 10.1093/jamia/ocad224 PMID: 38099504

Baskara, R., & Mukarto, M. (2023). Exploring the implications of ChatGPT for language learning in higher education. *Indonesian Journal of English Language Teaching and Applied Linguistics*, *7*(2), 343–358. DOI: 10.21093/ijeltal.v7i2.1387

Bastable, S. B., Sopczyk, D., Gramet, P., & Jacobs, K. (2019). *Health professional as educator: principles of teaching and learning: principles of teaching and learning*. Jones & Bartlett Learning.

Beatty, A. E., Esco, A., Curtiss, A. B., & Ballen, C. J. (2022). Students who prefer face-to-face tests outperform their online peers in organic chemistry. *Chemistry Education Research and Practice*, *23*(2), 464–474. DOI: 10.1039/D1RP00324K

Bedarf, P., Dutto, A., Zanini, M., & Dillenburger, B. (2021). Foam 3D printing for construction: A review of applications, materials, and processes. *Automation in Construction*, *130*, 103861. DOI: 10.1016/j.autcon.2021.103861

Benoit, B., Frédéric, B., & Jean-Charles, D. (2022). Current state of dental informatics in the field of health information systems: A scoping review. *BMC Oral Health*, *22*(1), 131. DOI: 10.1186/s12903-022-02163-9 PMID: 35439988

Bergeler, E., & Read, M. F. (2021). Comparing learning outcomes and satisfaction of an online algebra-based physics course with a face-to-face course. *Journal of Science Education and Technology*, *30*(1), 97–111. DOI: 10.1007/s10956-020-09878-w

Berlivet, L., & Löwy, I. (2020). Hydroxychloroquine controversies: Clinical trials, epistemology, and the democratization of science. *Medical Anthropology Quarterly*, *34*(4), 525–541. DOI: 10.1111/maq.12622 PMID: 33210338

Binks, A. P., LeClair, R. J., Willey, J. M., Brenner, J. M., Pickering, J. D., Moore, J. S., Huggett, K. N., Everling, K. M., Arnott, J. A., Croniger, C. M., Zehle, C. H., Kranea, N. K., & Schwartzstein, R. M. (2021). Changing medical education, overnight: The curricular response to COVID-19 of nine medical schools. *Teaching and Learning in Medicine*, *33*(3), 334–342. DOI: 10.1080/10401334.2021.1891543 PMID: 33706632

Blease, C., & Rodman, A. (2024). 2024/12/09). Generative Artificial Intelligence in Mental Healthcare: An Ethical Evaluation. *Current Treatment Options in Psychiatry*, *12*(1), 5. DOI: 10.1007/s40501-024-00340-x

Bonny, T., Al Nassan, W., Obaideen, K., Al Mallahi, M. N., Mohammad, Y., & El-Damanhoury, H. M. (2023). Contemporary Role and Applications of Artificial Intelligence in Dentistry. *F1000 Research*, *12*, 1179. DOI: 10.12688/f1000research.140204.1 PMID: 37942018

Boscardin, C. K., Gin, B., Golde, P. B., & Hauer, K. E. (2024). ChatGPT and Generative Artificial Intelligence for Medical Education: Potential Impact and Opportunity. *Academic Medicine*, *99*(1), 22–27. Advance online publication. DOI: 10.1097/ACM.0000000000005439 PMID: 37651677

Bouabdellah, M. (2023). Digital Innovation in Healthcare. In Bouarar, A., Mouloudj, K., & Martínez Asanza, D. (Eds.), *Integrating Digital Health Strategies for Effective Administration* (pp. 1–19). IGI Global., DOI: 10.4018/978-1-6684-8337-4.ch001

Bouarar, A. C., Asanza, D. M., Mouloudj, S., Bouarar, A., Mouloudj, K., & Bozorgi, M. (2024). Elderly's Intention to Use Teledentistry Services: Antecedents and Challenges. In Martínez Asanza, D. (Ed.), *Geriatric Dentistry in the Age of Digital Technology* (pp. 101–116). IGI Global., DOI: 10.4018/979-8-3693-0260-6.ch004

Boulos, M. N. K., Brewer, A. C., Karimkhani, C., Buller, D. B., & Dellavalle, R. P. (2014). Mobile medical and health apps: State of the art, concerns, regulatory control and certification. *Online Journal of Public Health Informatics*, *5*(3). Advance online publication. DOI: 10.5210/ojphi.v5i3.4814 PMID: 24683442

Bozkurt, A. (2021). *Surfing on three waves of MOOCs: An examination and snapshot of research in Massive Open Online Courses*. Open Praxis.

Bozkurt, A., Xiao, J., Farrow, R., Bai, J. Y. H., Nerantzi, C., Moore, S., Dron, J., Stracke, C. M., Singh, L., Crompton, H., Koutropoulos, A., Terentev, E., Pazurek, A., Nichols, M., Sidorkin, A. M., Costello, E., Watson, S., Mulligan, D., Honeychurch, S., & Asino, T. I. (2024). The Manifesto for Teaching and Learning in a Time of Generative AI: A Critical Collective Stance to Better Navigate the Future. *Open Praxis*, *16*(4), 487–513. DOI: 10.55982/openpraxis.16.4.777

Brand, G., Sheers, C., Wise, S., Seubert, L., Clifford, R., Griffiths, P., & Etherton-Beer, C. (2021). A research approach for co-designing education with healthcare consumers. *Medical Education*, *55*(5), 574–581. DOI: 10.1111/medu.14411 PMID: 33155301

Braunack-Mayer, A. J., Street, J. M., Tooher, R., Feng, X., & Scharling-Gamba, K. (2020). Student and staff perspectives on the use of big data in the tertiary education sector: A scoping review and reflection on the ethical issues. *Review of Educational Research*, *90*(6), 788–823. DOI: 10.3102/0034654320960213

Breton, M., Sullivan, E. E., & Deville-Stoetzel, N. (2021). *Telehealth challenges during COVID-19 as reported by primary healthcare physicians in Quebec and Massachusetts*. BMC Family. DOI: 10.1186/s12875-021-01543-4

Bugliarello, G. (2000). Reflections on technological literacy. *Bulletin of Science, Technology & Society*, *20*(2), 83–89. DOI: 10.1177/027046760002000201

Buja, L. M. (2019). Medical Education Today: All That Glitters is Not Gold. *BMC Medical Education*, *19*(1), 1–11. DOI: 10.1186/s12909-019-1535-9 PMID: 30991988

Busch, F., Hoffmann, L., Truhn, D., Ortiz-Prado, E., Makowski, M. R., Bressem, K. K., Adams, L. C., Abdala, N., Navarro, Á. A., Aerts, H. J. W. L., Águas, C., Aineseder, M., Alomar, M., Angkurawaranon, S., Angus, Z. G., Asouchidou, E., Bakhshi, S., Bamidis, P. D., Barbosa, P. N. V. P., & Zhang, L. (2024). Global cross-sectional student survey on AI in medical, dental, and veterinary education and practice at 192 faculties. *BMC Medical Education*, *24*(1), 1066. DOI: 10.1186/s12909-024-06035-4 PMID: 39342231

Cai, Y. Q., Gong, D. X., Tang, L. Y., Cai, Y., Li, H. J., Jing, T. C., Gong, M., Hu, W., Zhang, Z. W., Zhang, X., & Zhang, G. W. (2024). Pitfalls in Developing Machine Learning Models for Predicting Cardiovascular Diseases: Challenge and Solutions [Article]. *Journal of Medical Internet Research, 26*, e47645. Advance online publication. DOI: 10.2196/47645 PMID: 38869157

Çakmakkaya, Ö. S., Jaremko, K. M., Kitapçıoğlu, D., & Wolpaw, J. (2025). Orthopedic Anesthesia Training: A Narrative Review on Program Development [Article]. *Current Anesthesiology Reports*, *15*(1), 4. Advance online publication. DOI: 10.1007/s40140-024-00669-2

Campbell, S. D., Cooper, L., Craddock, H., Hyde, T. P., Nattress, B., Pavitt, S. H., & Seymour, D. W. (2017). Removable partial dentures: The clinical need for innovation. *The Journal of Prosthetic Dentistry*, *118*(3), 273–280. DOI: 10.1016/j.prosdent.2017.01.008 PMID: 28343666

Capuano, N., & Caballé, S. (2020). Adaptive Learning Technologies. *AI Magazine*, *41*(2), 96–98. DOI: 10.1609/aimag.v41i2.5317

Cardullo, V., Wang, C. H., Burton, M., & Dong, J. (2021). K-12 teachers' remote teaching self-efficacy during the pandemic. *Journal of Research in Innovative Teaching & Learning*, *14*(1), 32–45. DOI: 10.1108/JRIT-10-2020-0055

Carrillo, C., & Flores, M. A. (2020). COVID-19 and teacher education: A literature review of online teaching and learning practices. *European Journal of Teacher Education*, *43*(4), 466–487. DOI: 10.1080/02619768.2020.1821184

Carvalho, L. F. C. S., & Zanatta, R. F. (2024). Editorial: Technological innovation for improved prevention and diagnosis of oral disease. *Frontiers in Oral Health*, *5*(1481890), 1481890. Advance online publication. DOI: 10.3389/froh.2024.1481890 PMID: 39355782

Casola— Rivera, W. (2020). El papel de la didáctica en los proceso de enseñanza y aprendizaje universitarios. *Comunicación (Cartago)*, *29*(1), 38–51. DOI: 10.18845/rc.v29i11-2020.5258

Castellano, M. S., Contreras-McKay, I., Neyem, A., Farfán, E., Inzunza, O., Ottone, N. E., del Sol, M., Alario-Hoyos, C., Alvarado, M. S., & Tubbs, R. S. (2024). Empowering human anatomy education through gamification and artificial intelligence: An innovative approach to knowledge appropriation. *Clinical Anatomy (New York, N.Y.)*, *37*(1), 12–24. DOI: 10.1002/ca.24074 PMID: 37453079

Castro-Schez, J. J., Glez-Morcillo, C., Albusac, J., & Vallejo, D. (2021). An Intelligent Tutoring System for Supporting Active Learning: A Case Study on Predictive Parsing Learning. *Information Sciences*, *544*, 446–468. DOI: 10.1016/j.ins.2020.08.079 PMID: 32958966

Caviezel, C., Grünwald, R., Ehrenberg-Silies, S., Kind, S., Jetzke, T., & Bovenschulte, M. (2017). *Additive Fertigungsverfahren (3D-Druck)—Innovationsanalyse*. Berlin, Germany: TAB Arbeitsbereicht. Retrieved May 22, 2024, from https://www.google.com/scholar

Cecilio-Fernandes, D., Parisi, M. C. R., Santos, T. M., & Sandars, J. (2020). The COVID-19 pandemic and the challenge of using technology for medical education in low and middle income countries.

CEPAL. (2018). *La Agenda 2030 y los Objetivos de Desarrollo Sostenible: una oportunidad para América Latina y el Caribe*. https://repositorio.cepal.org/bitstream/handle/11362/40155/24/S1801141_es.pdf

Cervantes, J., Smith, B., Ramadoss, T., D'Amario, V., Shoja, M. M., & Rajput, V. (2024). Decoding Medical Educators' Perceptions on Generative Artificial Intelligence in Medical Education. *Journal of Investigative Medicine*, *72*(7), 633–639. DOI: 10.1177/10815589241257215 PMID: 38785310

Chaleta, E., Saraiva, M., Leal, F., Fialho, I., & Borralho, A. (2021). Higher education and sustainable development goals (SDG)—Potential contribution of the undergraduate courses of the school of social sciences of the University of Évora. *Sustainability (Basel)*, *13*(4), 1828. DOI: 10.3390/su13041828

Chan, C. K. Y. (2023). A comprehensive AI policy education framework for university teaching and learning. *International Journal of Educational Technology in Higher Education*, *20*(1), 38. DOI: 10.1186/s41239-023-00408-3

Chandra, A., Nongkynrih, B., & Gupta, S. K. (2019). Role of smartphone technology in medical education in India. *Indian Journal of Community and Family Medicine*, *5*(2), 103–107. DOI: 10.4103/IJCFM.IJCFM_42_19

Chan, K. S., & Zary, N. (2019). Applications and challenges of implementing artificial intelligence in medical education: Integrative review. *JMIR Medical Education*, *5*(1), e13930. https://preprints.jmir.org/preprint/13930. DOI: 10.2196/13930 PMID: 31199295

Chankseliani, M., & McCowan, T. (2021). Higher education and the sustainable development goals. *Higher Education*, *81*(1), 1–8. DOI: 10.1007/s10734-020-00652-w PMID: 33173242

Chase, T. J., Julius, A., Chandan, J. S., Powell, E., Hall, C. S., Phillips, B. L., Burnett, R., Gill, D., & Fernando, B. (2018). Mobile learning in medicine: An evaluation of attitudes and behaviours of medical students. *BMC Medical Education, 18*(1), 1–8. DOI: 10.1186/s12909-018-1264-5 PMID: 29945579

Chen, C. H., & Tsai, C. C. (2021). In-service teachers' conceptions of mobile technology-integrated instruction: Tendency towards student-centered learning. *Computers & Education, 170*, 104224. https://doi.org/doi:10.1016/j.compedu.2021.104224

Cheng, L., Varshney, K. R., & Liu, H. (2021). Socially responsible AI algorithms: Issues, purposes, and challenges. *Journal of Artificial Intelligence Research, 71*, 1137–1181. DOI: 10.1613/jair.1.12814

Chen, H., Gomez, C., Huang, C. M., & Unberath, M. (2022). Explainable medical imaging AI needs human-centered design: Guidelines and evidence from a systematic review. *NPJ Digital Medicine, 5*(1), 156. DOI: 10.1038/s41746-022-00699-2 PMID: 36261476

Chen, J., Zhao, L., & Zhou, K. (2022). Multi-jet fusion 3D voxel printing of conductive elastomers. *Advanced Materials, 34*(47), e2205909. DOI: 10.1002/adma.202205909 PMID: 36125341

Chen, M., Wang, R., Zhou, Y., He, Z., Liu, X., He, M., & Tao, G. (2022). Digital medical education empowered by intelligent fabric space. *National Science Open, 1*(1), 20220011. DOI: 10.1360/nso/20220011

Chen, Y., & Esmaeilzadeh, P. (2024). Generative AI in Medical Practice: In-Depth Exploration of Privacy and Security Challenges. *Journal of Medical Internet Research, 26*, 1–19. DOI: 10.2196/53008 PMID: 38457208

Cherkowski, S., Kutsyuruba, B., & Walker, K. (2020). Positive leadership: Animating purpose, presence, passion and play for flourishing in schools. *Journal of Educational Administration, 58*(4), 401–415. DOI: 10.1108/JEA-04-2019-0076

Chérrez-Ojeda, I., Vera, C., Vanegas, E., Gallardo, J. C., Felix, M., Espinoza-Fuentes, F., Chedraui, P., Gavilanes, A. W. D., & Mata, V. L. (2020). The use of information and communication technologies in Latin American dentists: A cross-sectional study from Ecuador. *BMC Oral Health, 20*(1), 146. DOI: 10.1186/s12903-020-01137-z PMID: 32429887

Chisadza, C., Clance, M., Mthembu, T., Nicholls, N., & Yitbarek, E. (2021). Online and face-to-face learning: Evidence from students' performance during the COVID-19 pandemic. *African Development Review*, *33*(S1), S114–S125. DOI: 10.1111/1467-8268.12520 PMID: 38607902

Chiu, T. K., Meng, H., Chai, C. S., King, I., Wong, S., & Yam, Y. (2021). Creation and evaluation of a pretertiary artificial intelligence (AI) curriculum. *IEEE Transactions on Education*, *65*(1), 30–39. DOI: 10.1109/TE.2021.3085878

Chowdhury, P. N., Vaish, A., Puri, B., & Vaishya, R. (2024). Medical education technology: Past, present and future. *Apollo Medicine*, *21*(4), 374–380. DOI: 10.1177/09760016241256202

Chu, H., Yang, W., Sun, L., Cai, S., Yang, R., Liang, W., Yu, H., & Liu, L. (2020). 4D printing: A review on recent progresses. *Micromachines*, *11*(796), 1–15. DOI: 10.3390/mi11090796 PMID: 32842588

Chu, S. L., Garcia, B. M., & Rani, N. (2023, November). Research on wearable technologies for learning: A systematic review. [). Frontiers Media SA.]. *Frontiers in Education*, *8*, 1270389.

Civaner, M. M., Uncu, Y., Bulut, F., Chalil, E. G., & Tatli, A. (2022). Artificial intelligence in medical education: A cross-sectional needs assessment. *BMC Medical Education*, *22*(1), 772. DOI: 10.1186/s12909-022-03852-3 PMID: 36352431

Coates, W. C. (2025). Precision education–a call to action to transform medical education. *International Journal of Emergency Medicine*, *18*(1), 21. DOI: 10.1186/s12245-025-00819-1 PMID: 39924527

Cobb, C. D., & Mayer, J. D. (2000). Emotional intelligence. *Educational Leadership*, *58*(3), 14–18. DOI: 10.2190/dugg-p24e-52wk-6cdg

Coccia, M. (2019). Artifical intelligence technology in cancer imaging: Clinical challenges for detection of lung and breast cancer. *Journal of Social and Administrative Sciences*, *6*(2), 82–98. DOI: 10.1453/jsas.v6i2.1888

Coghlan, S., Miller, T., & Paterson, J. (2021). Good proctor or "big brother"? Ethics of online exam supervision technologies. *Philosophy & Technology*, *34*(4), 1581–1606. DOI: 10.1007/s13347-021-00476-1 PMID: 34485025

Comisión Económica para América Latina y el Caribe. CEPAL. (2018). La Agenda 2030 y los Objetivos de Desarrollo Sostenible: una oportunidad para América Latina y el Caribe. Disponible en: https://repositorio.cepal.org/bitstream/handle/11362/40155/24/S1801141_es.pdf

Conard, S. (2019). Best practices in digital health literacy. *International Journal of Cardiology*, *292*, 277–279. DOI: 10.1016/j.ijcard.2019.05.070 PMID: 31230937

Cook, D. A. (2024). Creating Virtual Patients Using Large Language Models: Scalable, Global, and Low Cost. *Medical Teacher*, *47*(1), 40–42. DOI: 10.1080/0142159X.2024.2376879 PMID: 38992981

Corpman, D. W. (2013). Mobile health in China: A review of research and programs in medical care, health education, and public health. *Journal of Health Communication*, *18*(11), 1345–1367. DOI: 10.1080/10810730.2013.778370 PMID: 23915211

Cortes-Briones, J. A., Tapia-Rivas, N. I., D'Souza, D. C., & Estevez, P. A. (2022). Going deep into schizophrenia with artificial intelligence. *Schizophrenia Research*, *245*, 122–140. DOI: 10.1016/j.schres.2021.05.018 PMID: 34103242

Costa, E. D., Brasil, D. M., Santaella, G. M., Cascante-Sequeira, D., Ludovichetti, F. S., & Freitas, D. Q. (2021). Digital technology in dental education during COVID-19 pandemic: Worldwide experience of professors and students. *Odovtos*, *23*(3), 179–208. DOI: 10.15517/ijds.2021.47770

Cox, G., Willmers, M., Brown, R., & Held, M. (2024). Learning along the Way: A Case Study on a Pedagogically Innovative Approach to Engage Medical Students in the Creation of Open Educational Resources Using ChatGPT. *Mousaion: South African Journal of Information Studies*, *42*(1), 1–21. DOI: 10.25159/2663-659X/15331

Coyne, E., Calleja, P., Forster, E., & Lin, F. (2021). A review of virtual-simulation for assessing healthcare students' clinical competency. *Nurse Education Today*, *96*, 104623. DOI: 10.1016/j.nedt.2020.104623 PMID: 33125979

Cranfield, D. J., Tick, A., Venter, I. M., Blignaut, R. J., & Renaud, K. (2021). Higher education students' perceptions of online learning during COVID-19—A comparative study. *Education Sciences*, *11*(8), 403. DOI: 10.3390/educsci11080403

Criollo-C, S., Guerrero-Arias, A., Jaramillo-Alcázar, Á., & Luján-Mora, S. (2021). Mobile learning technologies for education: Benefits and pending issues. *Applied Sciences (Basel, Switzerland)*, *11*(9), 4111. DOI: 10.3390/app11094111

Crompton, H. (2013). A historical overview of mobile learning: Toward learner-centered education. In Berge, Z. L., & Muilenburg, L. Y. (Eds.), *Handbook of mobile learning* (pp. 3–14)., https://www.academia.edu/5601076/A_historical_overview_of_mobile_learning_Toward_learner_centered_education

Cross, J. L., Choma, M. A., & Onofrey, J. A. (2024). Bias in Medical AI: Implications for Clinical Decision-Making. *PLOS Digital Health*, *3*(11), 1–19. DOI: 10.1371/journal.pdig.0000651 PMID: 39509461

Cui, X., Zhao, Z., Zhang, T., Guo, W., Guo, W., Zheng, J., Zhang, J., Dong, C., Na, R., Zheng, L., Li, W., Liu, Z., Ma, J., Wang, J., He, S., Xu, Y., Si, P., Shen, Y., & Cai, C. (2021). A systematic review and meta-analysis of children with coronavirus disease 2019 (COVID-19). *Journal of Medical Virology*, *93*(2), 1057–1069. DOI: 10.1002/jmv.26398 PMID: 32761898

Currie, G., Robbie, S., & Tually, P. (2023). ChatGPT and Patient Information in Nuclear Medicine: GPT-3.5 Versus GPT-4 [Article]. *Journal of Nuclear Medicine Technology*, *51*(4), 307–313. DOI: 10.2967/jnmt.123.266151 PMID: 37699647

Curum, B., & Khedo, K. K. (2021). Cognitive load management in mobile learning systems: Principles and theories. *Journal of Computers in Education*, *8*(1), 109–136. DOI: 10.1007/s40692-020-00173-6

Daher, R., Ardu, S., di Bella, E., Krejci, I., & Duc, O. (2024). Efficiency of 3D printed composite resin restorations compared with subtractive materials: Evaluation of fatigue behavior, cost, and time of production. *The Journal of Prosthetic Dentistry*, *131*(5), 943–950. DOI: 10.1016/j.prosdent.2022.08.001 PMID: 36333176

Daher, R., Krejci, I., & Ardu, S. (2024). Time-and cost-effective 3-dimensional-printing workflow to rehabilitate worn dentitions: A clinical report. *The Journal of Prosthetic Dentistry*, *131*(6), 996–999. DOI: 10.1016/j.prosdent.2023.02.013 PMID: 36959005

Dai, C.-P., & Ke, F. (2022). Educational Applications of Artificial Intelligence in Simulation-Based Learning: A Systematic Mapping Review. *Computers and Education: Artificial Intelligence*, *3*, 1–17. DOI: 10.1016/j.caeai.2022.100087

Daniel, M., Gordon, M., Patricio, M., Hider, A., Pawlik, C., Bhagdev, R., Ahmad, S., Alston, S., Park, S., Pawlikowska, T., Rees, E., Doyle, A. J., Pammi, M., Thammasitboon, S., Haas, M., Peterson, W., Lew, M., Khamees, D., Spadafore, M., & Stojan, J. (2021). An update on developments in medical education in response to the COVID-19 pandemic: A BEME scoping review: BEME Guide No. 64. *Medical Teacher*, *43*(3), 253–271. DOI: 10.1080/0142159X.2020.1864310 PMID: 33496628

Dao, X.-Q., Le, N.-B., & Nguyen, T.-M.-T. (2021). AI-Powered MOOCs: Video Lecture Generation. *Proceedings of the 2021 3rd International Conference on Image, Video and Signal Processing*, 95–102. https://doi.org/DOI: 10.1145/3459212.3459227

Dash, S., Shakyawar, S. K., Sharma, M., & Kaushik, S. (2019). Big data in healthcare: Management, analysis and future prospects. *Journal of Big Data*, *6*(1), 1–25. DOI: 10.1186/s40537-019-0217-0

DaSilva, A.F., Robinson, M.A., Shi, W., & McCauley, L.K. (2022). The Forefront of Dentistry Promising Tech-Innovations and New Treatments. *JDR clinical and translational research*, 7(1-suppl), 16S-24S. https://doi.org/DOI: 10.1177/23800844221116850

Datta, R., Upadhyay, K. K., & Jaideep, C. N. (2012). Simulation and its role in medical education. *Medical Journal, Armed Forces India*, *68*(2), 167–172. DOI: 10.1016/S0377-1237(12)60040-9 PMID: 24623932

Daud, A., Matoug-Elwerfelli, M., Khalid, A., & Ali, K. (2024). The impact of virtual reality haptic simulators in pre-clinical restorative dentistry: A qualitative enquiry into dental students' perceptions. *BMC Oral Health*, *24*(1), 988. DOI: 10.1186/s12903-024-04704-w PMID: 39180025

Davies, E. (2024). Health simulation through the lens of self-determination theory — Opportunities and pathways for discovery. *Advances in Simulation (London, England)*, *9*(1), 31. DOI: 10.1186/s41077-024-00304-4 PMID: 39039553

Davis, F. D., Bagozzi, R. P., & Warshaw, P. R. (1989). User Acceptance of Computer Technology : A Comparison of Two Theoretical Models. *Management Science*, *35*(8), 982–1003. DOI: 10.1287/mnsc.35.8.982

Dawood, A., Marti, B., Sauret Jackson, V., & Darwood, A. (2015). 3D printing in dentistry. *British Dental Journal*, *219*(11), 521–529. DOI: 10.1038/sj.bdj.2015.914 PMID: 26657435

DeCook, R., Muffly, B. T., Mahmood, S., Holland, C. T., Ayeni, A. M., Ast, M. P., Bolognese, M. P., Guild, G. N.III, Sheth, N. P., Pean, C. A., & Premkumar, A. (2024). 2024/06/01/). AI-Generated Graduate Medical Education Content for Total Joint Arthroplasty: Comparing ChatGPT Against Orthopaedic Fellows. *Arthroplasty Today*, *27*, 101412. https://doi.org/https://doi.org/10.1016/j.artd.2024.101412. DOI: 10.1016/j.artd.2024.101412 PMID: 38912098

Dedeilia, A., Sotiropoulos, M. G., Hanrahan, J. G., Janga, D., Dedeilias, P., & Sideris, M. (2020). Medical and surgical education challenges and innovations in the COVID-19 era: A systematic review. *In Vivo (Athens, Greece)*, *34*(3, Suppl), 1603–1611. DOI: 10.21873/invivo.11950 PMID: 32503818

Della Bona, A., Cantelli, V., Britto, V. T., Collares, K. F., & Stansbury, J. W. (2021). 3D printing restorative materials using a stereolithographic technique: A systematic review. *Dental Materials*, *37*(2), 336–350. DOI: 10.1016/j.dental.2020.11.030 PMID: 33353734

Di Fede, O., La Mantia, G., Cimino, M. G. C. A., & Campisi, G. (2023). Protection of patient data in digital oral and general health care: A scoping review with respect to the current regulations.

Díaz Lozada, J. A., & de la Rúa Batistapau, M. (2022). Uso de las TIC en la preparación docente de profesores en condiciones de distanciamiento social. Mendive. *Review of Education*, *20*(1), 172–182.

Dickens, G. L., Watson, F., Schoultz, M., Kemp, C., Ion, R., Hallett, N., & Al Maqbali, M. (2024). Mental health risk assessment and safety planning during UK Covid-19 pandemic lockdown: Mixed methods survey and interview study. *Issues in Mental Health Nursing*, *45*(10), 1111–1119. DOI: 10.1080/01612840.2024.2415468 PMID: 39447076

Dixon, D., Sattar, H., Moros, N., Kesireddy, S. R., Ahsan, H., Lakkimsetti, M., Fatima, M., Doshi, D., Sadhu, K., & Junaid Hassan, M. (2024). Unveiling the Influence of AI Predictive Analytics on Patient Outcomes: A Comprehensive Narrative Review. *Cureus*, *16*(5), e59954. DOI: 10.7759/cureus.59954 PMID: 38854327

Dowling, M., & Cooney, A. (2012). Research approaches related to phenomenology: Negotiating a complex landscape. *Nurse Researcher*, *20*(2), 21–27. DOI: 10.7748/nr2012.11.20.2.21.c9440 PMID: 23316534

Doyumgaç, I., Tanhan, A., & Kiymaz, M. S. (2021). Understanding the most important facilitators and barriers for online education during COVID-19 through online photovoice methodology. *International Journal of Higher Education*, *10*(1), 166–190. DOI: 10.5430/ijhe.v10n1p166

Duchac, J. N., & Duchac, N. E. (2023). A servant leadership model of social awareness development in a higher education non-profit setting. *Emotional Intelligence in Organizational Leadership*, *13*(1), 67.

Dunn, P., & Hazzard, E. (2019). Technology approaches to digital health literacy. *International Journal of Cardiology*, *293*, 294–296. DOI: 10.1016/j.ijcard.2019.06.039 PMID: 31350037

Ebnali Harari, R., Altaweel, A., Ahram, T., Keehner, M., & Shokoohi, H. (2025). A randomized controlled trial on evaluating clinician-supervised generative AI for decision support [Article]. *International Journal of Medical Informatics*, *195*, 105701. Advance online publication. DOI: 10.1016/j.ijmedinf.2024.105701 PMID: 39631268

Elbanna, S., & Armstrong, L. (2024). Exploring the integration of ChatGPT in education: Adapting for the future. *Management & Sustainability: An Arab Review*, *3*(1), 16–29. DOI: 10.1108/MSAR-03-2023-0016

Elfirdoussi, S., Lachgar, M., Kabaili, H., Rochdi, A., Goujdami, D., & El Firdoussi, L. (2020). Assessing distance learning in higher education during the COVID-19 pandemic. *Education Research International, 2020*(1), 8890633. DOI: 10.1155/2020/8890633

Elhaddad, M., & Hamam, S. (2024). AI-Driven Clinical Decision Support Systems: An Ongoing Pursuit of Potential. *Cureus, 16*(4), 1–9. DOI: 10.7759/cureus.57728 PMID: 38711724

Ellis, L. D. (August 30, 2024). Exploring current trends in medical education. Harvard Medical School. https://postgraduateeducation.hms.harvard.edu/trends-medicine/benefits-latest-ai-technologies-patients-clinicians

El-Sofany, H., & El-Haggar, N. (2020). The effectiveness of using mobile learning techniques to improve learning outcomes in higher education. https://doi.org/DOI: 10.3991/ijim.v14i08.13125

Elundu, C., Amaechi, D. C., Okatta, A. U., Amaechi, E. C., Elundu, T. C., Ezeh, C. P., & Elundu, I. D. (2024). The impact of Simulation-based training in medical education. *Revista de Medicina (São Paulo), 103*(27), e38813. DOI: 10.1097/MD.0000000000038813 PMID: 38968472

Emosda, E., & Annisa, V. (2020, May). Digital literacy skills on the generation of digital immigrants. In *Proceeding of International Conference on Social Sciences* (pp. 81–88).

Enoch, L. C., Abraham, R. M., & Singaram, V. S. (2022). A comparative analysis of the impact of online, blended, and face-to-face learning on medical students' clinical competency in the affective, cognitive, and. *BMC Medical Education, 22*(1), 753. DOI: 10.1186/s12909-022-03777-x PMID: 36320031

Erdilek, D., Gümüştaş, B., & Güray Efes, B. (2023). Digitalization era of dental education: A systematic review. *Dental and Medical Problems, 60*(3), 513–525. DOI: 10.17219/dmp/156804 PMID: 37747703

Escobar-Taipe, A. M., Rivera-Marcatinco, M., Veliz-Vicharra, S., & Mattos-Vela, M. A. (2023). La digitalización en la formación odontológica. *Revista de la Facultad de Odontología Universidad de Antioquia, 35*(1), 62–75. DOI: 10.17533/udea.rfo.v35n1a5

Estes, J. S. (2017). Teacher preparation programs and learner-centred, technology-integrated instruction. In *Handbook of Research on Learner-centred Pedagogy in Teacher Education and Professional Development* (pp. 85–103). IGI Global. DOI: 10.4018/978-1-5225-0892-2.ch005

European Health Parliament. (2016). *Digital Skills for Health Professionals.* https://www.healthparliament.eu/wp-content/uploads/2017/09/Digital-skills-for-health-professionals.pdf

Evans, C., & Robertson, W. (2020). The four phases of the digital natives debate. *Human Behavior and Emerging Technologies, 2*(3), 269–277. DOI: 10.1002/hbe2.196

Eysenbach, G. (2023). The role of ChatGPT, generative language models, and artificial intelligence in medical education: A conversation with ChatGPT and a call for papers. *JMIR Medical Education, 9*, e46885. DOI: 10.2196/46885 PMID: 36863937

Farah, S., Anderson, D. G., & Langer, R. (2016). Physical and mechanical properties of PLA, and their functions in widespread applications—A comprehensive review. *Advanced Drug Delivery Reviews, 107*, 367–392. DOI: 10.1016/j.addr.2016.06.012 PMID: 27356150

Fariah, F., Mahato, S., Pattanaik, C. R., & Mohanty, S. N. (2024). Application of wearable devices in the medical domain. In *Reconnoiter*. Taylor & Francis., DOI: 10.1201/9781003401841-7

Fariani, R. I., Junus, K., & Santoso, H. B. (n.d.). A systematic literature review on personalised learning in the higher education context. *Technology*.

Fatima, N.. (2024). The role of feedback in enhancing creative writing skills in ELT contexts. *Remittances Review, 9*(3), 350–368.

Fatima, S., Haleem, A., Bahl, S., Javaid, M., Mahla, S. K., & Singh, S. (2021). Exploring the significant applications of internet of things (IoT) with 3D printing using advanced materials in medical field. *Materials Today: Proceedings, 45*(6), 4844–4851. DOI: 10.1016/j.matpr.2021.01.305

Faust, J. L., & Paulson, D. R. (1998). Active learning in the college classroom. *Journal on Excellence in College Teaching, 9*(2), 3–24.

Fawaz, M., El-Malti, W., Alreshidi, S. M., & Kavuran, E. (2025). Exploring Health Sciences Students' Perspectives on Using Generative Artificial Intelligence in Higher Education: A Qualitative Study [Article]. *Nursing & Health Sciences, 27*(1), e70030. Advance online publication. DOI: 10.1111/nhs.70030 PMID: 39797529

Fawns, T., Jones, D., & Aitken, G. (2020). Challenging assumptions about "moving online" in response to COVID-19, and some practical advice. *MedEdPublish*.

Feigerlova, E., Hani, H., & Hothersall-Davies, E. (2025). A Systematic Review of the Impact of Artificial Intelligence on Educational Outcomes in Health Professions Education. *BMC Medical Education*, *25*(1), 1–18. DOI: 10.1186/s12909-025-06719-5 PMID: 39871336

Fernández-Herrero, J. (2024). Evaluating Recent Advances in Affective Intelligent Tutoring Systems: A Scoping Review of Educational Impacts and Future Prospects [Review]. *Education Sciences*, *14*(8), 839. Advance online publication. DOI: 10.3390/educsci14080839

Ferrier, B., Lee, J., Mbuli, A., & James, D. A. (2022). Translational applications of wearable sensors in education: Implementation and efficacy. *Sensors (Basel)*, *22*(4), 1675. DOI: 10.3390/s22041675 PMID: 35214578

Fitria, T. N. (2021). *Artificial intelligence (AI) in education: Using AI tools for teaching and learning process*. Prosiding Seminar Nasional & Call for Paper STIE AAS.

Francis, N. J., Jones, S., & Smith, D. P. (2025). 2025-January-09). Generative AI in Higher Education: Balancing Innovation and Integrity [Review]. *British Journal of Biomedical Science*, *81*, 14048. Advance online publication. DOI: 10.3389/bjbs.2024.14048 PMID: 39850144

Franco D'Souza, R., Mathew, M., Mishra, V., & Mohan Surapaneni, K. (2024). Twelve tips for addressing ethical concerns in the implementation of artificial intelligence in medical education.

Franco D'Souza, R., Mathew, M., Mishra, V., & Surapaneni, K. M. (2024). Twelve tips for addressing ethical concerns in the implementation of artificial intelligence in medical education. *Medical Education Online*, *29*(1), 2330250. DOI: 10.1080/10872981.2024.2330250 PMID: 38566608

Freebody, P. (2003). *Qualitative Research in Education: Interaction and Practice*. SAGE Publications. DOI: 10.4135/9781849209670

Frenk, J., Chen, L. C., Chandran, L., Groff, E. O. H., King, R., Meleis, A., & Fineberg, H. V. (2022). Challenges and opportunities for educating health professionals after the COVID-19 pandemic. *Lancet*, *400*(10362), 1539–1556. DOI: 10.1016/S0140-6736(22)02092-X PMID: 36522209

Frenk, J., Chen, L., Bhutta, Z. A., Cohen, J., Crisp, N., Evans, T., Fineberg, H., Garcia, P., Ke, Y., Kelley, P., Kistnasamy, B., Meleis, A., Naylor, D., Pablos-Mendez, A., Reddy, S., Scrimshaw, S., Sepulveda, J., Serwadda, D., & Zurayk, H. (2010). Health professionals for a new century: Transforming education to strengthen health systems in an interdependent world. *Lancet*, *376*(9756), 1923–1958. DOI: 10.1016/S0140-6736(10)61854-5 PMID: 21112623

Froese, T., Richter, M., Hofmann, F., & Lüdeke-Freund, F. (2023). Degrowth-oriented organisational value creation: A systematic literature review of case studies. *Ecological Economics*, *207*, 107765. DOI: 10.1016/j.ecolecon.2023.107765

Fukuhara-Nakama, M., Chávez-Alayo, P., Flores-Mas, R., Fernández-Jacinto, L., Castilla-Camacho, M., Maldonado-Mendoza, M., & Loechle-Verde, O. (2023). Introducción de la tecnología CAD-CAM en la educación dental: Una mirada desde los estudiantes y los docentes. *Revista Estomatológica Herediana*, *33*(4), 372–376. DOI: 10.20453/reh.v33i4.5123

Fu, L., Wang, B., Yuan, T., Chen, X., Ao, Y., Fitzpatrick, T., Li, P., Zhou, Y., Lin, Y., Duan, Q., Luo, G., Fan, S., Lu, Y., Feng, A., Zhan, Y., Liang, B., Cai, W., Zhang, L., Du, X., & Zou, H. (2020). Clinical characteristics of coronavirus disease 2019 (COVID-19) in China: A systematic review and meta-analysis. *The Journal of Infection*, *80*(6), 656–665. DOI: 10.1016/j.jinf.2020.03.041 PMID: 32283155

Fu, Y., Chu, F., Lu, X., Wang, C., Xiao, N., Jiang, J., Zheng, J., & Jiang, H. (2024). Assessment and evaluation of online education and virtual simulation technology in dental education: A cross-sectional survey. *BMC Medical Education*, *24*(1), 191. DOI: 10.1186/s12909-024-05171-1 PMID: 38403582

Galante, R., Figueiredo-Pina, C. G., & Serro, A. P. (2019). Additive manufacturing of ceramics for dental applications: A review. *Dental Materials*, *35*(6), 825–846. DOI: 10.1016/j.dental.2019.02.026 PMID: 30948230

García-Ancira, C., & Treviño-Cubero, A. (2020). Las competencias universitarias y el perfil de egreso. *RevistaEstudios del desarrollo social: Cuba y América Latina,* 8 (1). http://scielo.sld.cu/scielo.php?script=sci_arttext&pid=S12308-013220200003&lng=es&tlng=es

Garcia, M. B., & Almeida, R. P. P. (2024). *Emerging technologies for health literacy and medical practice*. IGI Global., DOI: 10.4018/979-8-3693-1214-8

Garcia, M. B., Arif, Y. M., Khlaif, Z. N., Zhu, M., de Almeida, R. P., de Almeida, R. S., & Masters, K. (2024). Effective Integration of Artificial Intelligence in Medical Education: Practical Tips and Actionable Insights. In Garcia, M., & de Almeida, R. (Eds.), *Transformative Approaches to Patient Literacy and Healthcare Innovation* (pp. 1–19). IGI Global., DOI: 10.4018/979-8-3693-3661-8.ch001

Garcia, M. B., de Almeida, R. P. P., Arif, Y. M., Miranda, J. P. P., Tavares, D. P., Tariq, M. U., de Almeida, R. S., & López, M. (2025). Technology-Enhanced Learning in Health Professions Education: Current Trends and Applications. In Jesus, Â. (Ed.), *Technological Approaches to Medical and Pharmaceutical Education* (pp. 455–488). IGI Global., DOI: 10.4018/979-8-3373-1127-2.ch013

Garcia, M. B., Garcia, P. S., Maaliw, R. R.III, Lagrazon, P. G. G., Arif, Y. M., Ofosu-Ampong, K., Yousef, A. M. F., & Vaithilingam, C. A. (2024). Technoethical Considerations for Advancing Health Literacy and Medical Practice: A Posthumanist Framework in the Age of Healthcare 5.0. In *Emerging Technologies for Health Literacy and Medical Practice*. IGI Global., DOI: 10.4018/979-8-3693-1214-8.ch001

Garcia, P. P., Wambier, L. M., de Geus, J. L., da Cunha, L. F., Correr, G. M., & Gonzaga, C. C. (2019). Do anterior and posterior teeth treated with post-and-core restorations have similar failure rates? A systematic review and meta-analysis. *The Journal of Prosthetic Dentistry*, *121*(6), 887–894.e4. DOI: 10.1016/j.prosdent.2018.08.004 PMID: 30617032

Garg, T. (2020). Artificial intelligence in medical education. *The American Journal of Medicine*, *133*(2), e68. DOI: 10.1016/j.amjmed.2019.08.017 PMID: 31954481

Gaur, U., Majumder, M. A. A., Sa, B., Sarkar, S., Williams, A., & Singh, K. (2020). Challenges and opportunities of preclinical medical education: COVID-19 crisis and beyond. *SN Comprehensive Clinical Medicine*, *2*(11), 1992–1997. DOI: 10.1007/s42399-020-00528-1 PMID: 32984766

Gavali, M. Y., Khismatrao, D. S., Gavali, Y. V., & Patil, K. B. (2017). Smartphone, the new learning aid amongst medical students. *Journal of Clinical and Diagnostic Research : JCDR*, *11*(5), JC05–JC08. DOI: 10.7860/JCDR/2017/20948.9826 PMID: 28658804

Gawali, N., Shah, P. P., Gowdar, I. M., Bhavsar, K. A., Giri, D., & Laddha, R. (2024). The Evolution of Digital Dentistry: A Comprehensive Review. *Journal of Pharmacy & Bioallied Sciences*, *16*(Suppl 3), S1920–S1922. DOI: 10.4103/jpbs.jpbs_11_24 PMID: 39346228

Gellisch, M., Morosan-Puopolo, G., Brand-Saberi, B., & Schäfer, T. (2024). Adapting to new challenges in medical education: A three-step digitization approach for blended learning. *BMC Medical Education, 24*(1), 1–15. DOI: 10.1186/s12909-024-05503-1 PMID: 38807088

Genovese, A., Borna, S., Gomez-Cabello, C. A., Haider, S. A., Prabha, S., Forte, A. J., & Veenstra, B. R. (2024). Artificial Intelligence in Clinical Settings: A Systematic Review of Its Role in Language Translation and Interpretation. *Annals of Translational Medicine, 12*(6), 1–16. DOI: 10.21037/atm-24-162 PMID: 39817236

Georgieva-Tsaneva, G., Serbezova, I., & Beloeva, S. (2025). Application of virtual reality, artificial intelligence, and other innovative technologies in healthcare education (nursing and midwifery specialties): Challenges and strategies. *Education Sciences, 15*(1), 11. DOI: 10.3390/educsci15010011

Ghavami Hosein Pour, B., Karimian, Z., & Hatami Niya, N. (2025). A narrative review of advancing medical education through technology: The role of smart glasses in situated learning. *BMC Medical Education, 25*(1), 359. DOI: 10.1186/s12909-025-06949-7 PMID: 40065257

Giannakopoulos, K., Kavadella, A., Salim, A. A., Stamatopoulos, V., & Kaklamanos, E. G. (2023). Evaluation of the Performance of Generative AI Large Language Models ChatGPT, Google Bard, and Microsoft Bing Chat in Supporting Evidence-Based Dentistry: Comparative Mixed Methods Study [Article]. *Journal of Medical Internet Research, 25*(1), e51580. Advance online publication. DOI: 10.2196/51580 PMID: 38009003

Giannakos, M., Azevedo, R., Brusilovsky, P., Cukurova, M., Dimitriadis, Y., Hernandez-Leo, D., Järvelä, S., Mavrikis, M., & Rienties, B. (2024). The Promise and Challenges of Generative AI in Education. *Behaviour & Information Technology*, •••, 1–27. DOI: 10.1080/0144929X.2024.2394886

Gkrimpizi, T., Peristeras, V., & Magnisalis, I. (2023). Classification of barriers to digital transformation in higher education institutions: Systematic literature review. *Education Sciences, 13*(7), 746. DOI: 10.3390/educsci13070746

Gnaur, D., Svidt, K., & Thygesen, M. K. (2015). Developing students' collaborative skills in interdisciplinary learning environments. *International Journal of Engineering Education, 31*(1B), 257–266.

Goguta, L., Lungeanu, D., Negru, R., Birdeanu, M., Jivanescu, A., & Sinescu, C. (2021). Selective laser sintering versus selective laser melting and computer-aided design—Computer-aided manufacturing in double crowns retention. *Journal of Prosthodontic Research*, *65*(3), 371–378. DOI: 10.2186/jpr.JPOR_2019_556 PMID: 32981911

Goh, P. S., & Sandars, J. (2020). A vision of the use of technology in medical education after the COVID-19 pandemic. *MedEdPublish*. Advance online publication. DOI: 10.15694/mep.2020.000049.1 PMID: 38058893

Goisauf, M., & Cano Abadía, M. (2022). Ethics of AI in radiology: A review of ethical and societal implications. *Frontiers in Big Data*, *5*, 850383. DOI: 10.3389/fdata.2022.850383 PMID: 35910490

Gómez-González, E., Gomez, E., Márquez-Rivas, J., Guerrero-Claro, M., Fernández-Lizaranzu, I., Relimpio-López, M. I., & Capitán-Morales, L. (2020). Artificial intelligence in medicine and healthcare: A review and classification of current and near-future applications and their ethical and social. *Impact*. Advance online publication. arXiv2001.09778. DOI: 10.48550/arXiv.2001.09778

Gordon, M., Daniel, M., Ajiboye, A., Uraiby, H., Xu, N. Y., Bartlett, R., Hanson, J., Haas, M., Spadafore, M., Grafton-Clarke, C., Gasiea, R. Y., Michie, C., Corral, J., Kwan, B., Dolmans, D., & Thammasitboon, S. (2024). A Scoping Review of Artificial Intelligence in Medical Education: BEME Guide No. 84. *Medical Teacher*, *46*(4), 446–470. DOI: 10.1080/0142159X.2024.2314198 PMID: 38423127

Goulah-Pabst, D. M. (2023). Suicide loss survivors: Navigating social stigma and threats to social bonds. *Omega*, *87*(3), 769–792. DOI: 10.1177/00302228211026513 PMID: 34218692

Gracco, A., De Stefani, A., & Bruno, G. (2023). Influence of New Technology in Dental Care: A Public Health Perspective. *International Journal of Environmental Research and Public Health*, *20*(7), 5364. DOI: 10.3390/ijerph20075364 PMID: 37047978

Grant, M. C., Geoghegan, L., Arbyn, M., Mohammed, Z., McGuinness, L., Clarke, E. L., & Wade, R. G. (2020). The prevalence of symptoms in 24,410 adults infected by the novel coronavirus (SARS-CoV-2; COVID-19): A systematic review and meta-analysis of 148 studies from 9 countries. *PLoS One*, *15*(6), e0234765. DOI: 10.1371/journal.pone.0234765 PMID: 32574165

Grant, M. J., & Booth, A. (2009, June). A typology of reviews: An analysis of 14 review types and associated methodologies. *Health Information and Libraries Journal*, *26*(2), 91–108. DOI: 10.1111/j.1471-1842.2009.00848.x PMID: 19490148

Gravina, A. G., Pellegrino, R., Palladino, G., Imperio, G., Ventura, A., & Federico, A. (2024). 2024/08/01/). Charting new AI education in gastroenterology: Cross-sectional evaluation of ChatGPT and perplexity AI in medical residency exam. *Digestive and Liver Disease*, *56*(8), 1304–1311. https://doi.org/https://doi.org/10.1016/j.dld.2024.02.019. DOI: 10.1016/j.dld.2024.02.019 PMID: 38503659

Greenhow, C., & Galvin, S. (2020). Teaching with social media: Evidence-based strategies for making remote higher education less remote. *Information and Learning Science*, *121*(7/8), 513–524. DOI: 10.1108/ILS-04-2020-0138

Griffin, A. C., Wang, K. H., Leung, T. I., & Facelli, J. C. (2024). Recommendations to promote fairness and inclusion in biomedical AI research and clinical use [Article]. *Journal of Biomedical Informatics*, *157*, 104693. Advance online publication. DOI: 10.1016/j.jbi.2024.104693 PMID: 39019301

Grover, V., & Balusamy, B. MK, N., Anand, V., & Milanova, M. (Eds.). (2024). *Approaches to Human-centered AI in Healthcare*. IGI Global.

Grunhut, J., Marques, O., & Wyatt, A. T. (2022). Needs, challenges, and applications of artificial intelligence in medical education curriculum. *JMIR Medical Education*, *8*(2), e35587. DOI: 10.2196/35587 PMID: 35671077

Guan, C., Mou, J., & Jiang, Z. (2020). Artificial intelligence innovation in education: A twenty-year data-driven historical analysis. *International Journal of Innovation Studies*.

Gudmundsdottir, G. B., & Hatlevik, O. E. (2020). "I just Google it"–Developing professional digital competence and preparing student teachers to exercise responsible ICT use. [NJCIE]. *Nordic Journal of Comparative and International Education*, *4*(3), 39–55. DOI: 10.7577/njcie.3752

Guillodo, E., Lemey, C., Simonnet, M., Walter, M., Baca-García, E., Masetti, V., Moga, S., Larsen, M., Ropars, J., & Berrouiguet, S. (2020). Clinical applications of mobile health wearable–based sleep monitoring: Systematic review. *JMIR mHealth and uHealth*, *8*(4), e10733. DOI: 10.2196/10733 PMID: 32234707

Guraya, S. Y. (2024). Transforming Simulation in Healthcare to Enhance Interprofessional Collaboration Leveraging Big Data Analytics and Artificial Intelligence. *BMC Medical Education*, *24*(1), 941. Advance online publication. DOI: 10.1186/s12909-024-05916-y PMID: 39198809

Gurupur, V. P., Vu, G., Mayya, V., & King, C. (2024). The Need for Standards in Evaluating the Quality of Electronic Health Records and Dental Records: A Narrative Review. *Big Data and Cognitive Computing*, *8*(12), 168. DOI: 10.3390/bdcc8120168

Gu, T., Pan, W., Yu, J., Ji, G., Meng, X., Wang, Y., & Li, M. (2025). Mitigating bias in AI mortality predictions for minority populations: A transfer learning approach [Article]. *BMC Medical Informatics and Decision Making*, *25*(1), 30. Advance online publication. DOI: 10.1186/s12911-025-02862-7 PMID: 39825353

Gutierrez, G., Lunsky, I. O., Van Heer, S., Szulewski, A., & Chaplin, T. (2023). Cognitive load theory in action: E-learning modules improve performance in simulation-based education. A pilot study. *Canadian Journal of Emergency Medical Care*, *25*(11), 893–901. DOI: 10.1007/s43678-023-00586-z PMID: 37751082

Habs, M., Knecht, S., & Schmidt-Wilcke, T. (2025, 2025/03/18/). Using artificial intelligence (AI) for form and content checks of medical reports: Proofreading by ChatGPT4.0 in a neurology department. *Zeitschrift für Evidenz, Fortbildung und Qualität im Gesundheitswesen*. https://doi.org/https://doi.org/10.1016/j.zefq.2025.02.007

Haleem, A., Javaid, M. A., & Suman, R. (2022). Understanding the role of digital technologies in education: A review. *Sustainable Operations and Computers*, *3*, 275–285. DOI: 10.1016/j.susoc.2022.05.004

Hale, J., Alexander, S., Wright, S. T., & Gilliland, K. (2024). Generative AI in Undergraduate Medical Education: A Rapid Review. *Journal of Medical Education and Curricular Development*, *11*, 1–15. DOI: 10.1177/23821205241266697

Haltaufderheide, J., & Ranisch, R. (2024). The ethics of ChatGPT in medicine and healthcare: A systematic review on large language models (LLMs). *NPJ Digital Medicine*, *7*(1), 183. DOI: 10.1038/s41746-024-01157-x PMID: 38977771

Hanna, M. G., Pantanowitz, L., Jackson, B., Palmer, O., Visweswaran, S., Pantanowitz, J., Deebajah, M., & Rashidi, H. H. (2025). Ethical and Bias Considerations in Artificial Intelligence/Machine Learning. *Modern Pathology*, *38*(3), 1–13. DOI: 10.1016/j.modpat.2024.100686 PMID: 39694331

Han, Z., Battaglia, F., Udaiyar, A., Fooks, A., & Terlecky, S. R. (2024). An Explorative Assessment of ChatGPT as an Aid in Medical Education: Use It With Caution. *Medical Teacher*, *46*(5), 657–664. DOI: 10.1080/0142159X.2023.2271159 PMID: 37862566

Harari, G. M., Lane, N. D., Wang, R., Crosier, B. S., Campbell, A. T., & Gosling, S. D. (2016). Using smartphones to collect behavioral data in psychological science. *Perspectives on Psychological Science*, *11*(6), 838–854. DOI: 10.1177/1745691616650285 PMID: 27899727

Hardinata, S., Suchyadi, Y., & Wulandari, D. (2021). Strengthening technological literacy in junior high school teachers in the industrial revolution era 4.0. *Journal of Humanities and Social Studies*, *5*(3), 330–335.

Harries, A. J., Lee, C., Jones, L., Rodriguez, R. M., Davis, J. A., Boysen-Osborn, M., & Langsfeld, J. M. (2021). Effects of the COVID-19 pandemic on medical students: A multicenter quantitative study. *BMC Medical Education*, *21*(1), 1–8. DOI: 10.1186/s12909-020-02462-1 PMID: 33407422

Hasan, S. S., Woo, J. J., Cote, M. P., & Ramkumar, P. N. (2025). Generative Versus Nongenerative Artificial Intelligence [Article]. *Arthroscopy*, *41*(3), 545–546. DOI: 10.1016/j.arthro.2024.12.001 PMID: 39929595

Hattie, L. D., Sahlberg, C. W., & Comer, P. P. (2023). Impact of mobile learning apps on study habits and academic performance of college students in the United States: A review of literature. *Journal of Education*, *6*(3), 13–22. DOI: 10.53819/81018102t4182

Hayat, A. A., Keshavarzi, M. H., Zare, S., Bazrafcan, L., Rezaee, R., Faghihi, S. A., Amini, M., & Kojuri, J. (2021). Challenges and opportunities from the COVID-19 pandemic in medical education: A qualitative study. *BMC Medical Education*, *21*(1), 247. DOI: 10.1186/s12909-021-02682-z PMID: 33926439

Hays, R. B., Ramani, S., & Hassell, A. (2020). Healthcare systems and the sciences of health professional education. *Advances in Health Sciences Education : Theory and Practice*, *25*(5), 1149–1162. DOI: 10.1007/s10459-020-10010-1 PMID: 33206272

Hegedűs, M., Szivós, E., Adamopoulus, I., & Dávid, L. D. (2024). Hospital integration to improve the chances of recovery for decubitus (pressure ulcer) patients through centralised procurement procedures. *Journal of Infrastructure. Policy and Development*, *8*(10), 7273.

Hegedus, T., Kreuter, P., Kismarczi-Antalffy, A. A., Demeter, T., Banyai, D., Vegh, A., Geczi, Z., Hermann, P., Payer, M., Zsembery, A., Al-Hassiny, A., Mukaddam, K., Herber, V., Jakse, N., & Vegh, D. (2022). User experience and sustainability of 3D printing in dentistry. *International Journal of Environmental Research and Public Health*, *19*(4), 1921. DOI: 10.3390/ijerph19041921 PMID: 35206116

Hendricks, S., & Mwapwele, S. D. (2024). A systematic literature review on the factors influencing e-commerce adoption in developing countries. *Data and Information Management*, *8*(1), 100045. DOI: 10.1016/j.dim.2023.100045

Hensen, B., Mackworth-Young, C. R. S., Simwinga, M., Abdelmagid, N., Banda, J., Mavodza, C., Doyle, A. M., Bonell, C., & Weiss, H. A. (2021). Remote data collection for public health research in a COVID-19 era: Ethical implications, challenges and opportunities. *Health Policy and Planning*, *36*(3), 360–368. DOI: 10.1093/heapol/czaa158 PMID: 33881138

Herschdorfer, L., Negreiros, W., Gallucci, G., & Hamilton, A. (2020). Comparison of the accuracy of implants placed with CAD-CAM surgical templates manufactured with various 3D printers: An in vitro study. *The Journal of Prosthetic Dentistry*, *125*(6), 905–910. DOI: 10.1016/j.prosdent.2020.03.017 PMID: 32499166

Hilburg, R., Patel, N., Ambruso, S., Biewald, M. A., & Farouk, S. S. (2020). Medical education during the coronavirus disease-2019 pandemic: Learning from a distance. *Advances in Chronic Kidney Disease*, *27*(5), 412–417. DOI: 10.1053/j.ackd.2020.05.017 PMID: 33308507

Himi, S. T., Monalisa, N. T., Sultana, S., Afrin, A., & Hasib, K. M. (2024, 25-26 Sept. 2024). Automated Exam Script Checking using Zero-Shot LLM and Adaptive Generative AI. *2024 IEEE International Conference on Computing, Applications and Systems (COMPAS)*, 1-6. https://doi.org/DOI: 10.1109/COMPAS60761.2024.10795949

Hoffman, J., Wenke, R., Angus, R. L., Shinners, L., Richards, B., & Hattingh, L. (2025). Overcoming barriers and enabling artificial intelligence adoption in allied health clinical practice: A qualitative study. *Digital Health*, *11*, 20552076241311144. DOI: 10.1177/20552076241311144 PMID: 39906878

Hong, H., Dai, L., & Zheng, X. (2025). Advances in wearable sensors for learning analytics: Trends, challenges, and prospects. *Sensors (Basel)*, *25*(9), 2714. DOI: 10.3390/s25092714 PMID: 40363153

Horn, L. H., Jensen, C. G., Kjærgaard, T., Lukassen, B., Sørensen, I. M., Valbak-Andersen, C., & Bund-gaard, S. B. (2020). *White Paper on Reflective Practice-Based Learning*. University College of Northern Denmark.

Horn, T. J., & Harryson, O. L. A. (2012). Overview of current additive manufacturing technologies and selected applications. *Science Progress*, *95*(3), 255–282. DOI: 10.3184/003685012X13420984463047 PMID: 23094325

Hosen, M., Ogbeibu, S., Giridharan, B., Cham, T. H., Lim, W. M., & Paul, J. (2021). Individual motivation and social media influence on student knowledge sharing and learning performance: Evidence from an emerging economy. *Computers & Education*, *172*, 104262. DOI: 10.1016/j.compedu.2021.104262

Hossain, E., Rana, R., Higgins, N., Soar, J., Barua, P. D., Pisani, A. R., & Turner, K. (2023). Natural Language Processing in Electronic Health Records in Relation to Healthcare Decision-Making: A Systematic Review. *Computers in Biology and Medicine*, *155*, 1–24. DOI: 10.1016/j.compbiomed.2023.106649 PMID: 36805219

Hsiao, P. W., & Su, C. H. (2021). A study on the impact of STEAM education for sustainable development courses and its effects on student motivation and learning. *Sustainability (Basel)*, *13*(7), 3772. DOI: 10.3390/su13073772

Hsu, M. S., Yeh, C. L., Cheng, S. J., & Lin, C. P. (2025). Integrating digital technologies in dental technician education: A comparative study of national examination in Asian countries. *Journal of Dental Sciences*, *20*(1), 28–35. DOI: 10.1016/j.jds.2024.10.017 PMID: 39873091

Huang, L. (2023). *Ethics of artificial intelligence in education: Student privacy and data protection*. Science Insights Education Frontiers.

Huo, B., Boyle, A., Marfo, N., Tangamornsuksan, W., Steen, J. P., McKechnie, T., Lee, Y., Mayol, J., Antoniou, S. A., Thirunavukarasu, A. J., Sanger, S., Ramji, K., & Guyatt, G. (2025). Large Language Models for Chatbot Health Advice Studies: A Systematic Review. *JAMA Network Open*, *8*(2), e2457879–e2457879. DOI: 10.1001/jamanetworkopen.2024.57879 PMID: 39903463

Huo, W., Li, Q., Liang, B., Wang, Y., & Li, X. (2025). When healthcare professionals use AI: Exploring work well-being through psychological needs satisfaction and job complexity. *Behavioral Sciences (Basel, Switzerland)*, *15*(1), 88. DOI: 10.3390/bs15010088 PMID: 39851892

Hwang, G. J., & Chien, S. Y. (2022). Definition, roles, and potential research issues of the metaverse in education: An artificial intelligence perspective. *Computers and Education: Artificial Intelligence*.

Hwang, G. J., & Chang, S. C. (2021). Facilitating knowledge construction in mobile learning contexts: A bi-directional peer-assessment approach. *British Journal of Educational Technology*, *52*(1), 337–357. DOI: 10.1111/bjet.13001

IBM Data and AI Team. (2023). *Understanding the different types of artificial intelligence*. IBM. https://www.ibm.com/think/topics/artificial-intelligence-types

Ide, T., Bruch, C., Carius, A., Conca, K., Dabelko, G. D., Matthew, R., & Weinthal, E. (2021). The past and future (s) of environmental peacebuilding. *International Affairs*, *97*(1), 1–16. DOI: 10.1093/ia/iiaa177

Illers, K. (2007). *How We Learn: Learning and Non-Learning in School and Beyond*. Routledge. DOI: 10.4324/9780203939895

Ingerman, Å., & Collier-Reed, B. (2011). Technological literacy reconsidered: A model for enactment. *International Journal of Technology and Design Education, 21*(2), 137–148. DOI: 10.1007/s10798-009-9108-6

Irasuti, I., & Bachtiar, B. (2024). Empowering Indonesian EFL teachers: The transformative impact of visual literacy training on teaching materials. *International Journal of Learning. Teaching and Educational Research, 23*(8), 116–136.

Izard, S. G., Juanes, J. A., García Peñalvo, F. J., Estella, J. M. G., Ledesma, M. J. S., & Ruisoto, P. (2018). Virtual reality as an educational and training tool for medicine. *Journal of Medical Systems, 42*(3), 1–5. DOI: 10.1007/s10916-018-0900-2 PMID: 29392522

Jackson, P., Ponath Sukumaran, G., Babu, C., Tony, M. C., Jack, D. S., Reshma, V. R., Davis, D., Kurian, N., & John, A. (2024). Artificial Intelligence in Medical Education - Perception Among Medical Students. *BMC Medical Education, 24*(1), 1–9. DOI: 10.1186/s12909-024-05760-0 PMID: 38172860

Jang, H. W., & Kim, K. J. (2014). Use of online clinical videos for clinical skills training for medical students: Benefits and challenges. *BMC Medical Education, 14*(1), 1–6. DOI: 10.1186/1472-6920-14-56 PMID: 24650290

Janumpally, R., Nanua, S., Ngo, A., & Youens, K. (2024). Generative Artificial Intelligence in Graduate Medical Education. *Frontiers in Medicine, 11*, 1–9. DOI: 10.3389/fmed.2024.1525604 PMID: 39867924

Javaid, M., Haleem, A., Singh, R. P., Suman, R., & Gonzalez, E. S. (2022). Understanding the adoption of Industry 4.0 technologies in improving environmental sustainability. *Sustainable Operations and Computers, 3*, 203–217. DOI: 10.1016/j.susoc.2022.01.008

Jeong, K. O. (2022). Facilitating sustainable self-directed learning experience with the use of mobile-assisted language learning. *Sustainability (Basel), 14*(5), 2894. DOI: 10.3390/su14052894

Jha Kukreja, B., & Kukreja, P. (2025). Integration of Artificial Intelligence in Dentistry: A Systematic Review of Educational and Clinical Implications. *Cureus, 17*(2), e79350. DOI: 10.7759/cureus.79350 PMID: 40125123

Jha, S. (2022). Role of technology in medical education: SWOC analysis. *SBV Journal of Basic. Clinical and Applied Health Science, 5*(1), 19–21. DOI: 10.5005/jp-journals-10082-03131

Jiang, L., et al. (2021). Opportunities and challenges of artificial intelligence in the medical field: Current application, emerging problems, and problem-solving strategies. *Journal of International Medical Research, 49*(3), 030.

Jin, Q., Chen, F., Zhou, Y., Xu, Z., Cheung, J. M., Chen, R., Summers, R. M., Rousseau, J. F., Ni, P., Landsman, M. J., Baxter, S. L., Al'Aref, S. J., Li, Y., Chen, A., Brejt, J. A., Chiang, M. F., Peng, Y., & Lu, Z. (2024). Hidden Flaws Behind Expert-Level Accuracy of Multimodal GPT-4 Vision in Medicine. *npj. Digital Medicine, 7*(1), 1–6. DOI: 10.1038/s41746-024-01185-7 PMID: 38172429

Jones, K. M., Asher, A., Goben, A., Perry, M. R., Salo, D., Briney, K. A., & Robertshaw, M. B. (2020). "We're being tracked at all times": Student perspectives of their privacy in relation to learning analytics in higher education. *Journal of the Association for Information Science and Technology, 71*(9), 1044–1059. DOI: 10.1002/asi.24358

Jordan, R. A., & Micheelis, W. (2016). *Fünfte Deutsche Mundgesundheitsstudie (DMS V)*. Köln, Germany: Deutscher Zahnärzte Verlag. Retrieved December 10, 2020, from https://www.ncbi.nlm.nih.gov/pmc/

Juan, J., Gil, M. M., Rong, Z., Zhang, Y., Yang, H., & Poon, L. C. (2020). Effect of coronavirus disease 2019 (COVID-19) on maternal, perinatal and neonatal outcome: Systematic review. *Ultrasound in Obstetrics & Gynecology, 56*(1), 15–27. DOI: 10.1002/uog.22088 PMID: 32430957

Judson, E. (2010). Improving technology literacy: Does it open doors to traditional content? *Educational Technology Research and Development, 58*(3), 271–284. DOI: 10.1007/s11423-009-9135-8

Jumreornvong, O., Yang, E., Race, J., & Appel, J. (2020). Telemedicine and medical education in the age of COVID-19. *Academic Medicine.*

Jumreornvong, O., Yang, E., Race, J., & Appel, J. (2020). Telemedicine and medical education in the age of COVID-19. *Academic Medicine, 95*(12), 1838–1843. DOI: 10.1097/ACM.0000000000003711 PMID: 32889946

Jun, M.-K., Kim, J.-W., & Ku, H.-M. (2025). Three-dimensional printing in dentistry: A scoping review of clinical applications, advantages, and current limitations. *Oral, 5*(2), 24. DOI: 10.3390/oral5020024

Jurado, C. A., Tsujimoto, A., Punj, A., Aida, N., Miyazaki, M., & Watanabe, H. (2021). Successful of development and implementation of a digital dentistry curriculum at US dental School. *Journal of Oral Science, 63*(4), 358–360. DOI: 10.2334/josnusd.21-0070 PMID: 34497245

Kabongo, S., D'Souza, J., & Auer, S. (2021). Automated mining of leaderboards for empirical AI research. In *Towards Open and Trustworthy Digital Societies: 23rd International Conference on Asia-Pacific Digital Libraries, ICADL 2021*. Springer International Publishing. DOI: 10.1007/978-3-030-91669-5_35

Kabudi, T., Pappas, I., & Olsen, D. H. (2021). AI-Enabled Adaptive Learning Systems: A Systematic Mapping of the Literature. *Computers and Education: Artificial Intelligence*, *2*, 100017. DOI: 10.1016/j.caeai.2021.100017

Kalantarion, M., Sadoughi, M. M., Ahmady, S., Kallestrup, P., Katibeh, M., & Khajeali, N. (2022). Introducing a mobile learning model in medical education during COVID-19; a critical review. *Journal of Advances in Medical Education & Professionalism*, *10*(3), 145. DOI: 10.30476/JAMP.2022.93494.1534 PMID: 35910511

Kamalov, F., Santandreu Calonge, D., & Gurrib, I. (2023). New Era of Artificial Intelligence in Education: Towards a Sustainable Multifaceted Revolution. *Sustainability (Basel)*, *15*(16), 12451. Advance online publication. DOI: 10.3390/su151612451

Kanani, H., Khubchandani, M., Dangore-Khasbage, S., & Pandey, R. (2024). Teledentistry: A Comprehensive Review and Its Application in Pediatric Dental Care. *Cureus*, *16*(1), e52685. DOI: 10.7759/cureus.52685 PMID: 38384649

Kaplan, B. (2020). Revisiting health information technology ethical, legal, and social issues and evaluation: Telehealth/telemedicine and COVID-19. *International Journal of Medical Informatics*.

Karabacak, M., Ozkara, B. B., Margetis, K., Wintermark, M., & Bisdas, S. (2023). The advent of generative language models in medical education. *JMIR Medical Education*, *9*, e48163. DOI: 10.2196/48163 PMID: 37279048

Karataş, F., Eriçok, B., & Tanrikulu, L. (2024). Reshaping curriculum adaptation in the age of artificial intelligence: Mapping teachers' AI-driven curriculum adaptation patterns [Article]. *British Educational Research Journal*. Advance online publication. DOI: 10.1002/berj.4068

Karpouzis, K., Pantazatos, D., Taouki, J., & Meli, K. (2024, 8-11 May 2024). Tailoring Education with GenAI: A New Horizon in Lesson Planning. *2024 IEEE Global Engineering Education Conference (EDUCON)*, 1-10. https://doi.org/DOI: 10.1109/EDUCON60312.2024.10578690

Katz, M., & Nandi, N. (2021). Social media and medical education in the context of the COVID-19 pandemic: Scoping review. *JMIR Medical Education*, *7*(2), e25892. DOI: 10.2196/25892 PMID: 33755578

Katznelson, G., & Gerke, S. (2021). The need for health AI ethics in medical school education. *Advances in Health Sciences Education : Theory and Practice*, *26*(4), 1447–1458. DOI: 10.1007/s10459-021-10040-3 PMID: 33655433

Kaul, V., de Moraes, A. G., Khateeb, D., Greenstein, Y., Winter, G., Chae, J., & Dangayach, N. S. (2021). Medical education during the COVID-19 pandemic. *Chest*, *159*(5), 1949–1960. DOI: 10.1016/j.chest.2020.12.026 PMID: 33385380

Kay, A. C. (2011). A personal computer for children of all ages. *Proceedings of the ACM Annual Conference*- Volume 1.https://doi.org/DOI: 10.1145/800193.1971922

Kearney, M., Burden, K., & Schuck, S. (2020). Theorising and implementing mobile learning. *Springer Nature*, *10*, 978–981.

Kerimbayev, N., Umirzakova, Z., Shadiev, R., & Jotsov, V. (2023). *A student - centered approach using modern technologies in distance learning : a systematic review of the literature*. Smart Learning Environments., DOI: 10.1186/s40561-023-00280-8

Kernberg, A., Gold, J. A., & Mohan, V. (2024). Using ChatGPT-4 to Create Structured Medical Notes From Audio Recordings of Physician-Patient Encounters: Comparative Study [Article]. *Journal of Medical Internet Research*, *26*(1), e54419. Advance online publication. DOI: 10.2196/54419 PMID: 38648636

Kessler, A., Hickel, R., & Reymus, M. (2020). 3D printing in dentistry—State of the art. *Operative Dentistry*, *45*(1), 30–40. DOI: 10.2341/18-229-L PMID: 31172871

Khan, N. U., Wei, H., Yue, G., Nazir, N., & Zainol, N. R. (2021). Exploring themes of sustainable practices in manufacturing industry: Using thematic networks approach. *Sustainability (Basel)*, *13*(18), 10288. DOI: 10.3390/su131810288

Khan, R. A., Jawaid, M., Khan, A. R., & Sajjad, M. (2023). ChatGPT—Reshaping medical education and clinical management. *Pakistan Journal of Medical Sciences*, *39*(2), 605. DOI: 10.12669/pjms.39.2.7653 PMID: 36950398

Khan, S. A., Koc, M., & Al-Ghamdi, S. G. (2021). Sustainability assessment, potentials and challenges of 3D printed concrete structures: A systematic review for built environmental applications. *Journal of Cleaner Production*, *303*, 127027. DOI: 10.1016/j.jclepro.2021.127027

Khatoon, U. T., & Velidandi, A. (2025). An Overview on the Role of Government Initiatives in Nanotechnology Innovation for Sustainable Economic Development and Research Progress. *Sustainability (Basel)*, *17*(3), 1250. DOI: 10.3390/su17031250

Khlaif, Z. N., Ayyoub, A., Hamamra, B., Bensalem, E., Mitwally, M. A. A., Ayyoub, A., Hattab, M. K., & Shadid, F. (2024). University Teachers' Views on the Adoption and Integration of Generative AI Tools for Student Assessment in Higher Education [Article]. *Education Sciences, 14*(10), 1090. Advance online publication. DOI: 10.3390/educsci14101090

Khojasteh, L., Kafipour, R., Pakdel, F., & Mukundan, J. (2025). Empowering Medical Students With AI Writing Co-Pilots: Design and Validation of AI Self-Assessment Toolkit. *BMC Medical Education, 25*(1), 1–22. DOI: 10.1186/s12909-025-06753-3 PMID: 39891148

Khorsandi, D., Fahimipour, A., Abasian, P., Saber, S. S., Seyedi, M., Ghanavati, S., Ahmad, A., De Stephanis, A. A., Taghavinezhaddilami, F., Leonova, A., Mohammadinejad, R., Shabani, M., Mazzolai, B., Mattoli, V., Tay, F. R., & Makvandi, P. (2021). 3D and 4D printing in dentistry and maxillofacial surgery: Printing techniques, materials, and applications. *Acta Biomaterialia, 122*, 26–49. DOI: 10.1016/j.actbio.2020.12.044 PMID: 33359299

Khosravi, M., Zare, Z., Mojtabaeian, S. M., & Izadi, R. (2024). Artificial Intelligence and Decision-Making in Healthcare: A Thematic Analysis of a Systematic Review of Reviews. *Health Services Research and Managerial Epidemiology, 11*, 1–15. DOI: 10.1177/23333928241234863 PMID: 38449840

Kilag, O. K., Marquita, J., & Laurente, J. (2023). Teacher-led curriculum development: Fostering innovation in education. *Excellencia: International Multi-disciplinary Journal of Education (2994-9521), 1*(4), 223-237. https://multijournals.org/index.php/excellencia-imje/article/view/53

Kilag, O. K., Tokong, C., Enriquez, B., Deiparine, J., Purisima, R., & Zamora, M. (2023). School Leaders: The Extent of Management Empowerment and Its Impact on Teacher and School Effectiveness. *Excellencia: International Multi-disciplinary Journal of Education (2994-9521), 1*(1), 127-140. https://multijournals.org/index.php/excellencia-imje/article/view/13/12

Kim, J. W., Myung, S. J., Yoon, H. B., Moon, S. H., Ryu, H., & Yim, J. J. (2020). How medical education survives and evolves during [Our experience and future direction.]. *COVID, •••*, 19. PMID: 33338045

Kirby, S., Pesun, I., Nowakowski, A., & França, R. (2024). Effect of different post-curing methods on the degree of conversion of 3D-printed resin for models in dentistry. *Polymers, 16*(4), 549. DOI: 10.3390/polym16040549 PMID: 38399926

Kirchgasler, C., & Choi, S. (2024). Performing a global learning crisis: Citizen-led assessments, social accountability, and directing democracy. *Compare: A Journal of Comparative Education*, •••, 1–18. DOI: 10.1080/03057925.2024.2314015

Kirch, S. A., & Sadofsky, M. J. (2021). Medical Education From a Theory–Practice–Philosophy Perspective. *Academic Pathology*, *8*, 1–15. DOI: 10.1177/23742895211010236 PMID: 33959676

Kirovska-Simjanoska, D. (2021). Designing an ESP course for the 21st century students: The clash of the digital immigrants and natives. *Journal of Teaching English for Specific and Academic Purposes*, 17–30.

Klimova, B., & Polakova, P. (2020). Students' perceptions of an EFL vocabulary learning mobile application. *Education Sciences*, *10*(2), 37. DOI: 10.3390/educsci10020037

Koçak, B.. (2024). *Bias in artificial intelligence for medical imaging: Fundamentals, detection, avoidance, mitigation, challenges, ethics, and prospects*. Diagnostic and Interventional Radiology.

Kohnke, L., Moorhouse, B. L., & Zou, D. (2023). ChatGPT for language teaching and learning. *RELC Journal*, *54*(2), 537–550. DOI: 10.1177/00336882231162868

Kolb, A. Y., & Kolb, D. A. (2009). Experiential learning theory: a dynamic, holistic approach to management learning, education and development. In Armstrong, S. J., & Fukami, C. V. (Eds.), *The SAGE Handbook of Management Learning, Education and Development* (pp. 42–68). SAGE Publishing. DOI: 10.4135/9780857021038.n3

Kolb, D. A. (1984). *Experiential Learning: Experience as the Source of Learning and Development*. Prentice-Hall, Inc.

Konttila, J., Siira, H., Kyngäs, H., Lahtinen, M., Elo, S., Kääriäinen, M., Kaakinen, P., Oikarinen, A., Yamakawa, M., Fukui, S., Utsumi, M., Higami, Y., Higuchi, A., & Mikkonen, K. (2019). Healthcare professionals' competence in digitalisation: A systematic review. *Journal of Clinical Nursing*, *28*(5-6), 745–761. DOI: 10.1111/jocn.14710 PMID: 30376199

Krishnamurthy, K., Selvaraj, N., Gupta, P., Cyriac, B., Dhurairaj, P., Abdullah, A., Krishnapillai, A., Lugova, H., Haque, M., Xie, S., & Ang, E. T. (2022). Benefits of gamification in medical education. *Clinical Anatomy (New York, N.Y.)*, *35*(6), 795–807. DOI: 10.1002/ca.23916 PMID: 35637557

Krive, J., Isola, M., Chang, L., Patel, T., Anderson, M., & Sreedhar, R. (2023). Grounded in Reality: Artificial Intelligence in Medical Education. *JAMIA Open*, *6*(2), 1–7. DOI: 10.1093/jamiaopen/ooad037 PMID: 37273962

Kulkov, I., Kulkova, J., Rohrbeck, R., Menvielle, L., Kaartemo, V., & Makkonen, H. (2024). Artificial intelligence-driven sustainable development: Examining organizational, technical, and processing approaches to achieving global goals. *Sustainable Development (Bradford)*, *32*(3), 2253–2267. DOI: 10.1002/sd.2773

Kulkov, I., Tsvetkova, A., & Ivanova-Gongne, M. (2023). Identifying institutional barriers when implementing new technologies in the healthcare industry. *European Journal of Innovation Management*, *26*(4), 909–932. DOI: 10.1108/EJIM-02-2021-0093

Kumar, I., Yadav, N., & Verma, A. (2025). Navigating Artificial Intelligence in Scientific Manuscript Writing: Tips and Traps [Review]. *The Indian Journal of Radiology & Imaging*, *35*(1), S178–S186. DOI: 10.1055/s-0044-1800801 PMID: 39802715

La Bella, S., Attanasi, M., Porreca, A., Di Ludovico, A., Maggio, M. C., Gallizzi, R., La Torre, F., Rigante, D., Soscia, F., Ardenti Morini, F., Insalaco, A., Natale, M. F., Chiarelli, F., Simonini, G., De Benedetti, F., Gattorno, M., & Breda, L. (2024). Reliability of a generative artificial intelligence tool for pediatric familial Mediterranean fever: Insights from a multicentre expert survey [Article]. *Pediatric Rheumatology Online Journal*, *22*(1), 78. Advance online publication. DOI: 10.1186/s12969-024-01011-0 PMID: 39180115

Lajoie, S. P., & Gube, M. (2018). Adaptive Expertise in Medical Education: Accelerating Learning Trajectories by Fostering Self-Regulated Learning. *Medical Teacher*, *40*(8), 809–812. DOI: 10.1080/0142159X.2018.1485886 PMID: 30033791

Lakshminarayana, S., Ranganatha, M., Sun, Y., & Park, H. (2025). Smartphone enabled wearable diabetes monitoring system. *IEEE Access : Practical Innovations, Open Solutions*, *13*, 52324–52333. DOI: 10.1109/ACCESS.2025.3552731

Lalama, M., Rocha, M. G., O'Neill, E., & Zoidis, P. (2022). Polyetheretherketone (PEEK) post and core restorations: A 3D accuracy analysis between heat-pressed and CAD-CAM fabrication methods. *Journal of Prosthodontics*, *31*(5), 537–542. DOI: 10.1111/jopr.13452 PMID: 34755428

Langenfeld, T. (2020). Internet-based proctored assessment: Security and fairness issues. *Educational Measurement: Issues and Practice*, *39*(3), 24–27. DOI: 10.1111/emip.12359

Laouris, Y., & Eteokleous, N. (2005, October). We need an educationally relevant definition of mobile learning. In *Proceedings of mLearn* (Vol. 2005).

Larrazabal, A. J., Nieto, N., Peterson, V., Milone, D. H., & Ferrante, E. (2020, June 9). Gender imbalance in medical imaging datasets produces biased classifiers for computer-aided diagnosis. *Proceedings of the National Academy of Sciences of the United States of America, 117*(23), 12592–12594. DOI: 10.1073/pnas.1919012117 PMID: 32457147

Lassen, A. M., & Andersen, M. F. (2021). Valgfagsudvikling på to sundhedsuddannelser. I L. H. Horn, P. M. Pedersen, & M. Georgsen (red.), *Teori og Praksis i Professionsdidaktik: En Bog om Refleksiv Praksislæring* (pp. 171-182). Aalborg Universitetsforlag.

Lassen, A. M., & Kjærgaard, T. (2022). Teknologiforståelser i professionerne. Learning Tech – Tidsskrift for Læremidler. *Didaktik og Teknologi*, (11), 15–43.

Lave, J., & Wenger, E. (1991). *Situated Learning: Legitimate Peripheral Participation*. Cambridge University Press. DOI: 10.1017/CBO9780511815355

Lee, Y. C., Zheng, J., Kuo, J., Acosta-Vélez, G. F., Linsley, C. S., & Wu, B. M. (2022). Binder jetting of custom silicone powder for direct three-dimensional printing of maxillofacial prostheses. *3D Printing and Additive Manufacturing, 9,* 520-534. https://doi.org/DOI: 10.1089/3dp.2021.0099

Lee, J., Kim, H., Kim, K. H., Jung, D., Jowsey, T., & Webster, C. S. (2020). Effective virtual patient simulators for medical communication training: A systematic review. *Medical Education, 54*(9), 786–795. DOI: 10.1111/medu.14152 PMID: 32162355

Legg, M. (2021). The COVID-19 pandemic, the courts and online hearings: Maintaining open justice, procedural fairness and impartiality. *Federal Law Review*.

Leppink, J. (2017). Cognitive load theory: Practical implications and an important challenge. *Journal of Taibah University Medical Sciences, 12*(5), 385–391. DOI: 10.1016/j.jtumed.2017.05.003 PMID: 31435268

Levande, J. S. (2003). A Curricular and Instructional Challenge: Teaching and Learning for Technological Literacy/Capability. *The Journal of Technology Studies, 29*(2), 88–97. DOI: 10.21061/jots.v29i2.a.6

Levingston, H., Anderson, M. C., & Roni, M. A. (2024). From theory to practice: Artificial intelligence (AI) literacy course for first-year medical students. *Cureus, 16*(10), e70706. DOI: 10.7759/cureus.70706 PMID: 39493023

Li, N. (2023). Ethical considerations in artificial intelligence: A comprehensive discussion from the perspective of computer vision. *SHS Web of Conferences*.

Liaw, S. Y., Tan, J. Z., Lim, S., Zhou, W., Yap, J., Ratan, R., Ooi, S. L., Wong, S. J., Seah, B., & Chua, W. L. (2023). Artificial intelligence in virtual reality simulation for interprofessional communication training: Mixed method study. *Nurse Education Today, 122*, 105718. DOI: 10.1016/j.nedt.2023.105718 PMID: 36669304

Liberatore, G., Kim, A., Brenner, J., & Milanaik, R. (2025). Artificial intelligence impacts in education and pediatric mental health [Review]. *Current Opinion in Pediatrics*, Article . https://doi.org/DOI: 10.1097/MOP.0000000000001453

Lilhore, U. K., Simaiya, S., Poongodi, M., & Dutt, V. (2024). *Federated learning and privacy-preserving in healthcare AI* [Book]. IGI Global. https://doi.org/DOI: 10.4018/979-8-3693-1874-4

Lin, C.-C., Huang, A. Y. Q., & Lu, O. H. T. (2023). Artificial Intelligence in Intelligent Tutoring Systems Toward Sustainable Education: A Systematic Review. *Smart Learning Environments, 10*(1), 1–22. DOI: 10.1186/s40561-023-00260-y

Lin, G. S. S., Goh, S. M., & Halil, M. H. M. (2023). Unravelling the impact of dental workforce training and education programmes on policy evolution: Mixed-method study protocol. *Health Research Policy and Systems, 21*(95), 95. Advance online publication. DOI: 10.1186/s12961-023-01048-9 PMID: 37700266

Lin, H., & Chen, Q. (2024). Artificial Intelligence (AI) -Integrated Educational Applications and College Students' Creativity and Academic Emotions: Students and Teachers' Perceptions and Attitudes. *BMC Psychology, 12*(1), 1–16. DOI: 10.1186/s40359-024-01979-0 PMID: 39285268

Lin, P.-Y., Chen, T.-C., Lin, C.-J., Huang, C.-C., Tsai, Y.-H., Tsai, Y.-L., & Wang, C.-Y. (2024). The use of augmented reality (AR) and virtual reality (VR) in dental surgery education and practice: A narrative review. *Journal of Dental Sciences, 19*(Suppl 2), S91–S101. DOI: 10.1016/j.jds.2024.10.011 PMID: 39807259

Lintner, T. (2024, 2024/08/06). A systematic review of AI literacy scales. *npj Science of Learning, 9*(1), 50. https://doi.org/DOI: 10.1038/s41539-024-00264-4

Li, Q., & Qin, Y. (2023). AI in medical education: Medical student perception, curriculum recommendations and design suggestions. *BMC Medical Education, 23*(1), 1–18. DOI: 10.1186/s12909-023-04700-8 PMID: 37946176

Liu, C.-M., Su, N.-Y., Chen, Y.-T., Chiang, C.-P., & Yu, C.-H. (2024). Analysis of approved dental teaching projects in the teaching practice research program in 8 dental schools of Taiwan from 2018 to 2023. *Journal of Dental Sciences, 19*(2), 1083–1086. DOI: 10.1016/j.jds.2024.01.021 PMID: 38618124

Liu, F., Vyas, C., Poologasundarampillai, G., Pape, I., Hinduja, S., Mirihanage, W., & Bartolo, P. (2018). Structural evolution of PCL during melt extrusion 3D printing. *Macromolecular Materials and Engineering*, *303*(2), 1700494. DOI: 10.1002/mame.201700494

Liu, L. (2025). AI and the Crisis of Legitimacy in Higher Education. *American Journal of STEM Education*, *4*, 16–26. DOI: 10.32674/42qssk59

Liu, Y., Wang, D., Wu, S., Liu, X., & Xiao, C. (2024). Literature review of the clinical features of sulfasalazine-induced drug reaction with eosinophilia and systemic symptoms/drug-induced hypersensitivity syndrome. *Frontiers in Pharmacology*, *15*, 1488483. DOI: 10.3389/fphar.2024.1488483 PMID: 39687296

Lobo, M. D., Miravent, S., de Almeida, R. P. P., & Garcia, M. B. (2024). Advancing Precision in Physical Education and Sports Science: A Review of Medical Imaging Methods for Assessing Body Composition. In *Global Innovations in Physical Education and Health*. IGI Global., DOI: 10.4018/979-8-3693-3952-7.ch011

Locsin, R. C. (2017). The co-existence of technology and caring in the theory of technological competency as caring in nursing. *The Journal of Medical Investigation*, 64(1.2), 160-164.

Lombardi, B. M., Zerden, L. D. S., & Thyberg, C. (2022). Social work answers the (video) call: Tele-behavioral health use during COVID-19. *Journal of the Society for Social Work and Research*, *13*(1), 67–87. DOI: 10.1086/715621

Long, N. M. H., & Chung, W.-Y. (2021). Wearable noninvasive glucose estimation based on multi-wavelength reflective photoplethysmography. In *2021 IEEE Photonics Conference (IPC)* (pp. 1–2). IEEE. DOI: 10.1109/IPC48725.2021.9592997

LoPresti, M., & Igarashi, A. (2024). A pragmatic review of cost-effectiveness evaluations of reimbursed medical devices conducted for Japan. *Journal of Medical Economics*, *27*(1), 1456–1471. DOI: 10.1080/13696998.2024.2420542 PMID: 39436025

Loughlin, C., Lygo-Baker, S., & Lindberg-Sand, Å. (2021). Reclaiming constructive alignment. *European Journal of Higher Education*, *11*(2), 119–136. DOI: 10.1080/21568235.2020.1816197

Lovat, L. B. (2024). Artificial intelligence in gastroenterology: Where are we and where are we going? [Article]. *Gastrointestinal Nursing*, *22*(Sup3), S6–S13. DOI: 10.12968/gasn.2024.22.Sup3.S6

Luu, H. S. (2025). Laboratory Data as a Potential Source of Bias in Healthcare Artificial Intelligence and Machine Learning Models [Review]. *Annals of Laboratory Medicine*, *45*(1), 12–21. DOI: 10.3343/alm.2024.0323 PMID: 39444135

Ma, Y., Song, Y., Balch, J. A., Ren, Y., Vellanki, D., Hu, Z., Shickel, B. (2024). Promoting AI competencies for medical students: a scoping review on frameworks, programs, and tools. *arXiv preprint*:2407.18939. https://doi.org/10.48550/arXiv.2407.18939

Macanchí-Pico, M. L., Orozco-Castillo, B. M., & Campoverde-Encalada, M. A. (2020). Innovación educativa, pedagógica y didáctica. Concepciones para la práctica en la educación superior. *Revista Universidad y Sociedad, 12*(1), 396-403. http://scielo.sld.cu/scielo.php?script=sci_arttext&pid=S2218-36202020000100396&lng=es&tlng=es

MacPhail, A., Tannehill, D., Leirhaug, P. E., & Borghouts, L. (2023). Promoting instructional alignment in physical education teacher education. *Physical Education and Sport Pedagogy*, *28*(2), 153–164. DOI: 10.1080/17408989.2021.1958177

Madfa, A. A., Al-Ibrahim, I. K., Alshammary, F. L., Alharbi, S. M., & Alharbi, B. B. (2023). An audit of Saudi dental students' opinions and attitudes toward digital dentistry. *The Open Dentistry Journal*, *17*(1), e18742106276082. Advance online publication. DOI: 10.2174/0118742106276082231123053341

Mahajan, S., Thapa, P., Sharma, P., Tsirkas, P., Ali, G., & Adamopoulos, I. (2025). Prevalence and risk factors of nomophobia among students studying in private colleges. *Preprints*.

Mahato, S., Pathak, L. K., Sweta, S., & Choubey, D. K. (2024). Wearable smart technologies. In *Changing the future of healthcare*. Taylor & Francis., DOI: 10.1201/9781003388845-11

Mahmood, S. (2019). *The use of medical apps amongst doctors working in the Department of Paediatrics and child health of the University of the Witwatersrand, in Johannesburg South Africa* (Doctoral dissertation, Faculty of Health Sciences, University of the Witwatersrand, Johannesburg). https://wiredspace.wits.ac.za/server/api/core/bitstreams/740ff759-0b0a-4b0a-b1ec-0f3a231ec26a/content

MAI. (2025). All-in-One VR & MR Anatomy and Acupuncture Platform. https://www.mai.ai/

Mallakpour, S., Tabesh, F., & Hussain, C. M. (2021). 3D and 4D printing: From innovation to evolution. *Advances in Colloid and Interface Science*, *294*, 102482. DOI: 10.1016/j.cis.2021.102482 PMID: 34274721

Malone, D. M. (2020). Ethics education in teacher preparation: A case for stakeholder responsibility. *Ethics and Education*, *15*(1), 77–97. DOI: 10.1080/17449642.2019.1700447

Manyika, J. (2021). The Future of Think Tanks: Trends and Transformations. *The Future of Think Tanks and Policy Advice in the United States*, 139–143. https:// link .springer .com/ chapter/ _21DOI: 10.1007/978-3-030-60386-1

Manzer, J. L., Carrillo-Perez, A., Tingey, L., Ouellette, L., Hogan, C., Atkins, N., Carmichael, K., Ramirez, G. G., Magee, M. M., Miller, M. A., Nwankwo, C., Reid, S., Strelevitz, T., Taylor, V., Waddell, W., Wong, M., Yuksel, B., & Blum, J. (2024). Client perspectives on contraceptive care: A systematic review. *American Journal of Preventive Medicine*, *67*(6), S22–S31. DOI: 10.1016/j.amepre.2024.07.019 PMID: 39570202

Maqsoom, A., Zulqarnain, M., Irfan, M., Ullah, F., Alqahtani, F. K., & Khan, K. I. A. (2023). Drivers of, and barriers to, the adoption of mixed reality in the construction industry of developing countries. *Buildings (Basel, Switzerland)*, *13*(4), 872. DOI: 10.3390/buildings13040872

Marinucci, L., Mazzuca, C., & Gangemi, A. (2023). Exposing implicit biases and stereotypes in human and artificial intelligence: State of the art and challenges with a focus on gender. *AI & Society*, *38*(2), 747–761. DOI: 10.1007/s00146-022-01474-3

Martens, T., Beck, R. W., Bailey, R., Ruedy, K. J., Calhoun, P., Peters, A. L., Pop-Busui, R., Philis-Tsimikas, A., Bao, S., Umpierrez, G., Davis, G., Kruger, D., Bhargava, A., Young, L., McGill, J. B., Aleppo, G., Nguyen, Q. T., Orozco, I., Biggs, W., & Balo, A.MOBILE Study Group. (2021). Effect of continuous glucose monitoring on glycemic control in patients with type 2 diabetes treated with basal insulin: A randomized clinical trial. *Journal of the American Medical Association*, *325*(22), 2262–2272. DOI: 10.1001/jama.2021.7444 PMID: 34077499

Martin-Alguacil, N., Avedillo, L., Mota-Blanco, R., & Gallego-Agundez, M. (2024). Student-Centered Learning: Some Issues and Recommendations for Its Implementation in a Traditional Curriculum Setting in Health Sciences. *Education Sciences*, *14*(11), 1179. https://www.mdpi.com/2227-7102/14/11/1179. DOI: 10.3390/educsci14111179

Martínez Asanza, D. (2018). ¿Enseñanza tradicional en el siglo XXI? *Revista Neuronum*, *4*(1), 99–106. http://eduneuro.com/revista/index.php/revistaneuronum/article/view/108/98

Martínez- Asanza. D. (Ed.). (2024a). *Transforming Dental Health in Rural Communities: Digital Dentistry*. IGI Global. https://doi.org/DOI: 10.4018/979-8-3693-7165-7

Martínez- Asanza. D. (Ed.). (2024b). *Leveraging Digital Technology for Preventive Dentistry*. IGI Global. https://doi.org/DOI: 10.4018/979-8-3693-3872-8

Martínez- Asanza. D. (Ed.). (2024d). *Geriatric Dentistry in the Age of Digital Technology*. IGI Global. https://doi.org/DOI: 10.4018/979-8-3693-0260-6

Martínez- Asanza. D., Rojas Herrera, I. A., Njoku, A. U., Reyes Puig, A. C., Mouloudj, F., Capote, I. G., & Maupome, G. (2024c). Study Plans and Programs Supporting Geriatric Dentistry Teaching in Cuba: An Update. In D. Martínez Asanza (Ed.), *Geriatric Dentistry in the Age of Digital Technology* (pp. 174-191). IGI Global. https://doi.org/DOI: 10.4018/979-8-3693-0260-6.ch007

Martínez-Asanza, D. (2021). La visita a la familia en la carrera de Estomatología: una estructura didáctica [thesis]. La Habana: Universidad de Ciencias Médicas de La Habana. https://tesis.sld.cu/index.php?P=FullRecord&ID=1812

Martínez-Asanza, D. (2025). Emerging Trends and Future Perspectives in Digital Dentistry for Rural Areas: An Update. D. Asanza (Ed.), *Transforming Dental Health in Rural Communities: Digital Dentistry* (pp. 1-20). IGI Global. https://doi.org/DOI: 10.4018/979-8-3693-7165-7.ch001

Martínez-Asanza, D., Rojas-Herrera, I. A., Mouloudj, K., Garrido-Amable, O., & Muzzamil, M. (2024e). Impact of Digital Innovations in Preventive Dentistry: A Narrative Review. In Asanza, D. (Ed.), *Leveraging Digital Technology for Preventive Dentistry* (pp. 55–84). IGI Global., DOI: 10.4018/979-8-3693-3872-8.ch003

Martinez, C. (2022). Developing 21st century teaching skills: A case study of teaching and learning through project-based curriculum. *Cogent Education*, *9*(1), 2024936. DOI: 10.1080/2331186X.2021.2024936

Martin, F., Chen, Y., Moore, R. L., & Westine, C. D. (2020). Systematic Review of Adaptive Learning Research Designs, Context, Strategies, and Technologies from 2009 to 2018. *Educational Technology Research and Development*, *68*(4), 1903–1929. DOI: 10.1007/s11423-020-09793-2 PMID: 32837122

Masters, K. (2019). Artificial intelligence in medical education. *Medical Teacher*, *41*(9), 976–980. DOI: 10.1080/0142159X.2019.1595557 PMID: 31007106

Masters, K. (2023). Ethical use of artificial intelligence in health professions education: AMEE Guide No. 158. *Medical Teacher*, *45*(6), 574–584. DOI: 10.1080/0142159X.2023.2186203 PMID: 36912253

Mbakwe, A. B., Lourentzou, I., Celi, L. A., Mechanic, O. J., & Dagan, A. (2023). ChatGPT passing USMLE shines a spotlight on the flaws of medical education. *PLOS Digital Health*, *2*(2), e0000205. DOI: 10.1371/journal.pdig.0000205 PMID: 36812618

McClure, C., & Williams, P. (2021). Gather. town: An opportunity for self-paced learning in a synchronous, distance-learning environment. *Compass (Eltham)*, *14*(2). Advance online publication. DOI: 10.21100/compass.v14i2.1232

McGee, R. G., Wark, S., Mwangi, F., Drovandi, A., Alele, F., & Malau-Aduli, B. S.ACHIEVE Collaboration. (2024). Digital learning of clinical skills and its impact on medical students' academic performance: A systematic review. *BMC Medical Education*, *24*(1), 1477. DOI: 10.1186/s12909-024-06471-2 PMID: 39696150

McGraw, D., & Mandl, K. D. (2021). 2021/01/04). Privacy protections to encourage use of health-relevant digital data in a learning health system. *npj. Digital Medicine*, *4*(1), 2. DOI: 10.1038/s41746-020-00362-8 PMID: 33398052

McKenney, S., & Reeves, T. C. (2021). Educational design research: Portraying, conducting, and enhancing productive scholarship. *Medical Education*, *55*(1), 82–92. DOI: 10.1111/medu.14280 PMID: 32564385

McLennan, S., Fiske, A., Tigard, D., Müller, R., Haddadin, S., & Buyx, A. (2022). Embedded ethics: A proposal for integrating ethics into the development of medical AI. *BMC Medical Ethics*, *23*(1), 6. DOI: 10.1186/s12910-022-00746-3 PMID: 35081955

McMahon, G. T. (2024). The Risks and Challenges of Artificial Intelligence in Endocrinology [Article]. *The Journal of Clinical Endocrinology and Metabolism*, *109*(6), e1468–e1471. DOI: 10.1210/clinem/dgae017 PMID: 38471009

Meaney, M. (2021). Essays on the design of inclusive learning in Massive Open Online Courses, and implications for educational futures.

Mejeh, M., & Rehm, M. (2024). 2024/06/01). Taking adaptive learning in educational settings to the next level: Leveraging natural language processing for improved personalization. *Educational Technology Research and Development*, *72*(3), 1597–1621. DOI: 10.1007/s11423-024-10345-1

Memarian, B., & Doleck, T. (2023). Fairness, accountability, transparency, and ethics (FATE) in artificial intelligence (AI), and higher education: A systematic review. *Computers and Education: Artificial Intelligence*.

Mergen, M., Graf, N., & Meyerheim, M. (2024). Reviewing the current state of virtual reality integration in medical education—A scoping review. *BMC Medical Education*, *24*(1), 788. DOI: 10.1186/s12909-024-05777-5 PMID: 39044186

Meschede, C. (2020). The sustainable development goals in scientific literature: A bibliometric overview at the meta-level. *Sustainability (Basel)*, *12*(11), 4461. DOI: 10.3390/su12114461

Mhlongo, S., Mbatha, K., Ramatsetse, B., & Dlamini, R. (2023). Challenges, opportunities, and prospects of adopting and using smart digital technologies in learning environments: An iterative review. *Heliyon*, *9*(6), e16348. DOI: 10.1016/j.heliyon.2023.e16348 PMID: 37274691

Michel-Villarreal, R., Vilalta-Perdomo, E., Salinas-Navarro, D. E., Thierry-Aguilera, R., & Gerardou, F. S. (2023). Challenges and opportunities of Generative AI for Higher education as explained by ChatGPT. *Education Sciences*, *13*(9), 856. DOI: 10.3390/educsci13090856

Mihan, A., Pandey, A., & Van Spall, H. G. (2024). Mitigating the risk of artificial intelligence bias in cardiovascular care [Review]. *The Lancet. Digital Health*, *6*(10), e749–e754. DOI: 10.1016/S2589-7500(24)00155-9 PMID: 39214762

Mijwil, M. (2024). M., Adamopoulos, I., & Pudasaini, P. (2024). Machine learning Helps in Quickly Diagnosis Cases of "New Corona". *Mesopotamian Journal of Artificial Intelligence in Healthcare*, *16–19*. Advance online publication. DOI: 10.58496/MJAIH/2024/003

Mirchi, N., Ledwos, N., & Del Maestro, R. F. (2020). Intelligent Tutoring Systems: Re-Envisioning Surgical Education in Response to COVID-19. *The Canadian Journal of Neurological Sciences*, *48*(2), 198–200. DOI: 10.1017/cjn.2020.202 PMID: 32907644

Mir, M. M., Mir, G. M., Raina, N. T., Mir, S. M., Mir, S. M., Miskeen, E., Alharthi, M. H., & Alamri, M. M. S. (2023). Application of Artificial Intelligence in Medical Education: Current Scenario and Future Perspectives. *Journal of Advances in Medical Education & Professionalism*, *11*(3), 133–140. DOI: 10.30476/jamp.2023.98655.1803 PMID: 37469385

Mistry, D., Brock, C. A., & Lindsey, T. (2023). The present and future of virtual reality in medical education: A narrative review. *Cureus*, *15*(12), e51124. DOI: 10.7759/cureus.51124 PMID: 38274907

Mitra, N. K., & Chitra, E. (2024). Glimpses of the Use of Generative AI and ChatGPT in Medical Education [Review]. *Education in Medicine Journal, 16*(2), 155–164. DOI: 10.21315/eimj2024.16.2.11

Mohammed, A., Li, S., & Liu, X. (2024). Exploring the potentials of wearable technologies in managing vestibular hypofunction. *Bioengineering (Basel, Switzerland), 11*(7), 641. DOI: 10.3390/bioengineering11070641 PMID: 39061723

Mohsin Khan, M., Shah, N., Shaikh, N., Thabet, A., alrabayah, T., & Belkhair, S. (2025). Towards secure and trusted AI in healthcare: A systematic review of emerging innovations and ethical challenges [Review]. *International Journal of Medical Informatics, 195*, 105780. Advance online publication. DOI: 10.1016/j.ijmedinf.2024.105780 PMID: 39753062

Molina, W. P. C., Caisaguano, J. W. R., & Núñez, M. A. R. (2023). Utilidad de la tecnología CAD/CAM en la fabricación de prótesis dentales. *Medisur, 21*(6), 1305–1311. http://scielo.sld.cu/scielo.php?script=sci_arttext&pid=S1727-897X2023000601305&lng=es&tlng=es

Monib, W. K., Qazi, A., De Silva, L., & Mahmud, M. M. (2024). Exploring Learners' Experiences with ChatGPT in Personalized Learning. *2024 6th International Workshop on Artificial Intelligence and Education (WAIE)*, 66-70. https://doi.org/ DOI: 10.1109/WAIE63876.2024.00019

Monib, W. K. (2023). Implementation of 21st Century Skills in EFL Classroom: Perceptions of Lecturers and Students. [IJonSES]. *International Journal on Social & Education Sciences, 5*(3), 536–559. https://doi.org/https://doi.org/10.46328/ijonses.544. DOI: 10.46328/ijonses.544

Monib, W. K., Qazi, A., Apong, R. A., Azizan, M. T., De Silva, L., & Yassin, H. (2024). Generative AI and future education: A review, theoretical validation, and authors' perspective on challenges and solutions. *PeerJ. Computer Science, 10*, e2105. DOI: 10.7717/peerj-cs.2105 PMID: 39650462

Monib, W. K., Qazi, A., & Mahmud, M. M. (2025). 2025/01/01). Exploring learners' experiences and perceptions of ChatGPT as a learning tool in higher education. *Education and Information Technologies, 30*(1), 917–939. DOI: 10.1007/s10639-024-13065-4

Moore, C. M. (2022). 2022/01/01/). The challenges of health inequities and AI. *Intelligence-Based Medicine, 6*, 100067. https://doi.org/https://doi.org/10.1016/j.ibmed.2022.100067. DOI: 10.1016/j.ibmed.2022.100067

Moran, J., Briscoe, G., & Peglow, S. (2018). Current technology in advancing medical education: Perspectives for learning and providing care. *Academic psychiatry: the journal of the American Association of Directors of Psychiatric Residency Training and the Association for Academic Psychiatry, 42*(6), 796–799. https://doi.org/DOI: 10.1007/s40596-018-0946-y

Morawska, L., & Milton, D. K. (2020). It is time to address airborne transmission of COVID-19. *Clinical Infectious Diseases: An Official Publication of the Infectious Diseases Society of America.*

Moudatsou, M., Stavropoulou, A., Philalithis, A., & Koukouli, S. (2020, January). The role of empathy in health and social care professionals. [). MDPI.]. *Health Care, 8*(1), 26. PMID: 32019104

Mouloudj, K. LE, V. L., Bouarar, A., Bouarar, A. C., Martínez-Asanza, D., & Srivastava, M. (2024). Adopting Artificial Intelligence in Healthcare: A Narrative Review. In S. Teixeira & J. Remondes (Eds.). *The Use of Artificial Intelligence in Digital Marketing: Competitive Strategies and Tactics* (pp. 1-20). IGI Global. https://doi.org/DOI: 10.4018/978-1-6684-9324-3.ch001

Mouloudj, F., Aljaeed, S. A., & Asanza, D. M. (2025). Understanding Students' Intentions to Use AI for English Language Learning. In Ali, M., Anwar, M., Fazal, S., & Ayyaz, S. (Eds.), *AI Applications for English Language Learning* (pp. 157–178). IGI Global., DOI: 10.4018/979-8-3693-9077-1.ch007

Mouloudj, K., Bouarar, A. C., Martínez Asanza, D. A., & Dimitrova, M. (2025b). Understanding Customers' Intentions to use Digital Dental Health Services: An Expanded Technology Acceptance Model. In Martínez Asanza, D. (Ed.), *Transforming Dental Health in Rural Communities: Digital Dentistry* (pp. 173–194). IGI Global., DOI: 10.4018/979-8-3693-7165-7.ch007

Mousavinasab, E., Zarifsanaiey, N., & Niakan Kalhori, R., S., Rakhshan, M., Keikha, L., & Ghazi Saeedi, M. (. (2018). Intelligent Tutoring Systems: A Systematic Review of Characteristics, Applications, and Evaluation Methods. *Interactive Learning Environments, 29*(1), 142–163. DOI: 10.1080/10494820.2018.1558257

Mpuangnan, K. N. (2024). Teacher preparedness and professional development needs for successful technology integration in teacher education. *Cogent Education, 11*(1), 2408837. Advance online publication. DOI: 10.1080/2331186X.2024.2408837

Mullen, C. A. (2020). Does modality matter? A comparison of aspiring leaders' learning online and face-to-face. *Journal of Further and Higher Education, 44*(5), 670–688. DOI: 10.1080/0309877X.2019.1576859

Mun, M., Byrne, S., Shaw, L., & Lyons, K. (2025). Digital dentists: A curriculum for the 21st century. *JMIR Medical Education, 11*(1), e54153. DOI: 10.2196/54153 PMID: 39789757

Mustafa, M. Y., Tlili, A., Lampropoulos, G., Huang, R., Jandrić, P., Zhao, J., Salha, S., Xu, L., Panda, S., Kinshuk, , López-Pernas, S., & Saqr, M. (2024). A Systematic Review of Literature Reviews on Artificial Intelligence in Education (AIED): A Roadmap to a Future Research Agenda. *Smart Learning Environments, 11*(1), 1–33. DOI: 10.1186/s40561-024-00350-5

Mustapa, M., Shaharuddin, S., Wisman, M., Hamid, A., Noorul, N., & Mohamed, S. (2022). Student-Centred Approach in Medical Education : A Review of the Teaching- Student - Centred Approach In Medical Education : A Review of the Teaching - Learning Activities and the Perceptions of Educators on the Students Engagement and Performance At the Faculty of Medicine and Defence Health. *National Defence University of Malaysia.*, (May). Advance online publication. DOI: 10.4103/aihb.aihb

Mutimukwe, C., Viberg, O., Oberg, L. M., & Cerratto-Pargman, T. (2022). Students' privacy concerns in learning analytics: Model development. *British Journal of Educational Technology, 53*(4), 932–951. DOI: 10.1111/bjet.13234

Muzammil, M. A., Javid, S., Afridi, A. K., Siddineni, R., Shahabi, M., Haseeb, M., Fariha, F. N. U., Kumar, S., Zaveri, S., & Nashwan, A. J. (2024). 2024/03/01/). Artificial intelligence-enhanced electrocardiography for accurate diagnosis and management of cardiovascular diseases. *Journal of Electrocardiology, 83*, 30–40. https://doi.org/https://doi.org/10.1016/j.jelectrocard.2024.01.006. DOI: 10.1016/j.jelectrocard.2024.01.006 PMID: 38301492

Μαλχανγι, Γ., Πατανο, Α., Μορολλα, Ρ., Δε Σαντισ, Μ., Πιρασ, Φ., Σετταννι, ς., Μανχινι, Α., Δι ςενερε, Δ., Ινχηινγολο, Φ., Ινχηινγολο, Α. Δ., Διπαλμα, Γ., & Ινχηινγολο, Α. Μ. (2023). Αναλψσισ οφ δενταλ εναμελ ρεμινεραλιζατιον: Α σψστεματιχ ρεϖιεω οφ τεχηνιθυε χομπαρισονσ. *Βιοενγινεερινγ (Βασελ, Σωιτζερλανδ)*, 10(4), 472. ηττπσ:// ωωω .μδπι .χομ/ 2306 – 5354/ 10/ 4/ 472. ΔΟΙ: ΠΜΙΔ: 37106659DOI: 10.3390/βιοενγινεερινγ10040472

Μανσκι, Ρ. ϑ., & Μεψερηοεφερ, Χ. Δ. (2017). Προφεχτινγ τηε δεμανδ φορ δενταλ χαρε ιν 2040. *ϑουρναλ οφ Δενταλ Εδυχατιον*, 81(8), eS133–eS145. https:// onlinelibrary .wiley .com/ doi/ abs/ . DOI: PMID: 28765465DOI: 10.21815/JDE.017.020

Naeem, N. K., Hadie, S. N. H., Ismail, I. M., Ullah, S., & Yusoff, M. S. B. (2024). Buzz or fuss: Gauging the online learning environments in undergraduate medical education—A mixed-method study. *Education in Medicine Journal, 16*(2), 63–83. DOI: 10.21315/eimj2024.16.2.5

Nagi, F., Salih, R., Alzubaidi, M., Shah, H., Alam, T., Shah, Z., & Househ, M. (2023). Applications of artificial intelligence (AI) in medical education: A scoping review. *Studies in Health Technology and Informatics, 305*, 648–651. DOI: 10.3233/SHTI230581 PMID: 37387115

Naik, N., Hameed, B. M. Z., Shetty, D. K., Swain, D., Shah, M., Paul, R., Aggarwal, K., Ibrahim, S., Patil, V., Smriti, K., Shetty, S., Rai, B. P., Chlosta, P., & Somani, B. K. (2022). Legal and ethical consideration in Artificial Intelligence in healthcare: Who takes responsibility? *Frontiers in Surgery, 9*, 862322. DOI: 10.3389/fsurg.2022.862322 PMID: 35360424

Najeeb, M., & Islam, S. (2025). Artificial intelligence (AI) in restorative dentistry: Current trends and future prospects. *BMC Oral Health, 25*(1), 592. DOI: 10.1186/s12903-025-05989-1 PMID: 40251567

Narayanan, S., Ramakrishnan, R., Durairaj, E., & Das, A. (2023). Artificial Intelligence Revolutionizing the Field of Medical Education. *Cureus*. Advance online publication. DOI: 10.7759/cureus.49604 PMID: 38161821

Naseer, M. A., Saeed, S., Afzal, A., Ali, S., & Malik, M. G. R. (2025). Navigating the integration of artificial intelligence in the medical education curriculum: A mixed-methods study exploring the perspectives of medical students and faculty in Pakistan. *BMC Medical Education, 25*(1), 273. DOI: 10.1186/s12909-024-06552-2 PMID: 39979912

Nasra, M., Jaffri, R., Pavlin-Premrl, D., Kok, H. K., Khabaza, A., Barras, C., Slater, L. A., Yazdabadi, A., Moore, J., Russell, J., Smith, P., Chandra, R. V., Brooks, M., Jhamb, A., Chong, W., Maingard, J., & Asadi, H. (2025). Can artificial intelligence improve patient educational material readability? A systematic review and narrative synthesis [Review]. *Internal Medicine Journal, 55*(1), 20–34. DOI: 10.1111/imj.16607 PMID: 39720869

Nassani, L. M., Bencharit, S., Schumacher, F., Lu, W.-E., Resende, R., & Fernandes, G. V. O. (2024). The Impact of Technology Teaching in the Dental Predoctoral Curriculum on Students' Perception of Digital Dentistry. *Dentistry Journal, 12*(3), 75. DOI: 10.3390/dj12030075 PMID: 38534299

Nassar, A., & Kamal, M. (2021). Ethical dilemmas in AI-powered decision-making: A deep dive into big data-driven ethical considerations. *International Journal of Responsible Artificial Intelligence*, *11*(8).

Naveen, P., & Trojovský, P. (2024). Overview and Challenges of Machine Translation for Contextually Appropriate Translations. *iScience*, *27*(10), 1–25. DOI: 10.1016/j.isci.2024.110878 PMID: 39391737

Nennig, H. T., Idárraga, K. L., Salzer, L. D., Bleske-Rechek, A., & Theisen, R. M. (2020). Comparison of student attitudes and performance in an online and a face-to-face inorganic chemistry course. *Chemistry Education Research and Practice*, *21*(1), 168–177. DOI: 10.1039/C9RP00112C

Newman, P. A., Guta, A., & Black, T. (2021). Ethical considerations for qualitative research methods during the COVID-19 pandemic and other emergency situations: Navigating the virtual field. *International Journal of Qualitative Methods*, *20*, 16094069211047823. DOI: 10.1177/16094069211047823

Ngenzi, J. L., Scott, R. E., & Mars, M. (2021). Information and communication technology to enhance continuing professional development (CPD) and continuing medical education (CME) for Rwanda: A scoping review of reviews. *BMC Medical Education*, *21*(1), 245. DOI: 10.1186/s12909-021-02607-w PMID: 33926419

Nguyen, A., Ngo, H. N., Hong, Y., Dang, B., & Nguyen, B.-P. T. (2023). Ethical principles for artificial intelligence in education. *Education and Information Technologies*, *28*(4), 4221–4241. DOI: 10.1007/s10639-022-11316-w PMID: 36254344

Nguyen, T. (2024). ChatGPT in Medical Education: A Precursor for Automation Bias? *JMIR Medical Education*, *10*, e50174. DOI: 10.2196/50174 PMID: 38231545

Nikolopoulou, K. (2020). Secondary education teachers' perceptions of mobile phone and tablet use in classrooms: Benefits, constraints and concerns. *Journal of Computers in Education*, *7*(2), 257–275. DOI: 10.1007/s40692-020-00156-7

Nishant, R., Schneckenberg, D., & Ravishankar, M. N. (2024). The formal rationality of artificial intelligence-based algorithms and the problem of bias. *Journal of Information Technology*, *39*(1), 19–40. DOI: 10.1177/02683962231176842

Nissen, L., Rother, J. F., Heinemann, M., Reimer, L. M., Jonas, S., & Raupach, T. (2025). A Randomised Cross-Over Trial Assessing the Impact of AI-Generated Individual Feedback on Written Online Assignments for Medical Students. *Medical Teacher*, •••, 1–7. DOI: 10.1080/0142159X.2025.2451870 PMID: 39831699

Nissen, R. D., & Andersen, A. H. (2021). Addressing religion in secular healthcare: Existential communication and the post-secular negotiation. *Religions, 13*(1), 34. DOI: 10.3390/rel13010034

Nonaka, I., & Konno, N. (1998). The concept of 'Ba': Building a foundation for knowledge creation. *California Management Review, 40*(3), 40–54. DOI: 10.2307/41165942

Norori, N., Hu, Q., Aellen, F. M., Faraci, F. D., & Tzovara, A. (2021). Addressing bias in big data and AI for health care: A call for open science. *Patterns (New York, N.Y.), 2*(10), 100347. Advance online publication. DOI: 10.1016/j.patter.2021.100347 PMID: 34693373

Norris, T. (2023). Educational futures after [Big tech and pandemic profiteering versus education for democracy. *Policy Futures in Education.*]. *COVID*, •••, 19.

Ogden, K., Kilpatrick, S., & Elmer, S. (2023). Examining the Nexus Between Medical Education and Complexity: A Systematic Review to Inform Practice and Research. *BMC Medical Education, 23*(1), 1–15. DOI: 10.1186/s12909-023-04471-2 PMID: 37408005

Oh, K., Choi, J. K., Park, H., & Lee, S. (2025). Personalized ensemble based stress detection using wearable sensor data. In *2025 27th International Conference on Advanced Communications Technology (ICACT)* (pp. 470–475). IEEE. DOI: 10.23919/ICACT63878.2025.10936652

Oke, A. E., & Arowoiya, V. A. (2022). Critical barriers to augmented reality technology adoption in developing countries: A case study of Nigeria. *Journal of Engineering. Defence Technology, 20*(5), 1320–1333.

Öncül, G. (2021). Defining the need: Digital literacy skills for first-year university students. *Journal of Applied Research in Higher Education.*

Osasona, F.. (2024). Reviewing the ethical implications of AI in decision-making processes. *International Journal of Management & Entrepreneurship Research, 6*(2), 322–335. DOI: 10.51594/ijmer.v6i2.773

Owoc, M. L., Sawicka, A., & Weichbroth, P. (2021). Artificial intelligence technologies in education: Benefits, challenges and strategies of implementation. In *IFIP advances in information and communication technology.* Springer International Publishing.

Oyedotun, T. D. (2020). *Sudden change of pedagogy in education driven by COVID-19: Perspectives and evaluation from a developing country.* Research in Globalization.

Page, M. J., McKenzie, J. E., Bossuyt, P. M., Boutron, I., Hoffmann, T. C., Mulrow, C. D., Shamseer, L., Tetzlaff, J. M., Akl, E. A., Brennan, S. E., Chou, R., Glanville, J., Grimshaw, J. M., Hróbjartsson, A., Lalu, M. M., Li, T., Loder, E. W., Mayo-Wilson, E., McDonald, S., & Moher, D. (2021). The PRISMA 2020 statement: An updated guideline for reporting systematic reviews. *BMJ (Clinical Research Ed.), 372*(71), n71. Advance online publication. DOI: 10.1136/bmj.n71 PMID: 33782057

Page, , McKenzie, J. E., Bossuyt, P. M., Boutron, I., Hoffmann, T. C., Mulrow, C. D., Shamseer, L., Tetzlaff, J. M., Akl, E. A., Brennan, S. E., Chou, R., Glanville, J., Grimshaw, J. M., Hróbjartsson, A., Lalu, M. M., Li, T., Loder, E. W., Mayo-Wilson, E., McDonald, S., & Alonso-Fernández, S. (2021). Declaración PRISMA 2020: Una guía actualizada para la publicación de revisiones sistemáticas. *Revista Española de Cardiología, 74*(9), 790–799. DOI: 10.1016/j.recesp.2021.06.016 PMID: 34446261

Pakdel, F., Khojasteh, L., Kafipour, R., & Shahsavar, Z. (2025). Navigating AI writing tools in medical education: A SWOT analysis of L2 academic writing perspectives [Article]. *Language Teaching Research*, 13621688251322953. Advance online publication. DOI: 10.1177/13621688251322953

Palacios-Núñez, M. L., Toribio-López, A., & Deroncele-Acosta, A. (2021). Innovación educativa en el desarrollo de aprendizajes relevantes: una revisión sistemática de literatura. *Revista Universidad y Sociedad, 13*(5), 134-145.http://scielo.sld.cu/scielo.php?script=sci_arttext&pid=S2218-36202021000500134&lng=es&tlng=es

Palantza, E., Sykaras, N., Zoidis, P., & Kourtis, S. (2024). *In vitro* comparison of accuracy between conventional and digital impression using elastomeric materials and two intraoral scanning devices. *Journal of Esthetic and Restorative Dentistry, 36*(8), 1179–1198. DOI: 10.1111/jerd.13227 PMID: 38534043

Pandey, N., de Coninck, H., & Sagar, A. D. (2022). Beyond technology transfer: Innovation cooperation to advance sustainable development in developing countries. *Wiley Interdisciplinary Reviews. Energy and Environment, 11*(2), e422. DOI: 10.1002/wene.422

Pankajavalli, P. B., & Karthick, G. S. (Eds.). (2020). *Incorporating the Internet of Things in healthcare applications and wearable devices*. IGI Global., DOI: 10.4018/978-1-7998-1090-2

Papapanou, M., Routsi, E., Tsamakis, K., Fotis, L., Marinos, G., Lidoriki, I., Karamanou, M., Papaioannou, T. G., Tsiptsios, D., Smyrnis, N., Rizos, E., & Schizas, D. (2022). Medical education challenges and innovations during COVID-19 pandemic. *Postgraduate Medical Journal, 98*(1159), 321–327. DOI: 10.1136/postgradmedj-2021-140032 PMID: 33782202

Parmentola, A., Petrillo, A., Tutore, I., & De Felice, F. (2022). Is blockchain able to enhance environmental sustainability? A systematic review and research agenda from the perspective of Sustainable Development Goals (SDGs). *Business Strategy and the Environment*, *31*(1), 194–217. DOI: 10.1002/bse.2882

Patel, M. S., Asch, D. A., & Volpp, K. G. (2015). Wearable devices as facilitators, not drivers, of health behavior change. *Journal of the American Medical Association*, *313*(5), 459–460. DOI: 10.1001/jama.2014.14781 PMID: 25569175

Patel, R. H., Foltz, E. A., Witkowski, A., & Ludzik, J. (2023, September 23). Analysis of Artificial Intelligence-Based Approaches Applied to Non-Invasive Imaging for Early Detection of Melanoma: A Systematic Review. *Cancers (Basel)*, *15*(19), 4694. Advance online publication. DOI: 10.3390/cancers15194694 PMID: 37835388

Patel, V. L., Yoskowitz, N. A., & Arocha, J. F. (2009). Towards effective evaluation and reform in medical education: A cognitive and learning sciences perspective. *Advances in Health Sciences Education : Theory and Practice*, *14*(5), 791–812. DOI: 10.1007/s10459-007-9091-1 PMID: 18214707

Paul, J., Ueno, A., & Dennis, C. (2023). ChatGPT and consumers: Benefits, pitfalls and future research agenda. *International Journal of Consumer Studies*, *47*(4), 1213–1225. DOI: 10.1111/ijcs.12928

Payne, K. F. B., Wharrad, H., & Watts, K. (2012). Smartphone and medical related App use among medical students and junior doctors in the United Kingdom (UK): A regional survey. *BMC Medical Informatics and Decision Making*, *12*(1), 1–11. DOI: 10.1186/1472-6947-12-121 PMID: 23110712

PCS. (2025). PCS: Patient Communication Simulators. https://www.pcs.ai/alex/

Perle, J. G., Chandran, D. N., Brezler, E., Coleman, M., Deziel, J., Nahhas, P., McDonald, G., & Jent, J. F. (2025). Technology-enhanced practice competencies: Scoping review and novel model development. *Frontiers in Digital Health*, *7*, 1571518. DOI: 10.3389/fdgth.2025.1571518 PMID: 40352328

Petraki, E., & Khat, K. (2022). Challenges and constraints in the design of an ESP course in Cambodia: Implications for higher education institutions. *Asia Pacific Journal of Education*, *42*(2), 260–275. DOI: 10.1080/02188791.2020.1798738

Phuangsuwan, P., Siripipatthanakul, S., Limna, P., & Pariwongkhuntorn, N. (2024). The Impact of Google Maps Application on the Digital Economy. *Phuangsuwan, P., Siripipatthanakul, S., Limna, P., & Pariwongkhuntorn*, 192-203. https://papers.ssrn.com/sol3/papers.cfm?abstract_id=4785205

Piedra Cascon, W., Parra Nunez, A., Charlen Diez, I., & Revilla León, M. (2019). Laboratory workflow to obtain long-term injected resin composite interim restorations from an additive manufactured esthetic diagnostic template. *Journal of Esthetic and Restorative Dentistry*, *31*(1), 13–19. DOI: 10.1111/jerd.12419 PMID: 30367695

Pillai, A. S. (2021). Utilizing deep learning in medical image analysis for enhanced diagnostic accuracy and patient care: Challenges, opportunities, and ethical implications. *Journal of Deep Learning in Genomic Data Analysis*.

Pirri, C., Stecco, C., Porzionato, A., Boscolo-Berto, R., Fortelny, R. H., Macchi, V., Konschake, M., Merigliano, S., & De Caro, R. (2021). Forensic Implications of Anatomical Education and Surgical Training With Cadavers. *Frontiers in Surgery*, *8*, 1–10. DOI: 10.3389/fsurg.2021.641581 PMID: 34250002

Piwek, L., Ellis, D. A., Andrews, S., & Joinson, A. (2016). The rise of consumer health wearables: Promises and barriers. *PLoS Medicine*, *13*(2), e1001953. DOI: 10.1371/journal.pmed.1001953 PMID: 26836780

Poblete, P., McAleer, S., & Mason, A. G. (2020). 3D Technology Development and Dental Education: What Topics Are Best Suited for 3D Learning Resources? *Dentistry Journal*, *8*(3), 95. DOI: 10.3390/dj8030095 PMID: 32882795

Pokhrel, N. B., Khadayat, R., & Tulachan, P. (2020). Depression, anxiety, and burnout among medical students and residents of a medical school in Nepal: A cross-sectional study. *BMC Psychiatry*, *20*(1), 298. DOI: 10.1186/s12888-020-02645-6 PMID: 32539732

Potter, L., & Jefferies, C. (2024). Enhancing Communication and Clinical Reasoning in Medical Education: Building Virtual Patients With Generative AI. *Future Healthcare Journal*, *11*, 100043. DOI: 10.1016/j.fhj.2024.100043

Powell, K. R. (2017). Patient-perceived facilitators of and barriers to electronic portal use: A systematic review. *CIN: Computers, Informatics. Computers, Informatics, Nursing*, *35*(11), 565–573. DOI: 10.1097/CIN.0000000000000377 PMID: 28723832

Prakash, J., Shenoy, M., Alhasmi, A., Al Saleh, A. A., Shivakumar, G. C., & Shivakumar, S. (2024). Biocompatibility of 3D-printed dental resins: A systematic review. *Cureus*, *16*, e51721. DOI: 10.7759/cureus.51721 PMID: 38318586

Pregowska, A., & Perkins, M. (2023). Artificial Intelligence in medical education: Technology and ethical risk. *Available at SSRN* 4643763. DOI: 10.2139/ssrn.4643763

Preiksaitis, C., & Rose, C. (2023). Opportunities, challenges, and future directions of generative artificial intelligence in medical education: Scoping review. *JMIR Medical Education*, *9*, e48785. DOI: 10.2196/48785 PMID: 37862079

Punj, A., Negassa, A., Gutierrez, A. K., Ch'en, P., & Jariwala, S. (2025). Technology enhanced medical education using smart glasses for oral and dental examinations: An observational pilot study. *BMC Medical Education*, *25*(1), 252. DOI: 10.1186/s12909-025-06853-0 PMID: 39962453

Puras, D. (2022). *Report of the Special Rapporteur on the right of everyone to the enjoyment of the highest attainable standard of physical and mental health*. Phil. LJ.

Qizi, R. S. S., Shukhratovna, T. S., & Karamatovna, M. A. (2024). Implementation of education and protection of children's rights in the age of technology.

Quinn, T. P., & Coghlan, S. (2021). Readying medical students for medical AI: The need to embed AI ethics education. *arXiv preprint arXiv:2109.02866*.

Radwan, H. A., Alsharif, A. T., Alsharif, M. T., Aloufi, M. R., & Alshammari, B. S. (2023). Digital technologies in dentistry in Saudi Arabia: Perceptions, practices and Challenges. *Digital Health*, *9*, 20552076231197095. DOI: 10.1177/20552076231197095 PMID: 37662673

Rahiem, M. D. (2020). The emergency remote learning experience of university students in Indonesia amidst the COVID-19 crisis. *International Journal of Learning. Teaching and Educational Research*, *19*(6), 1–26. DOI: 10.26803/ijlter.19.6.1

Rajab, M. H., Gazal, A. M., & Alkattan, K. (2020). Challenges to online medical education during the COVID-19 pandemic.

Raman, R., Pattnaik, D., Hughes, L., & Nedungadi, P. (2024). Unveiling the dynamics of AI applications: A review of reviews using scientometrics and BERTopic modeling. *Journal of Innovation & Knowledge*, *9*(3), 100517. DOI: 10.1016/j.jik.2024.100517

Rampton, V., Mittelman, M., & Goldhahn, J. (2020). Implications of artificial intelligence for medical education. *The Lancet. Digital Health*, *2*(3), e111–e112. DOI: 10.1016/S2589-7500(20)30023-6 PMID: 33328081

Ranuharja, F., Rizal, F., Langeveldt, D., Ejjami, R., Torres-Toukoumidis, A., & Jalinus, N. (2025). Relevance and Impact of Generative AI in Vocational Instructional Material Design: A Systematic Literature Review [Review]. *Salud, Ciencia y Tecnología*, *5*, 1336. Advance online publication. DOI: 10.56294/saludcyt20251336

Rapanta, C., Botturi, L., Goodyear, P., Guàrdia, L., & Koole, M. (2021). Balancing technology, pedagogy and the new normal: Post-pandemic challenges for higher education. *Postdigital Science and Education*, *3*(3), 715–742. DOI: 10.1007/s42438-021-00249-1

Rashid, A. B., & Kausik, M. D. A. K. (2024, 2024/12/01/). AI revolutionizing industries worldwide: A comprehensive overview of its diverse applications. *Hybrid Advances, 7*, 100277. https://doi.org/https://doi.org/10.1016/j.hybadv.2024.100277

Rathee, M., Alam, M., Divakar, S., & Malik, S. (2022). Resin-bonded bridge as a simplified approach to restore missing teeth in esthetic zone by conventional and digital techniques. *Dental Research Journal (Isfahan), 19*(1), 92. DOI: 10.4103/1735-3327.361341 PMID: 36605148

Rawas, S. (2024). ChatGPT: Empowering lifelong learning in the digital age of higher education. *Education and Information Technologies, 29*(6), 6895–6908. DOI: 10.1007/s10639-023-12114-8

Ray, P. P. (2023). ChatGPT: A comprehensive review on background, applications, key challenges, bias, ethics, limitations and future scope. *Internet of Things and Cyber-Physical Systems, 3*, 121–154. DOI: 10.1016/j.iotcps.2023.04.003

Reddy, P., Chaudhary, K., Sharma, B., & Chand, R. (2020, December). Digital literacy: A catalyst for the 21st-century education. In *2020 IEEE Asia-Pacific Conference on Computer Science and Data Engineering (CSDE)* (pp. 1–6).

Reddy, S. (2024). Generative AI in healthcare: An implementation science informed translational path on application, integration and governance [Article]. *Implementation Science : IS, 19*(1), 27. Advance online publication. DOI: 10.1186/s13012-024-01357-9 PMID: 38491544

Regmi, K., & Jones, L. (2020). A systematic review of the factors–enablers and barriers–affecting e-learning in health sciences education. *BMC Medical Education, 20*(1), 91. DOI: 10.1186/s12909-020-02007-6 PMID: 32228560

Reid, L., Button, D., & Brommeyer, M. (2023). Challenging the myth of the digital native: A narrative review. *Nursing Reports, 13*(2), 573–600. DOI: 10.3390/nursrep13020052 PMID: 37092480

Remtulla, R. (2020). The present and future applications of technology in adapting medical education amidst the COVID-19 pandemic. *JMIR Medical Education, 6*(2), e20190. DOI: 10.2196/20190 PMID: 32634107

Resnik, D. B., & Hosseini, M. (2024). The Ethics of Using Artificial Intelligence in Scientific Research: New Guidance Needed for a New Tool. *AI and Ethics*, •••, 1–23. DOI: 10.1007/s43681-024-00493-8 PMID: 40337745

Reuben, J. S., Meiri, H., & Arien-Zakay, H. (2024). AI's pivotal impact on redefining stakeholder roles and their interactions in medical education and health care [Article]. *Frontiers in Digital Health, 6*, 1458811. Advance online publication. DOI: 10.3389/fdgth.2024.1458811 PMID: 39564581

Rhoney, D. H., Singleton, S., Nelson, N. R., Anderson, S. M., & Hubal, R. (2021). Forces driving change in pharmacy education: Opportunities to take academic, social, technological, economic, and political into the future [Article]. *Journal of the American College of Clinical Pharmacy: JAACP, 4*(5), 639–651. DOI: 10.1002/jac5.1407

Riddle, E. W., Kewalramani, D., Narayan, M., & Jones, D. B. (2024). Surgical Simulation: Virtual Reality to Artificial Intelligence. *Current Problems in Surgery, 61*(11), 1–55. DOI: 10.1016/j.cpsurg.2024.101625 PMID: 39477664

Robbins, D., & Dunn, P. (2019). Digital health literacy in a person-centric world. *International Journal of Cardiology, 290*, 154–155. DOI: 10.1016/j.ijcard.2019.05.033 PMID: 31130277

Robinson, J. R., Stey, A., Schneider, D. F., Kothari, A. N., Lindeman, B., Kaafarani, H. M., & Haines, K. L. (2025, 2025/02/10/). Generative Artificial Intelligence in Academic Surgery: Ethical Implications and Transformative Potential. *Journal of Surgical Research*. https://doi.org/https://doi.org/10.1016/j.jss.2024.12.059

Robson, J., Rung, A., McCusker, M., Grant, G., & George, R. (2024). A systematic review of methodology for the creation of virtual 3D models for use in dental education and a narrative review. *International Journal of Computerized Dentistry, 27*(4), 337–343. DOI: 10.3290/j.ijcd.b4224867 PMID: 37477083

Rolfe, G., & Freshwater, D. (2020). *Critical Reflection in Practice: Generating Knowledge for Care*. Blooms-bury Publishing.

Rožanec, J. M., Novalija, I., Zajec, P., Kenda, K., Tavakoli Ghinani, H., Suh, S., Veliou, E., Papamartzivanos, D., Giannetsos, T., Menesidou, S. A., Alonso, R., Cauli, N., Meloni, A., Recupero, D. R., Kyriazis, D., Sofianidis, G., Theodoropoulos, S., Fortuna, B., Mladenić, D., & Soldatos, J. (2023). Human-centric artificial intelligence architecture for industry 5.0 applications. *International Journal of Production Research, 61*(20), 6847–6872. DOI: 10.1080/00207543.2022.2138611

Rubach, C., & Lazarides, R. (2021). Addressing 21st-century digital skills in schools–Development and validation of an instrument to measure teachers' basic ICT competence beliefs. *Computers in Human Behavior, 118*, 106636. DOI: 10.1016/j.chb.2020.106636

Rubinstein, I., & Margulies, P. (2022). *Risk and rights in transatlantic data transfers: EU privacy law, US surveillance, and the search for common ground*. L. Rev.

Ruschel, G. H., Gomes, É. A., Silva-Sousa, Y. T., Pinelli, R. G. P., Sousa-Neto, M. D., Pereira, G. K. R., & Spazzin, A. O. (2018). Mechanical properties and superficial characterization of a milled CAD-CAM glass fiber post. *Journal of the Mechanical Behavior of Biomedical Materials, 82*, 187–192. DOI: 10.1016/j.jmbbm.2018.03.035 PMID: 29609139

Russell, S. J., & Norvig, P. (2021). *Artificial Intelligence: A Modern Approach* (4th ed.). Pearson.

Ru, Z. J., Panchal, O., Chen, C. T., Jonnagaddala, J., Dai, H. J., & Hsueh, S. C. (2025). Utilizing Large Language Models for Privacy Protection and Advancing Medical Digitization [Conference paper]. *Communications in Computer and Information Science, 2148*, 177–188. DOI: 10.1007/978-981-97-7966-6_13

Sadowsky, S. J. (2021). Comments regarding: Batista V. E. S., Bitencourt S. B., Bastos N. A., Pellizzer E. P., Goiato M. C., Dos Santos D. M. Influence of the ferrule effect on the failure of fiber-reinforced composite post-and-core restorations: A systematic review and meta-analysis. *The Journal of Prosthetic Dentistry, 125*(5), 554. DOI: 10.1016/j.prosdent.2020.02.036 PMID: 32807404

Safranek, C. W., Sidamon-Eristoff, A. E., Gilson, A., & Chartash, D. (2023). The role of large language models in medical education: Applications and implications. *JMIR Medical Education, 9*, e50945. DOI: 10.2196/50945 PMID: 37578830

Sahi, P. K., Mishra, D., & Singh, T. (2020). Medical education amid the COVID-19 pandemic. *Indian Pediatrics, 57*(7), 652–657. DOI: 10.1007/s13312-020-1894-7 PMID: 32412913

Saikat, S., Dhillon, J. S., Wan Ahmad, W. F., & Jamaluddin, R. A. D. (2021). A systematic review of the benefits and challenges of mobile learning during the COVID-19 pandemic. *Education Sciences, 11*(9), 459. DOI: 10.3390/educsci11090459

Saini, K. S., Tagliamento, M., Lambertini, M., McNally, R., Romano, M., Leone, M., Curigliano, G., & de Azambuja, E. (2020). Mortality in patients with cancer and coronavirus disease 2019: A systematic review and pooled analysis of 52 studies. *European Journal of Cancer, 139*, 43–50. DOI: 10.1016/j.ejca.2020.08.011 PMID: 32971510

Saleem, N., Mufti, T., Sohail, S. S., & Madsen, D. Ø. (2024). ChatGPT as an Innovative Heutagogical Tool in Medical Education. *Cogent Education, 11*(1), 1–10. DOI: 10.1080/2331186X.2024.2332850

Sallam, M., Salim, N. A., Barakat, M., & Ala'a, B. (2023). ChatGPT applications in medical, dental, pharmacy, and public health education: A descriptive study highlighting the advantages and limitations. *Narra J*, *3*(1), e103. DOI: 10.52225/narra.v3i1.103 PMID: 38450035

Salloum, A., Alfaisal, R., & Salloum, S. A. (2024). Revolutionizing Medical Education: Empowering Learning with ChatGPT. In *Studies in Big Data* (Vol. 144, pp. 79-90). Springer Science and Business Media Deutschland GmbH. https://doi.org/ DOI: 10.1007/978-3-031-52280-2_6

Sami, A., Tanveer, F., Sajwani, K., Kiran, N., Javed, M. A., Ozsahin, D. U., Muhammad, K., & Waheed, Y. (2025). Medical students' attitudes toward AI in education: Perception, effectiveness, and its credibility. *BMC Medical Education*, *25*(1), 1–12. DOI: 10.1186/s12909-025-06704-y PMID: 39833834

Samuel, J., Brennan-Tonetta, M., Samuel, Y., Subedi, P., & Smith, J. (2021). Strategies for democratization of supercomputing: Availability, accessibility and usability of high performance computing for education and practice of big data analytics. *arXiv preprint arXiv:2104.09091.*

Sanchez, T. W., Brenman, M., & Ye, X. (2024). The ethical concerns of artificial intelligence in urban planning. *Journal of the American Planning Association*, •••, 1–14.

Santamato, V., Tricase, C., Faccilongo, N., Iacoviello, M., & Marengo, A. (2024). Exploring the Impact of Artificial Intelligence on Healthcare Management: A Combined Systematic Review and Machine-Learning Approach. *Applied Sciences (Basel, Switzerland)*, *14*(22), 10144. DOI: 10.3390/app142210144

Sapci, A. H., & Sapci, H. A. (2020). Artificial intelligence education and tools for medical and health informatics students: Systematic review. *JMIR Medical Education*, *6*(1), e19285. DOI: 10.2196/19285 PMID: 32602844

Sarkar, U., Lee, J. E., Nguyen, K. H., Lisker, S., & Lyles, C. R. (2021). Barriers and facilitators to the implementation of virtual reality as a pain management modality in academic, community, and safety-net settings: Qualitative analysis. *Journal of Medical Internet Research*, *23*(9), e26623. DOI: 10.2196/26623 PMID: 34550074

Satapathy, P., Hermis, A. H., Rustagi, S., Pradhan, K. B., Padhi, B. K., & Sah, R. (2023). Artificial Intelligence in Surgical Education and Training: Opportunities, Challenges, and Ethical Considerations – Correspondence. *International Journal of Surgery*, *109*(5), 1543–1544. DOI: 10.1097/JS9.0000000000000387 PMID: 37037597

Sato, S. N., Condes Moreno, E., Rubio-Zarapuz, A., Dalamitros, A. A., Yañez-Sepulveda, R., Tornero-Aguilera, J. F., & Clemente-Suárez, V. J. (2024). Navigating the New Normal: Adapting Online and Distance Learning in the Post-Pandemic Era. *Education Sciences*, *14*(1), 19. DOI: 10.3390/educsci14010019

Sauder, M., Tritsch, T., Rajput, V., Schwartz, G., & Shoja, M. M. (2024, January). Exploring Generative Artificial Intelligence-Assisted Medical Education: Assessing Case-Based Learning for Medical Students. *Cureus*, *16*(1), e51961. DOI: 10.7759/cureus.51961 PMID: 38333501

Scherr, R., Halaseh, F. F., Spina, A., Andalib, S., & Rivera, R. (2023). ChatGPT interactive medical simulations for early clinical education: Case study. *JMIR Medical Education*, *9*, e49877. DOI: 10.2196/49877 PMID: 37948112

Schlenz, M. A., Michel, K., Wegner, K., Schmidt, A., Rehmann, P., & Wöstmann, B. (2020). Undergraduate dental students' perspective on the implementation of digital dentistry in the preclinical curriculum: A questionnaire survey. *BMC Oral Health*, *20*(1), 78. DOI: 10.1186/s12903-020-01071-0 PMID: 32188456

Schön, D. (1983). *The Reflective Practitioner: How Professionals Think in Action*. Basic Books.

Schön, D. (1987). *Educating the Reflective Practitioner: toward a New Design for Teaching and Learning in the Professions*. Jossey-Bass.

Schön, D. A. (1992). The theory of inquiry: Dewey's legacy to education. *Curriculum Inquiry*, *22*(2), 119–139. DOI: 10.1080/03626784.1992.11076093

Schubert, T., Oosterlinck, T., Stevens, R. D., Maxwell, P. H., & van der Schaar, M. (2025). AI Education for Clinicians. *EClinicalMedicine*, *79*, 1–7. DOI: 10.1016/j.eclinm.2024.102968 PMID: 39720600

Schünemann, W. J., & Windwehr, J. (2021). Towards a 'gold standard for the world'? The European General Data Protection Regulation between supranational and national norm entrepreneurship. *Journal of European Integration*, *43*(7), 859–874. DOI: 10.1080/07036337.2020.1846032

Schwartz, R.. (2022). *Towards a standard for identifying and managing bias in artificial intelligence* (Vol. 3). U.S. Department of Commerce, National Institute of Standards and Technology. DOI: 10.6028/NIST.SP.1270

Schweiger, J., & Güth, J. F. (2020). Neue Entwicklungen in der additiven und subtraktiven Fertigung. *Teamwork Journal of Continuing Dental Education, 23*, 82–90. Retrieved December 10, 2020, from https://www.google.com/scholar

Schweiger, J., Edelhoff, D., & Güth, J. F. (2020). Update digitale Zahnheilkunde 2020—Aktuelle Möglichkeiten und Limitationen. *Bayerisches Zahnärzte Blatt, 57*, 42–52. Retrieved May 12, 2024, from https://www.google.com/scholar

Sengar, S. S., Hasan, A. B., Kumar, S., & Carroll, F. (2024). 2024/08/14). Generative artificial intelligence: A systematic review and applications. *Multimedia Tools and Applications*. Advance online publication. DOI: 10.1007/s11042-024-20016-1

Sermonesi, G., Bertelli, R., Pieracci, F. M., Balogh, Z. J., Coimbra, R., Galante, J. M., Hecker, A., Weber, D., Bauman, Z. M., Kartiko, S., Patel, B., Whitbeck, S. A. S., White, T. W., Harrell, K. N., Perrina, D., Rampini, A., Tian, B., Amico, F., Beka, S. G., & Catena, F. (2024). Surgical stabilization of rib fractures (SSRF): The WSES and CWIS position paper. *World Journal of Emergency Surgery; WJES, 19*(1), 33. DOI: 10.1186/s13017-024-00559-2 PMID: 39425134

Serrano, D. R., Luciano, F. C., Anaya, B. J., Ongoren, B., Kara, A., Molina, G., Ramirez, B. I., Sánchez-Guirales, S. A., Simon, J. A., Tomietto, G., Rapti, C., Ruiz, H. K., Rawat, S., Kumar, D., & Lalatsa, A. (2024). Artificial Intelligence (AI) Applications in Drug Discovery and Drug Delivery: Revolutionizing Personalized Medicine. *Pharmaceutics, 16*(10), 1–27. DOI: 10.3390/pharmaceutics16101328 PMID: 39458657

Sezer, H., & Gül, A. (2024). Health sciences students' perspectives on metaverse and digital technology use: Cross-sectional descriptive study. *BMC Nursing, 23*(1), 656. DOI: 10.1186/s12912-024-02309-w PMID: 39278911

Shachak, A., Monkman, H., Lesselroth, B., Lee, W. W., & Alkureishi, M. L. A. (2024). Technological literacy as a framework for health professions education in the digital era. In *Digital Health and Informatics Innovations for Sustainable Health Care Systems* (pp. 1500–1504). IOS Press. DOI: 10.3233/SHTI240699

Shafik, W. (2024). Wearable medical electronics in artificial intelligence of medical things. In *Artificial Intelligence of Medical Things*. Taylor & Francis., DOI: 10.1201/9781003370321-2

Shah, S., Diwan, S., Kohan, L., Rosenblum, D., Gharibo, C., Soin, A., Sulindro, A., Quinn, N., & Provenzano, D. A. (2020). The technological impact of COVID-19 on the future of education and health care delivery. *Pain Physician, 23*(23, 4S), S367–S380. DOI: 10.36076/ppj.2020/23/S367 PMID: 32942794

Shamsuzzoha, A., Nieminen, J., Piya, S., & Rutledge, K. (2021). *Smart city for sustainable environment: A comparison of participatory strategies from Helsinki*. Cities.

Sharma, P., Adamopoulos, I. P., Syrou, N. F., Budhathoki, C. B., & Thapa, P. P. (2025). The impact of health-caregivers emotional nurturance on cognitive development in preschoolers: A nationwide public health cross-sectional study. *EJGM*, *22*(3), em643. DOI: 10.29333/ejgm/16184

Shcherbina, A., Mattsson, C. M., Waggott, D., Salisbury, H., Christle, J. W., Hastie, T., Wheeler, M. T., & Ashley, E. (2017). Accuracy in wrist-worn, sensor-based measurements of heart rate and energy expenditure in a diverse cohort. *Journal of Personalized Medicine*, *7*(2), 3. DOI: 10.3390/jpm7020003 PMID: 28538708

Shetty, A., Shetty, A. D., Pai, R. Y., Rao, R. R., Bhandary, R., Shetty, J., Nayak, S., Keerthi Dinesh, T., & Dsouza, K. J. (2022). Blockchain application in insurance services: A systematic review of the evidence. *SAGE Open*, *12*(1), 21. DOI: 10.1177/21582440221079877

Shin, E., Hartman, M., & Ramanathan, M. (2024). Performance of the ChatGPT large language model for decision support in community pharmacy [Article]. *British Journal of Clinical Pharmacology*, *90*(12), 3320–3333. DOI: 10.1111/bcp.16215 PMID: 39191671

Shorey, S., & Ng, E. D. (2021). The use of virtual reality simulation among nursing students and registered nurses: A systematic review. *Nurse Education Today*, *98*, 104662. DOI: 10.1016/j.nedt.2020.104662 PMID: 33203545

Silva-Velasco, E., López-Aballe, M., & Mayedo-Núñez, Y. (2023). La Educación Médica y su papel en la formación clínica de los estudiantes de Medicina. *Luz, 22*(3), 150-160. http://scielo.sld.cu/scielo.php?script=sci_arttext&pid=S1814-151X2023000300150&lng=es&tlng=es

Simms, R. C. (2025). 2025/03/01/). Generative artificial intelligence (AI) literacy in nursing education: A crucial call to action. *Nurse Education Today*, *146*, 106544. https://doi.org/https://doi.org/10.1016/j.nedt.2024.106544. DOI: 10.1016/j.nedt.2024.106544 PMID: 39708405

Simpson, D. D. (2011). A framework for implementing sustainable oral health promotion interventions. *Journal of Public Health Dentistry*, *71*(s1), S84–S94. DOI: 10.1111/j.1752-7325.2011.00234.x PMID: 21499507

Singh, V. K., & Ali, Z. (2025). *Design and Simulation of Wearable Antennas for Healthcare*. IGI Global. https://www.igi-global.com/book/design-simulation-wearable-antennas-healthcare/338208

Singh, N., Gunjan, V. K., & Nasralla, M. M. (2022). A Parametrized Comparative Analysis of Performance Between Proposed Adaptive and Personalized Tutoring System "Seis Tutor" With Existing Online Tutoring System. *IEEE Access : Practical Innovations, Open Solutions, 10*, 39376–39386. DOI: 10.1109/ACCESS.2022.3166261

Sirko, J., & Shi, W. (2024). Disruptive innovation events in dentistry. *JADA Foundational Science, 3*(100036), 100036. DOI: 10.1016/j.jfscie.2024.100036 PMID: 39384257

Solomonides, A. E., Koski, E., Atabaki, S. M., Weinberg, C., & Lehmann, C. U. (2022). Defining AMIA's artificial intelligence principles. *Journal of the American Medical Informatics Association : JAMIA, 29*(4), 585–591. DOI: 10.1093/jamia/ocac006 PMID: 35190824

Sophonhiranrak, S. (2021). Features, barriers, and influencing factors of mobile learning in higher education: A systematic review. *Heliyon, 7*(4), e06696. Advance online publication. DOI: 10.1016/j.heliyon.2021.e06696 PMID: 33869873

Southworth, J., Migliaccio, K., Glover, J., Reed, D., McCarty, C., Brendemuhl, J., & Thomas, A. (2023). Developing a model for AI across the curriculum: Transforming the higher education landscape via innovation in AI literacy. *Artificial Intelligence, 4*, 100127.

Souza, A. D., & Vaswani, V. (2020). Diversity in approach to teaching and assessing ethics education for medical undergraduates: A scoping review. *Annals of Medicine and Surgery (London), 56*, 178–185. DOI: 10.1016/j.amsu.2020.06.028 PMID: 32642060

Spencer, D., & Temple, T. (2021). Examining students' online course perceptions and comparing student performance outcomes in online and face-to-face classrooms.

Spielman, A. I. (2024). Dental education and practice: Past, present, and future trends. *Frontiers in Oral Health, 5*, 1368121. DOI: 10.3389/froh.2024.1368121 PMID: 38694791

Sridharan, K., & Sequeira, R. P. (2024). Artificial intelligence and medical education: Application in classroom instruction and student assessment using a pharmacology & therapeutics case study [Article]. *BMC Medical Education, 24*(1), 431. Advance online publication. DOI: 10.1186/s12909-024-05365-7 PMID: 38649959

Stahl, B. C., & Eke, D. (2024). The ethics of ChatGPT–Exploring the ethical issues of an emerging technology. *International Journal of Information Management, 74*, 102700. DOI: 10.1016/j.ijinfomgt.2023.102700

Steinhubl, S. R., Muse, E. D., & Topol, E. J. (2015). The emerging field of mobile health. *Science Translational Medicine*, *7*(283), 283rv3. Advance online publication. DOI: 10.1126/scitranslmed.aaa3487 PMID: 25877894

Stevens, G. J., Bienz, T., Wali, N., Condie, J., & Schismenos, S. (2021). Online university education is the new normal: But is face-to-face better? *Interactive Technology and Smart Education*, *18*(3), 278–297. DOI: 10.1108/ITSE-08-2020-0181

Stogiannos, N., Georgiadou, E., Rarri, N., & Malamateniou, C. (2025). 2025/01/01/). Ethical AI: A qualitative study exploring ethical challenges and solutions on the use of AI in medical imaging. *European Journal of Radiology Artificial Intelligence*, *1*, 100006. https://doi.org/https://doi.org/10.1016/j.ejrai.2025.100006. DOI: 10.1016/j.ejrai.2025.100006

Stretton, B., Kovoor, J., Arnold, M., & Bacchi, S. (2024). ChatGPT-Based Learning: Generative Artificial Intelligence in Medical Education. *Medical Science Educator*, *34*(1), 215–217. DOI: 10.1007/s40670-023-01934-5 PMID: 38510403

Strielkowski, W., Grebennikova, V., Lisovskiy, A., Rakhimova, G., & Vasileva, T. (2024). AI-Driven Adaptive Learning for Sustainable Educational Transformation. *Sustainable Development*. Advance online publication. DOI: 10.1002/sd.3221

Sui, A., Sui, W., Liu, S., & Rhodes, R. (2023). Ethical considerations for the use of consumer wearables in health research. *Digital Health*, *9*, 20552076231153740. Advance online publication. DOI: 10.1177/20552076231153740 PMID: 36756643

Su, J.-M., Hsu, S.-Y., Fang, T.-Y., & Wang, P.-C. (2024). 2024/08/01/). Developing and validating a knowledge-based AI assessment system for learning clinical core medical knowledge in otolaryngology. *Computers in Biology and Medicine*, *178*, 108765. https://doi.org/https://doi.org/10.1016/j.compbiomed.2024.108765. DOI: 10.1016/j.compbiomed.2024.108765 PMID: 38897143

Suliman, M. A. E.. (2024). Medical student's acceptance of mobile learning: Integrating TAM model with perceived reusability. *Education and Information Technologies*, *1*(24). Advance online publication. DOI: 10.1007/s10639-024-12917-3

Sumanasena, V., Rajabipour, A., Bazli, M., Kutay, C., & Guo, D. (2022). Strength and erosion resistance of mudbrick as an alternative local material for Australia's Northern Territory remote housing. *Case Studies in Construction Materials*, *16*, e01023. DOI: 10.1016/j.cscm.2022.e01023

Sun, C., & Harris, S. L. (2024). Reducing bias in healthcare artificial intelligence: A white paper [Article]. *Health Informatics Journal*, *30*(4), 14604582241291410. Advance online publication. DOI: 10.1177/14604582241291410 PMID: 39541598

Sun, J. C. (2023). Gaps, guesswork, and ghosts lurking in technology integration: Laws and policies applicable to student privacy. *British Journal of Educational Technology, 54*(6), 1604–1618. DOI: 10.1111/bjet.13379

Sun, L., He, L., Han, L., Yu, B., & Lin, J. (2025). Self-powered piezoelectric wearable sensor with motion recognition capability. *IEEE Sensors Journal, 25*(9), 14760–14769. Advance online publication. DOI: 10.1109/JSEN.2025.3549451

Sun, L., Yin, C., Xu, Q., & Zhao, W. (2023). Artificial intelligence for healthcare and medical education: A systematic review. *American Journal of Translational Research, 15*(7), 4820–4828. PMID: 37560249

Sun, W., Jiang, X., Dong, X., Yu, G., Feng, Z., & Shuai, L. (2024). The Evolution of Simulation-Based Medical Education Research: From Traditional to Virtual Simulations. *Heliyon, 10*(15), 1–14. DOI: 10.1016/j.heliyon.2024.e35627 PMID: 39170203

Sun, X., Zhou, J., Wang, Q., Shi, J., & Wang, H. (2022). PVA fibre reinforced high-strength cementitious composite for 3D printing: Mechanical properties and durability. *Additive Manufacturing, 49*, 102500. Advance online publication. DOI: 10.1016/j.addma.2021.102500

Swan, M. (2012). Health 2050: The realization of personalized medicine through crowdsourcing, the quantified self, and the participatory biocitizen. *Journal of Personalized Medicine, 2*(3), 93–118. DOI: 10.3390/jpm2030093 PMID: 25562203

Sweller, J. (1988). Cognitive Load During Problem Solving. *Effects on Learning., 285*, 257–285. DOI: 10.1207/s15516709cog1202

Syauqi, K., Munadi, S., & Triyono, M. B. (2020). Students' perceptions toward vocational education on online learning during the COVID-19 pandemic. *International Journal of Evaluation and Research in Education, 9*(4), 881–886. DOI: 10.11591/ijere.v9i4.20766

Syed, F. M., & ES, F. K. (2024). AI-powered security for Internet of Medical Things (IoMT) devices. *Revista de Inteligencia Artificial en Medicina.*

Syed, S. A., Sheikh, M., Syed, F. A., Atif, S., Iqbal, A., & Zeeshan, G. (2024). Comparison of virtual clinical scenario and role play in learning oral pathology among dental students. *PLoS One, 19*(7), e0306712. DOI: 10.1371/journal.pone.0306712 PMID: 38976658

Tabatabai, S. (2020). COVID-19 impact and virtual medical education. *Journal of Advances in Medical Education & Professionalism, 8*(3), 140. PMID: 32802908

Tahayeri, A., Morgan, M., Fugolin, A. P., Bompolaki, D., Athirasala, A., Pfeifer, C. S., Ferracane, J. L., & Bertassoni, L. E. (2018). 3D printed versus conventionally cured provisional crown and bridge dental materials. *Dental Materials*, *34*(2), 192–200. DOI: 10.1016/j.dental.2017.10.003 PMID: 29110921

Takeuchi, Y., Koizumi, H., Furuchi, M., Sato, Y., Ohkubo, C., & Matsumura, H. (2018). Use of digital impression systems with intraoral scanners for fabricating restorations and fixed dental prostheses. *Journal of Oral Science*, *60*(1), 1–7. DOI: 10.2334/josnusd.17-0444 PMID: 29576569

Tan, O. S. (2009). *Problem-Based Learning and Creativity*. Cengage: Learning Asia Pte Ltd: Singapore.

Tang, Y. M., Chau, K. Y., Kwok, A. P. K., Zhu, T., & Ma, X. (2022). A Systematic Review of Immersive Technology Applications for Medical Practice and Education - Trends, Application Areas, Recipients, Teaching Contents, Evaluation Methods, and Performance. *Educational Research Review*, *35*, 1–22. DOI: 10.1016/j.edurev.2021.100429

Teele, S. A., Sindelar, A., Brown, D., Kane, D. A., Thatte, N., Williams, R. J., Gueverra, J., & Wolbrink, T. A. (2021). Online education in a hurry: Delivering pediatric graduate medical education during COVID-19. *Progress in Pediatric Cardiology*, *60*, 101320. DOI: 10.1016/j.ppedcard.2020.101320 PMID: 33169056

Teixeira, K. N., Duque, T. M., Maia, H. P., & Gonçalves, T. (2020). Fracture resistance and failure mode of custom-made post-and-cores of polyetheretherketone and nano-ceramic composite. *Operative Dentistry*, *45*(5), 506–515. DOI: 10.2341/19-080-L PMID: 32101501

Tekin, P., Ilgaz, H., Adanır, G., Yıldırım, D., & Gülbahar Güven, Y. (2020). Flipping e-learning for teaching medical terminology: A study of learners' online experiences and perceptions. *Online Learning : the Official Journal of the Online Learning Consortium*, *24*(2), 76–93. DOI: 10.24059/olj.v24i2.2030

Templin, T., Perez, M. W., Sylvia, S., Leek, J., & Sinnott-Armstrong, N. (2024, May). Addressing 6 challenges in generative AI for digital health: A scoping review. *PLOS Digital Health*, *3*(5), e0000503. DOI: 10.1371/journal.pdig.0000503 PMID: 38781686

Temsah, O., Khan, S. A., Chaiah, Y., Senjab, A., Alhasan, K., Jamal, A., Aljamaan, F., Malki, K. H., Halwani, R., Al-Tawfiq, J. A., Temsah, M.-H., & Al-Eyadhy, A. (2023). Overview of early ChatGPT's presence in medical literature: Insights from a hybrid literature review by ChatGPT and human experts. *Cureus*, *15*(4). Advance online publication. DOI: 10.7759/cureus.37281 PMID: 37038381

Ten Cate, O. T. J., Kusurkar, R. A., & Williams, G. C. (2011). How self-determination theory can assist our understanding of the teaching and learning processes in medical education. AMEE guide No. 59. *Medical Teacher, 33*(12), 961–973. DOI: 10.3109/0142159X.2011.595435 PMID: 22225433

Teo, Z. L., Quek, C. W. N., Wong, J. L. Y., & Ting, D. S. W. (2024). 2024/07/01/). Cybersecurity in the generative artificial intelligence era. *Asia-Pacific Journal of Ophthalmology, 13*(4), 100091. https://doi.org/https://doi.org/10.1016/j.apjo.2024.100091. DOI: 10.1016/j.apjo.2024.100091 PMID: 39209217

Thaichana, P., Oo, M. Z., Thorup, G. L., Chansakaow, C., Arworn, S., & Rerkasem, K. (2025). Integrating Artificial Intelligence in Medical Writing: Balancing Technological Innovation and Human Expertise, with Practical Applications in Lower Extremity Wounds Care [Review]. *The International Journal of Lower Extremity Wounds*, 15347346241312814. Advance online publication. DOI: 10.1177/15347346241312814 PMID: 39801150

Thai, N. T. T., De Wever, B., & Valcke, M. (2020). Face-to-face, blended, flipped, or online learning environment? Impact on learning performance and student cognitions. *Journal of Computer Assisted Learning, 36*(3), 397–411. DOI: 10.1111/jcal.12423

Thapa, P., Adamopoulos, I. P., Sharma, P., & Lordkipanidze, R. (2024). Public hygiene and the awareness of beauty parlor: A study of consumer perspective. *European Journal of Environment and Public Health, 8*(2), em0157. DOI: 10.29333/ejeph/14738

Thapa, P., Rijal, A., Sharma, P., Tsirkas, P., Valamontes, A., & Adamopoulos, I. (2025). Impact of mobile phone use on distracted driving and the moderating role of self-regulatory skills. *Preprints*.

Thapa, P., Sharma, P., Goundar, S., Tsirkas, P., Valamontes, A., & Adamopoulos, I. (2025). Digital distractions in the classroom among students: A cross-sectional study. *Preprints*. DOI: 10.20944/preprints202502.1931.v1

Thayyib, P. V., Mamilla, R., Khan, M., Fatima, H., Asim, M., Anwar, I., Shamsudheen, M. K., & Khan, M. A. (2023). State-of-the-Art of Artificial Intelligence and Big Data Analytics Reviews in Five Different Domains: A Bibliometric Summary. *Sustainability (Basel), 15*(5), 4026. https://www.mdpi.com/2071-1050/15/5/4026. DOI: 10.3390/su15054026

Thomae, A. V., Witt, C. M., & Barth, J. (2024). Integration of ChatGPT Into a Course for Medical Students: Explorative Study on Teaching Scenarios, Students' Perception, and Applications. *JMIR Medical Education, 10*, 1–10. DOI: 10.2196/50545 PMID: 39177012

Thurzo, A., Strunga, M., Urban, R., Surovková, J., & Afrashtehfar, K. I. (2023). Impact of Artificial Intelligence on Dental Education: A Review and Guide for Curriculum Update. *Education Sciences*, *13*(2), 150. DOI: 10.3390/educsci13020150

Thurzo, A., Strunga, M., Urban, R., Surovková, J., & Afrashtehfar, K. I. (2023). *Impact of artificial intelligence on dental education: A review and guide for curricυλυμ υπδατε. Εδυχατιον Σχιενχεσ, 13(2), 150. ηττπσ:// ωωω. μδπι. χομ/ 2227 – 7102/ 13/ 2/ 150.* ΔΟΙ., DOI: 10.3390/εδυχσχι13020150

Tian, Y., Chen, C., Xu, X., Wang, J., Hou, X., Li, K., Lu, X., Shi, H., Lee, E., & Jiang, H. (2021). A review of 3D printing in dentistry: Technologies, affecting factors, and applications. *Scanning*, *9950131*, 1–19. Advance online publication. DOI: 10.1155/2021/9950131 PMID: 34367410

Tierney, A. A., Mosqueda, M., Cesena, G., Frehn, J. L., Payan, D. D., & Rodriguez, H. P. (2024). Telemedicine implementation for safety net populations: A systematic review. *Telemedicine Journal and e-Health*, *30*(3), 622–641. DOI: 10.1089/tmj.2023.0260 PMID: 37707997

Tiol-Carrillo, A. (2021). Aplicación de las tecnologías en la educación en odontología durante la pandemia por COVID-19. *Revista ADM*, *78*(3), 155–161. DOI: 10.35366/100073

Tiwari, A., Kumar, A., Jain, S., Dhull, K. S., Sajjanar, A., Puthenkandathil, R., Paiwal, K., & Singh, R. (2023). Implications of ChatGPT in public health dentistry: A systematic review. *Cureus*, *15*(6). Advance online publication. DOI: 10.7759/cureus.40367 PMID: 37456464

Tkachuk, V., Yechkalo, Y., Semerikov, S., Kislova, M., & Hladyr, Y. (2020, October). Using mobile ict for online learning during covid-19 lockdown. In *International Conference on Information and Communication Technologies in Education, Research, and Industrial Applications* (pp. 46-67). Cham: Springer International Publishing. DOI: 10.1007/978-3-030-77592-6_3

Tlili, A., Huang, R., Shehata, B., Liu, D., Zhao, J., Metwally, A. H. S., Wang, H., Denden, M., Bozkurt, A., Lee, L.-H., Beyoglu, D., Altinay, F., Sharma, R. C., Altinay, Z., Li, Z., Liu, J., Ahmad, F., Hu, Y., Salha, S., & Burgos, D. (2022). Is Metaverse in education a blessing or a curse: A combined content and bibliometric analysis. *Smart Learning Environments*, *9*(1), 1–31. DOI: 10.1186/s40561-022-00205-x

Tokuç, B., & Varol, G. (2023). Medical Education in the Era of Advancing Technology. *Balkan Medical Journal*, *40*(6), 395–399. DOI: 10.4274/balkanmedj.galenos.2023.2023-7-79 PMID: 37706676

Tolsgaard, M. G., Pusic, M. V., Sebok-Syer, S. S., Gin, B., Svendsen, M. B., Syer, M. D., Brydges, R., Cuddy, M. M., & Boscardin, C. K. (2023). The fundamentals of Artificial Intelligence in medical education research: AMEE Guide No. 156. *Medical Teacher*, *45*(6), 565–573. DOI: 10.1080/0142159X.2023.2180340 PMID: 36862064

Tonino, R., Larimer, K., Eissen, O., & Schipperus, M. R. (2019). Remote Patient Monitoring in Adults Receiving Transfusion or Infusion for Hematological Disorders Using the VitalPatch and accelerateIQ Monitoring System: Quantitative Feasibility Study. *Journal of Medical Internet Research*, *22*(7), e15103. DOI: 10.2196/15103 PMID: 31789596

Tozsin, A., Ucmak, H., Soyturk, S., Aydin, A., Gozen, A. S., Fahim, M. A., Güven, S., & Ahmed, K. (2024). The role of artificial intelligence in medical education: A systematic review. *Surgical Innovation*, *31*(4), 415–423. DOI: 10.1177/15533506241248239 PMID: 38632898

Tran, T., Ho, M. T., Pham, T. H., Nguyen, M. H., Nguyen, K. L. P., Vuong, T. T., Nguyen, T. H. T., Nguyen, T. D., Nguyen, T. L., Khuc, Q., La, V. P., & Vuong, Q.-H. (2020). How digital natives learn and thrive in the digital age: Evidence from an emerging economy. *Sustainability (Basel)*, *12*(9), 3819. DOI: 10.3390/su12093819

Traxler, J. (2005, June). Defining mobile learning. In IADIS international conference mobile learning (Vol. 261, p. 266).

Tripathi, S., Manoharan, P. S., & Nagda, S. (2024). Developing an instructional module of "digital dentistry" for undergraduate prosthodontics curriculum. *Journal of Oral Biology and Craniofacial Research*, *14*(1), 44–48. DOI: 10.1016/j.jobcr.2023.12.001 PMID: 38188908

Trocin, C., Mikalef, P., Papamitsiou, Z., & Conboy, K. (2023). Responsible AI for digital health: A synthesis and a research agenda. *Information Systems Frontiers*, *25*(6), 2139–2157. DOI: 10.1007/s10796-021-10146-4

Turner, L., Hashimoto, D. A., Vasisht, S., & Schaye, V. (2024). Demystifying AI: Current State and Future Role in Medical Education Assessment [Article]. *Hepatology (Baltimore, Md.)*, *99*(4), S42–S47. DOI: 10.1097/ACM.0000000000005598 PMID: 38166201

Tzimas, D., & Demetriadis, S. (2021). Ethical issues in learning analytics: A review of the field. *Educational Technology Research and Development*, *69*(2), 1101–1133. DOI: 10.1007/s11423-021-09977-4

Ταvγ, Ω. Λ., Χηαο, Ξ. Ψ., Ψε, Ζ., Λιυ, Μ. Ω., & ϑιαvγ, Η. (2024). Τηε υσε οφ δψvαμιχ vαϖιγατιοv σψστεμσ ασ α χομποvεvτ οφ διγιταλ δεvτιστρψ. *ϑουρvαλ οφ Δεvταλ Ρεσεαρχη*, 103(2), 119–128. https:// journals .sagepub .com/ doi/ abs/ . DOI: PMID: 38098369DOI: 10.1177/00220345231212811

Uctasli, S., Boz, Y., Sungur, S., Vallittu, P. K., Garoushi, S., & Lassila, L. (2021). Influence of post-core and crown type on the fracture resistance of incisors submitted to quasistatic loading. *Polymers*, *13*(7), 1130. DOI: 10.3390/polym13071130 PMID: 33918203

Uribe, S. E., Maldupa, I., & Schwendicke, F. (2025). Integrating Generative AI in Dental Education: A Scoping Review of Current Practices and Recommendations [Article]. *European Journal of Dental Education*, *29*(2), 341–355. Advance online publication. DOI: 10.1111/eje.13074 PMID: 39891376

Usman, M. (2024). Integration of Three-Dimensional Scanning and Computer-Aided Design/ Computer-Aided Manufacturing (CAD//CAM) Technology in Routine Prosthodontic Practice: A Cross-Sectional Study in Kerala. *Cureus*, *16*(12), e76409. DOI: 10.7759/cureus.76409 PMID: 39867077

Valcárcel-Izquierdo, N., & Díaz-Díaz, A. A. (2019). *Epistemología de las Ciencias de la Educación Médica*. Universidad de Ciencias Médicas de La Habana., http:// bvs.sld.cu/libros/epistemologia_ciencias_educacion_medica/epistemologia_ciencias _educacion.pdf

Valenti, C., Isabella Federici, M., Masciotti, F., Marinucci, L., Xhimitiku, I., Cianetti, S., & Pagano, S. (2022). Mechanical properties of 3D-printed prosthetic materials compared with milled and conventional processing. *The Journal of Prosthetic Dentistry*. Advance online publication. DOI: 10.1016/j.prosdent.2022.05.004 PMID: 35934576

Vallée, A., Blacher, J., Cariou, A., & Sorbets, E. (2020). Blended learning compared to traditional learning in medical education: Systematic review and meta-analysis. *Journal of Medical Internet Research*, *22*(8), e16504. DOI: 10.2196/16504 PMID: 32773378

Vallurupalli, S., Paydak, H., Agarwal, S. K., Agrawal, M., & Assad-Kottner, C. (2013). Wearable technology to improve education and patient outcomes in a cardiology fellowship program: A feasibility study. *Health and Technology*, *3*(4), 267–270. DOI: 10.1007/s12553-013-0065-4

Valverde-Berrocoso, J., Garrido-Arroyo, M. C., Burgos-Videla, C., & Morales-Cevallos, M. B. (2020). Trends in educational research about e-learning: A systematic literature review. *Sustainability (Basel)*, *12*(12), 5153. DOI: 10.3390/su12125153 van der Kruk, S. R., Zielinski, R., MacDougall, H., Hughes-Barton, D., & Gunn, K. M. (2022). Virtual reality as a patient education tool in healthcare: A scoping review. *Patient Education and Counseling, 105*(7), 1928–1942. DOI: 10.1016/j.pec.2022.02.005 PMID: 35168856

van der Niet, A. G., & Bleakley, A. (2021). Where medical education meets artificial intelligence: "Does technology care?". *Medical Education, 55*(1), 30–36. DOI: 10.1111/medu.14131 PMID: 32078175

Van Noort, R. (2012). The future of dental devices is digital. *Dental Materials, 28*(1), 3–12. DOI: 10.1016/j.dental.2011.10.014 PMID: 22119539

Van Veen, D., Van Uden, C., Blankemeier, L., Delbrouck, J.-B., Aali, A., Bluethgen, C., Pareek, A., Polacin, M., Reis, E. P., Seehofnerová, A., Rohatgi, N., Hosamani, P., Collins, W., Ahuja, N., Langlotz, C. P., Hom, J., Gatidis, S., Pauly, J., & Chaudhari, A. S. (2024). 2024/04/01). Adapted large language models can outperform medical experts in clinical text summarization. *Nature Medicine, 30*(4), 1134–1142. DOI: 10.1038/s41591-024-02855-5 PMID: 38413730

VanTassel-Baska, J., & Wood, S. M. (2023). The integrated curriculum model. In *Systems and models for developing programs for the gifted and talented* (pp. 655–691). Routledge. DOI: 10.4324/9781003419426-24

Varkey, B. (2021). Principles of clinical ethics and their application to practice. *Medical Principles and Practice : International Journal of the Kuwait University, Health Science Centre, 30*(1), 17–28. DOI: 10.1159/000509119 PMID: 32498071

Vasamsetty, P., Pss, T., Kukkala, D., Singamshetty, M., & Gajula, S. (2020). 3D printing in dentistry—Exploring the new horizons. *Materials Today: Proceedings, 26*, 838–841. DOI: 10.1016/j.matpr.2020.01.049

Vaughn, J., Ford, S. H., Scott, M., Jones, C., & Lewinski, A. (2024). Enhancing Healthcare Education: Leveraging ChatGPT for Innovative Simulation Scenarios. *Clinical Simulation in Nursing, 87*, 101487. DOI: 10.1016/j.ecns.2023.101487

Venkatesh, K. P., Raza, M. M., Nickel, G., Wang, S., & Kvedar, J. C. (2024). 2024/02/10). Deep learning models across the range of skin disease. *npj. Digital Medicine, 7*(1), 32. DOI: 10.1038/s41746-024-01033-8 PMID: 38341516

Vera-Carrasco, O. (2024). La educación médica en principios éticos, bioéticos, deontológicos, valores y actitudes. *Revista Médica La Paz, 30*(2), 63-68. http://www.scielo.org.bo/scielo.php?script=sci_arttext&pid=S1726-89582024000200063&lng=es&tlng=es

Verband Deutscher Zahntechniker-Innungen (VDZI). (2024). Betriebe—Beschäftigte—Auszubildende im Zahntechniker-Handwerk. Retrieved May 20, 2024, from https://www.vdzi.de/statistik.html

Vu Lan Oanh, L., Tettamanzi, P., Tien Minh, D., Comoli, M., Mouloudj, K., Murgolo, M., & Dang Thu Hien, M. (2024). How ethical behavior is considered in different contexts: A bibliometric analysis of global research trends. *Administrative Sciences, 14*(9), 200. DOI: 10.3390/admsci14090200

Wahlgren, B., Høyrup, S., Pedersen, K., & Rattleff, P. (2002). *Refleksion og Læring: Kompetenceudvikling i Arbejdslivet*. Samfundslitteratur.

Wallace, S., Clark, M., & White, J. (2012). 'It's on my iPhone': Attitudes to the use of mobile computing devices in medical education, a mixed-methods study. *BMJ Open, 2*(4), e001099. DOI: 10.1136/bmjopen-2012-001099 PMID: 22923627

Walsh, K. (2015). Mobile learning in medical education. *Ethiopian Journal of Health Sciences, 25*(4), 363–366. DOI: 10.4314/ejhs.v25i4.10 PMID: 26949301

Wang, Y., Kala, M. P., & Jafar, T. H. (2020). Psychological distress during the coronavirus disease 2019 (COVID-19) pandemic on the predominantly general population: A systematic review and meta-analysis. *PLOS ONE*.

Wang, B., Rau, P.-L. P., & Yuan, T. (2023). 2023/07/04). Measuring user competence in using artificial intelligence: Validity and reliability of artificial intelligence literacy scale. *Behaviour & Information Technology, 42*(9), 1324–1337. DOI: 10.1080/0144929X.2022.2072768

Wang, X., Young, G. W., Iqbal, M. Z., & Guckin, C. M. (2023). The potential of extended reality in rural education's future – perspectives from rural educators. *Education and Information Technologies, 29*(7), 8987–9011. DOI: 10.1007/s10639-023-12169-7

Wang, Y., Liu, C., Zhou, K., Zhu, T., & Han, X. (2024). Towards regulatory generative AI in ophthalmology healthcare: A security and privacy perspective [Review]. *The British Journal of Ophthalmology, 108*(10), 1349–1353. DOI: 10.1136/bjo-2024-325167 PMID: 38834290

Wanjari, N. D., & Patil, S. C. (2016). Wearable devices. In *2016 IEEE International Conference on Advances in Electronics, Communication and Computer Technology (ICAECCT)* (pp. 287–290). IEEE. DOI: 10.1109/ICAECCT.2016.7942600

Watari, T., Tokuda, Y., Owada, M., & Onigata, K. (2020). The utility of virtual patient simulations for clinical reasoning education. *International Journal of Environmental Research and Public Health, 17*(15), 5325. DOI: 10.3390/ijerph17155325 PMID: 32722097

Wenger, E. (1998). *Communities of practice: Learning, Meaning, and Identity.* Cambridge University Press. DOI: 10.1017/CBO9780511803932

Wesemann, C., Spies, B. C., Sterzenbach, G., Beuer, F., Kohal, R., Wemken, G., Krügel, M., & Pieralli, S. (2021). Polymers for conventional, subtractive, and additive manufacturing of occlusal devices differ in hardness and flexural properties but not in wear resistance. *Dental Materials, 37*(3), 432–442. DOI: 10.1016/j.dental.2020.11.020 PMID: 33288324

Wijaya, T. T., Yu, Q., Cao, Y., He, Y., & Leung, F. K. S. (2024). Latent Profile Analysis of AI Literacy and Trust in Mathematics Teachers and Their Relations with AI Dependency and 21st-Century Skills [Article]. *Behavioral Sciences (Basel, Switzerland), 14*(11), 1008. Advance online publication. DOI: 10.3390/bs14111008 PMID: 39594308

Wilcha, R. J. (2020). Effectiveness of virtual medical teaching during the COVID-19 crisis: Systematic review. *JMIR Medical Education, 6*(2), e20963. DOI: 10.2196/20963 PMID: 33106227

Williams, D. P. (2024). Disabling AI: Biases and values embedded in artificial intelligence. In *Handbook on the ethics of artificial intelligence.*

Williams, G. C., Saizow, R. B., & Ryan, R. M. (1999). The importance of self-determination theory for medical education. *Academic Medicine, 74*(9), 992–995. DOI: 10.1097/00001888-199909000-00010 PMID: 10498090

Winter, E., Costello, A., O'Brien, M., & Hickey, G. (2021). Teachers' use of technology and the impact of Covid-19. *Irish Educational Studies, 40*(2), 235–246. DOI: 10.1080/03323315.2021.1916559

Winterhalter, L., Kofler, F., Ströbele, D. A., Othman, A., & von See, C. (2024). AI-Assisted Diagnostics in Dentistry: An Eye-Tracking Study on User Behavior. *Journal of Clinical and Experimental Dentistry, 16*(5), e547–e555. DOI: 10.4317/jced.61491 PMID: 38988762

Wong, B. K. M., Vengusamy, S., & Bastrygina, T. (2024). Healthcare digital transformation through the adoption of artificial intelligence. In *Artificial Intelligence, big data, blockchain, and 5G for the digital transformation of the healthcare industry* (pp. 87–110). Academic Press., DOI: 10.1016/B978-0-443-21598-8.00014-2

World Health Organization. (2021). Global strategy on digital health 2020-2025. https://www.who.int/docs/default-source/documents/gs4hdaa2a9f352b0445bafbc79ca799dce4d.pdf

Wu, K. (2022). First Generation Asian Americans obstacles to seeking mental health services.

Wu, D., Xiang, Y., Wu, X., Yu, T., Huang, X., Zou, Y., Liu, Z., & Lin, H. (2020, June). Artificial intelligence-tutoring problem-based learning in ophthalmology clerkship. *Annals of Translational Medicine*, *8*(11), 700. DOI: 10.21037/atm.2019.12.15 PMID: 32617320

Wuersching, S. N., Hickel, R., Edelhoff, D., & Kollmuss, M. (2022). Initial biocompatibility of novel resins for 3D-printed fixed dental prostheses. *Dental Materials*, *38*(10), 1587–1597. DOI: 10.1016/j.dental.2022.08.001 PMID: 36008188

Wu, Z., Liu, Z., & Zhang, Z. (2024). Research on the current situation and future governance of artificial intelligence in the field of medical education [Article]. *Chinese Medical Ethics*, *37*(9), 1093–1100. DOI: 10.12026/j.issn.1001-8565.2024.09.12

Xiao, J., Bozkurt, A., Nichols, M., Pazurek, A., Stracke, C. M., Bai, J. Y. H., Farrow, R., Mulligan, D., Nerantzi, C., Sharma, R. C., Singh, L., Frumin, I., Swindell, A., Honeychurch, S., Bond, M., Dron, J., Moore, S., Leng, J., van Tryon, P. J. S., & Themeli, C. (2025). Venturing into the Unknown: Critical Insights into Grey Areas and Pioneering Future Directions in Educational Generative AI Research. *TechTrends*. Advance online publication. DOI: 10.1007/s11528-025-01060-6

Xia, Q., Weng, X., Ouyang, F., Lin, T. J., & Chiu, T. K. F. (2024). A Scoping Review on How Generative Artificial Intelligence Transforms Assessment in Higher Education. *International Journal of Educational Technology in Higher Education*, *21*(1), 40. Advance online publication. DOI: 10.1186/s41239-024-00468-z

Xu, A., Baysari, M. T., Stocker, S. L., Leow, L. J., Day, R. O., & Carland, J. E. (2020). Researchers' views on, and experiences with, the requirement to obtain informed consent in research involving human participants: A qualitative study. *BMC Medical Ethics*, *21*(1), 1–11. DOI: 10.1186/s12910-020-00538-7 PMID: 33008387

Xu, T., Weng, H., Liu, F., Yang, L., Luo, Y., Ding, Z., & Wang, Q. (2024). Current status of ChatGPT use in medical education: Potentials, challenges, and strategies. *Journal of Medical Internet Research*, *26*, e57896. DOI: 10.2196/57896 PMID: 39196640

Yamashiro, J. R., & de Riese, W. T. W. (2021). Any correlation between prostate volume and incidence of prostate cancer: A review of reported data for the last thirty years. *Research and Reports in Urology, 13*, 749–757. DOI: 10.2147/RRU.S331506 PMID: 34676178

Yang, W. (2022). Artificial Intelligence education for young children: Why, what, and how in curriculum design and implementation. *Computers and Education: Artificial Intelligence*.

Yang, J., Li, H., Xu, L., & Wang, Y. (2022). Selective laser sintering versus conventional lost-wax casting for single metal copings: A systematic review and meta-analysis. *The Journal of Prosthetic Dentistry, 128*(5), 897–904. DOI: 10.1016/j.prosdent.2021.02.011 PMID: 33789799

Yang, Y.-Y., & Shulruf, B. (2019). An Expert-Led and Artificial Intelligence System-Assisted Tutoring Course to Improve the Confidence of Chinese Medical Interns in Suturing and Ligature Skills: A Prospective Pilot Study. *Journal of Educational Evaluation for Health Professions, 16*, 7. DOI: 10.3352/jeehp.2019.16.7 PMID: 30986892

Yan, L., Sha, L., Zhao, L., Li, Y., Martinez-Maldonado, R., Chen, G., Li, X., Jin, Y., & Gašević, D. (2024). Practical and ethical challenges of large language models in education: A systematic scoping review. *British Journal of Educational Technology, 55*(1), 90–112. DOI: 10.1111/bjet.13370

Yates, A., Starkey, L., Egerton, B., & Flueggen, F. (2021). High school students' experience of online learning during Covid-19: The influence of technology and pedagogy. *Technology, Pedagogy and Education, 30*(1), 59–73. DOI: 10.1080/1475939X.2020.1854337

Yazdani, S., & Abardeh, M. H. (2019). Five Decades of Research and Theorization on Clinical Reasoning: A Critical Review. *Advances in Medical Education and Practice, 10*, 703–716. DOI: 10.2147/AMEP.S213492 PMID: 31695548

Yazdanpanahi, F., Shahi, M., & Davaridolatabadi, N. (2022). Investigating the application of new technologies in dental education: A systematic review. *Acta Medica Iranica*. Advance online publication. DOI: 10.18502/acta.v60i8.10830

Yeung, W.-L., & Ng, O.-L. (2024). Using empathy maps to support design-thinking enhanced transdisciplinary STEM innovation in K-12 setting. *International Journal of Technology and Design Education, 34*(4), 1325–1350. DOI: 10.1007/s10798-023-09861-7

Yim, D., Khuntia, J., Parameswaran, V., & Meyers, A. (2024). Preliminary Evidence of the Use of Generative AI in Health Care Clinical Services: Systematic Narrative Review [Article]. *JMIR Medical Informatics*, *12*, e52073. Advance online publication. DOI: 10.2196/52073 PMID: 38506918

Young, A. T., Cole, J. R., & Denton, D. (2002). Improving technological literacy. *Issues in Science and Technology*, *18*(4), 73–79.

Young, J. Q., Van Merrienboer, J., Durning, S., & Ten Cate, O. (2014). Cognitive load theory: implications for medical education: AMEE Guide No. 86. *Medical Teacher*, *36*(5), 371–384. DOI: 10.3109/0142159X.2014.889290 PMID: 24593808

Zalat, M. M., Hamed, M. S., & Bolbol, S. A. (2021). The experiences, challenges, and acceptance of e-learning as a tool for teaching during the COVID-19 pandemic among university medical staff.

Zamiri, M., & Esmaeili, A. (2024). Methods and Technologies for Supporting Knowledge Sharing within Learning Communities: A Systematic Literature Review. *Administrative Sciences*, *14*(1), 17. DOI: 10.3390/admsci14010017

Zarei, M., Eftekhari Mamaghani, H., Abbasi, A., & Hosseini, M.-S. (2024). Application of Artificial Intelligence in Medical Education: A Review of Benefits, Challenges, and Solutions. *Medicina Clínica Práctica*, *7*(2), 1–5. DOI: 10.1016/j.mcpsp.2023.100422

Zhai, C., Wibowo, S., & Li, L. D. (2024). The Effects of Over-Reliance on AI Dialogue Systems on Students' Cognitive Abilities: A Systematic Review. *Smart Learning Environments*, *11*(1), 1–37. DOI: 10.1186/s40561-024-00316-7

Zhang, Y., Liang, S., Feng, Y., Wang, Q., Sun, F., Chen, S., Yang, Y., He, X., Zhu, H., & Pan, H. (2022). Automation of literature screening using machine learning in medical evidence synthesis: A diagnostic test accuracy systematic review protocol [Review]. *Systematic Reviews*, *11*(1), 11. Advance online publication. DOI: 10.1186/s13643-021-01881-5 PMID: 35031074

Zhang, Z., Cajochen, C., & Khatami, R. (2019). Social jetlag and chronotypes in the Chinese population: Analysis of data recorded by wearable devices. *Journal of Medical Internet Research*, *21*(6), e13482. DOI: 10.2196/13482 PMID: 31199292

Zhong, W., Schröder, T., & Bekkering, J. (2022). Biophilic design in architecture and its contributions to health, well-being, and sustainability: A critical review. *Frontiers of Architectural Research*, *11*(1), 114–141. DOI: 10.1016/j.foar.2021.07.006

Zhou, C., & Lassen, A. M. (2024). Improving Technology Literacy among Health Professional Students. In *Proceedings of Nordic Education Research Association Conference 2024*. Malmö University.

Zhou, C. (2012). Learning engineering knowledge and creativity by solving projects. *International Journal of Engineering Pedagogy*, *2*(1), 26–31. DOI: 10.3991/ijep.v2i1.1873

Zhou, C., Michael Rosenberg Petri, S., & Bhattacharyya, S. (2025). AI Literacy and Professional Development in STEM Education. In Papadakis, S. (Ed.), *AI Roles and Responsibilities in Education*. Springer.

Zhou, J., Müller, H., Holzinger, A., & Chen, F. (2024). Ethical ChatGPT: Concerns, challenges, and commandments. *Electronics (Basel).*

Zhu, E., Hadadgar, A., Masiello, I., & Zary, N. (2014). Augmented reality in healthcare education: An integrative review. *PeerJ*, *2*, e469. DOI: 10.7717/peerj.469 PMID: 25071992

Zhu, W., Ma, X., Gou, M., Mei, D., Zhang, K., & Chen, S. (2016). 3D printing of functional biomaterials for tissue engineering. *Current Opinion in Biotechnology*, *40*, 103–112. DOI: 10.1016/j.copbio.2016.03.014 PMID: 27043763

Zidoun, Y., & Mardi, A. E. L. (2024). Artificial Intelligence (AI)-Based Simulators Versus Simulated Patients in Undergraduate Programs: A Protocol for a Randomized Controlled Trial. *BMC Medical Education*, *24*(1), 1–7. DOI: 10.1186/s12909-024-06236-x PMID: 39501219

Zitzmann, N. U., Matthisson, L., Ohla, H., & Joda, T. (2020). Digital Undergraduate Education in Dentistry: A Systematic Review. *International Journal of Environmental Research and Public Health*, *17*(9), 3269. DOI: 10.3390/ijerph17093269 PMID: 32392877

About The Contributors

Dachel Martínez Asanza is a senior researcher and distinguished academic with extensive expertise in medical education, geriatric dentistry and gerodontology. She is currently affiliated with the National School of Public Health (ENSAP) and the University of Medical Sciences of Havana, Cuba. With over 19 years of experience in dental surgery, 15 years as a Comprehensive Dentistry Specialist, and 14 years in medical education, Professor Martínez Asanza earned her PhD in Medical Education Sciences in 2021 and was appointed Full Professor at Havana Dental School in 2022. Her scholarly contributions include editing several influential books on digital dentistry, preventive dentistry and geriatric dentistry, such as Geriatric Dentistry in the Age of Digital Technology (2023), Transforming Dental Health in Rural Communities: Digital Dentistry (2024), and Leveraging Digital Technology for Preventive Dentistry (2024). She has also authored 12 book chapters, published 21 peer-reviewed journal articles and presented at numerous international conferences, establishing herself as a leading voice in digital health and dental education. Professor Martínez Asanza's editorial expertise and academic leadership make her a valuable contributor to advancing research and innovation in dental sciences.

***

Dharel P. Acut is a licensed professional teacher and a Science Education instructor at Cebu Technological University in Cebu City, Philippines. He holds a bachelor's degree in Secondary Education, majoring in General Science, from MSU-Iligan Institute of Technology. Currently, he is completing his master's degree in Science Education at Cebu Normal University. As an Associate Member of the National Research Council of the Philippines (DOST-NRCP), his research interests focus on science education, STEM education, systematic literature reviews, education for sustainable development, science instrumentation, and educational technology.

Murtala Ismail Adakawa, CLN, has been a practicing librarian for a decade. He is currently working at the University Library, Bayero University Kano. He has participated in various committees at different capacities. He has attended many international and local conferences and published several journal articles. He is currently a research fellow at the Department of Studies in Library and Information Science, University of Mysore, Manasagangothri, Mysuru, Karnataka, India.

Ioannis Adamopoulos, are: Postdoc Researcher in Department of Public Health Policy, Sector of Occupational & Environmental Health, School of Public Health, University of West Attica. Public Health and Environmental Inspector at Region of Attica, Department of Environmental Hygiene and Public Health Inspections. Member of the International Association: ICOH, EUPHA, UK & Ireland Occupational and Environmental Epidemiology Society, MEDICHEM, and Humanitarian Network of Experts. For the last few years, I have been working as an Inspector of Public Health and Safety, in the Ministry of Health & Unified Food Control Agency (EFET) & Prefectures local governance in Greece until now in the Region of Attica. Also, assigned to 2019 as a registered main teaching staff of the National School of Public Administration (E.S.D.D.A), National Center of Public Administration and Self-Government (E.K.D.D.A.), and Training Institute (IN. EP.). Register Main Instructor of Trainers and Operators in food hygiene and safety, H.A.C.C.P. system, in United Food Control Agency in Greece (E.F.E.T.) for the last 14 years. Researcher - also an associate member (in good standing) and scientific collaborator of the International Commission of Occupational Health (ICOH) and at three (3) scientific committees: 1) Accident Prevention 2) Epidemiology in Occupational Health 3) Occupational Medicine in Occupational Health of ICOH. Member of the UK & Ireland Occupational and Environmental Epidemiology Society. Member of the International Association MEDICHEM. Finally, Author and Reviewer-Assistant of Editors in Scientific Journals, Elsevier Journals, Safety Science, Health and Safety at @Work, PlosOne, International Research Journal of Pharmacy and Medical Sciences, European Journal of Environment and Public Health, Academia, European Journal of Investigation in Health Psychology and Education, Psychology Research and Behavior Management, and finally at Ergonomics Journal. Editorial Board Member-Assistant Editor in: 1) World Journal of Public Health, and 2)Journal of Health and Environmental Research(Science Publishing Group (SciencePG) in the USA). Associate Editor in: Epidemiology International Journal. (EIJ) ISSN:2639-2038-Medwin Publishers, Detroit, United States of America. Editor in: BMC Public Health journal ISSN: 1471-2458. Springer Nature, U.K.

Adrián Alvarez Pérez is a Professor at the National School of Public Health (ENSAP). He is a First Degree Specialist in General Integral Medicine and Biostatistics, and holds a Master's degree in Health Sciences Education.

Balakiruthiga's research interests are broad and include Networks, Distributed Computing, Software-Defined Networks, Network Routing and Traffic Management, Distributed Intelligence, and IoT-based AI applications. Currently, she is guiding several student projects in cutting-edge areas such as federated learning for IoT applications, Digital Twin applications in 5G and 6G, and Quality of Service Optimization in data centre networks.

Baiju B V is currently an Assistant Professor Senior Grade at the School of Computer Science and Engineering, Vellore Institute of Technology, Vellore, Tamil Nadu. He holds a B.E. in Computer Science and Engineering, M.E. in Computer Science and Engineering, and Ph.D. in Computer Science and Engineering. Dr. Baiju B V has over 17 years of experience in teaching and research. His domains of interest include Artificial Intelligence, Networks, Software Engineering, and IoT. He has published over 38 papers in national and international journals and conferences.

Rui de Almeida, In 2009, he completed the Degree in Radiology at the University of Algarve (Portugal). He holds a Master's Degree in Quality Management of Health Services from the Faculty of Medicine of the University of Murcia (2015) and a PhD in Health Science from the International Doctoral School of the University of Murcia (Spain, 2020). He is currently Professor in the Medical Imaging and Radiotherapy Department at the University of Algarve. Also, he is an Integrated Researcher at Comprehensive Health Research Center (CHRC) and CES-ESSUALG (Center for Studies and Development in Health); Member of the Editorial Board of the University of Algarve Publisher. Member of the youth club committee of EuSoMII (European Society of Medical Imaging Informatics). Currently, his research interests are in the area of Health Sciences, particularly in the fields of Allied Health Professions Education, Quality Management, Health Services and Policies, and Artificial intelligence applied to medicine.

Mariya Dimitrova, DMD, PhD was born in Plovdiv on October 5, 1990. She completed her secondary education at the Ivan Vazov Language High School with an emphasis on German, Russian, and English in 2009. In 2015, she graduated from the Faculty of Dental Medicine at the Medical University of Plovdiv with a degree in "Dental Medicine." Since 2018, she has been practicing her profession in her own private dental practice. She is a regular member of the Bulgarian Dental Association (BDS) and the Union of Scientists – Plovdiv. In 2020, she was appointed as an assistant professor after a competition. In 2023, she successfully defended her PhD dissertation, and in 2024, she obtained a specialization in prosthetic dental medicine. In the same year, she was appointed as a senior assistant professor at the Department of prosthetic dentistry of the Faculty of Dental Medicine - Plovdiv, Bulgaria.

Manuel B. Garcia is a professor of information technology and the founding director of the Educational Innovation and Technology Hub (EdITH) at FEU Institute of Technology, Manila, Philippines. He holds a Doctor of Information Technology degree from the University of the East and is currently pursuing a Doctor of Philosophy in Education at the University of the Philippines. His interdisciplinary research interests include topics that, individually or collectively, span the disciplines of education and information technology. He is a licensed professional teacher and a proud member of the National Research Council of the Philippines – an attached agency to the country's Department of Science and Technology (DOST-NRCP). Dr. Garcia is the first-ever recipient of the Ramon Dimacali Award for Information Technology, conferred by the Philippine Association for the Advancement of Science and Technology, and has been recognized as one of the World's Top 2% Scientists for 2023 and 2024 by Elsevier.

Precious S. Garcia is currently affiliated with the College of Nursing and Health Sciences at Jose Rizal University, Philippines. Her interests include nursing education, patient safety, clinical practice, and healthcare leadership.

Adania Siva Guanche Martínez is a Full Professor and Consultant at the University of Medical Sciences of Havana. She holds a Ph.D. in Educational Sciences and is the author of several books.

Flaka Hoti is a dedicated nurse with extensive experience in both clinical practice and academic research. With a strong foundation in nursing care, she has developed a deep interest in public health and evidence-based practice. Her research has focused on critical issues in nursing and public health, including the quality of care in long-term care institutions, elderly care, and the role of healthcare professionals in improving community health outcomes. Committed to lifelong learning and professional development, she continues to contribute to the advancement of nursing knowledge through applied research and collaborative projects.

Doruntina Kabashi, I was born in Peja on April 24, 1993. I completed my primary education in my hometown and attended the Medical High School in Peja from 2008 to 2012. I graduated with a Bachelor's degree in Physiotherapy from the Faculty of Medicine at the University of Prishtina in the period 2012–2016. Later, I pursued my Master's studies in Health Management at the Faculty of Medicine,

“Fehmi Agani” University in Gjakova (2022–2024). Currently, I serve as the Project Coordinator and Physiotherapist within the project “Health and Wellbeing of Students in the Municipality of Peja”. Additionally, I work as a Physiotherapist at Fizioterapia Kabashi in Klinë.

Sajeer Karattil is currently working as senior lecturer in the Engineering Department, Electrical and Electronics Section, University of Technology and Applied Sciences – Al Musanna, Al Muladdah, Sultanate of Oman . Previously he worked as Assistant Professor in Information and Technology Department, Hindustan University, Chennai, Tamil Nadu, India. He finished B.Tech in Computer Science and Engineering from School of Engineering Cusat, Kochi and M.Tech in Software Engineering from SRM University, Chennai, India. He completed PhD in Computer Science from Bharathiar University, Coimbatore, Tamilnadu, India. He has more than 15 years of academic and industry experience and his area of expertise include Software Engineering and speech processing.

Anna Marie Lassen, PhD, Associate Professor, is affiliated with the Occupational Therapy Education Programme and the two research centres: The Centre for Profession Studies and the Centre for Health and Applied Technology at University College Northern Denmark (UCN). Anna Marie’s research is situated within the Science and Technology Studies (STS) field, with a particular focus on the role of welfare technology in practice. Her work explores the implications of technology implementation in professional work routines, as well as how technology influences the autonomy and independence of citizens and patients with support from healthcare staff. She is particularly interested in how citizens/patients, professionals, and students learn about and through technology.

Mohammed Mubarak Mohammed Al Araimi, Experienced Senior Lecturer with a demonstrated history of working in the higher education industry. Skilled in Lecturing, Educational Technology.

Farida Mouloudj is an Assistant Professor in the Faculty of Letters and Languages at University of Medea, Algeria. Her academic and research have focused primarily on contrastive studies between Arabic and English. She earned her Bachelor and Master in Arabic literature from University of Medea, and Doctor of comparative linguistics from University of Blida 2, Algeria. She has over 5 years of teaching experience. She has 10 publications.

Kamel Mouloudj is a Professor at the College of Economics at the University of Medea in Algeria, specializing in research areas such as individual behavior prediction (including customers, employees, and students), marketing, waste management, sustainability, and green start-ups. He holds a Doctorate in Marketing from the University of Algiers 3 and has over 20 years of teaching experience. With more than 50 published works, Professor Mouloudj is also serving as the Chair of the Doctoral Training Committee in the Department of Commercial Sciences from 2019 to 2026. Additionally, he has actively participated in over 20 local and international conferences, contributing his expertise to a wide range of academic discussions.

Hayatullah Niazai holds an MD from Ahmad Shah Abdali Medical College, Afghanistan. He is an active physician at a private clinic, with professional interests in clinical practice, healthcare, and medical education. He is committed to evidence-based care and actively participates in community health outreach initiatives to enhance patient well-being.

Alisha Rijal, MSc, MA, is a psychiatric nurse, faculty teacher, researcher. She is Assistant Professor of Psychiatric nursing at Yeti Health Science Academy affiliated to Purvanchal University, Nepal. Mrs. Rijal has worked in various province of Nepal researching and aiding psychiatric services. She has worked in various Nursing colleges of Kathmandu tutoring on psychiatric nursing, research and biostatistics. She had worked as psychiatric nurse in Centre for Mental Health and Counseling-Nepal (CMC-Nepal), Pratiman-Neema Memorial Foundation (PNMF), Transcultural Psychosocial Organization Nepal (TPO Nepal). Mrs. Rijal's work focuses on positive psychology, psychoeducation and stigma reduction. She is member secretary of IRC-YHSA. She has written a Textbook of Biostatistics for Bachelor level Nursing program for Nepalese Students.

S.A. Angayarkanni, M.E., Ph.D, is an Assistant Professor in Department of Networking and Communication, with total teaching experience of 17 years. She obtained her B.Tech. (Information Technology) and M.E. (Wireless Technologies) from Anna University in 2005 and 2008. She scored 91.89 percentile in GATE – IT 2006 Examination. She completed her Ph.D in 2021 from Anna University. Her research domain is Intelligent Transportation Systems. Her area of interest includes Networking, Wireless Technologies and Intelligent Road Traffic System for Indian Roads. She has published 19 scopus indexed papers in International Journals and Conferences, out of which 3 are SCI indexed. She is a Life time Member of The Institution of Engineers (India) – IEI and Indian Society of Technical Education (ISTE).

Raquel holds a PhD in Psychology and a Master's in Psychosocial Rehabilitation and Mental Health. She holds postgraduate qualifications in Digital Health and in Pedagogical Innovation and Educational Change. Currently, she serves as a Senior Lecturer at the School of Health of the Polytechnic of Porto. As a researcher at the

Psychosocial Rehabilitation Laboratory – Research Center for Rehabilitation, she has published numerous book chapters and articles in the field of digital mental health, focusing particularly on virtual reality, digital platforms and mobile applications for mental health literacy, well-being, and mental health support.

Eleonora Stefani is a radiology technician at AULSS 2 Marca Trevigiana and corporate teaching tutor in the Bachelor's Degree Program in Medical Imaging and Radiotherapy at the University of Padua, Treviso, Italy. She is also the Erasmus coordinator for the program. She is actively involved in the development of peer education projects and interprofessional simulation training for healthcare students. Her work focuses on the use of AI and digital tools to enhance learning in radiological sciences.

Niki Syrou has a Bachelor's Degree in Nursing from the National and Kapodistrian University of Athens (1996-2000) and a Master's Degree in "Public Health" (MPH) from the National School of Public Health (2008-10) with a final grade of "excellent". Her postgraduate course is in "Health Standards and Behaviors" and her Diploma Thesis is titled "Genetically Modified Foods and Genetically Modified Organisms".She also has a Doctor of Philosophy (Ph.D.) in Public Health (2010-14) of the National and Kapodistrian University of Athens with a final grade of "excellent". Her Ph.D. thesis is about school safety and hygiene, and its title is: "Development, implementation, and evaluation of a program to modify risk factors for health and safety in Schools". Additionally, Dr Niki Syrou has a Post-Doctoral Research Certificate (2021-23) from the Athens Medical School regarding physicians' perceptions of physical activity and its role in chronic diseases. She has a certified knowledge of computer science and of 2 foreign languages, English (level C2) and French (level B2). She worked as a Registered Nurse (RN) in the Surgery and Intensive Care Unit (ICU) from 2000 until 2004. She worked as a School Nurse at Special Education and Training from 2004 until 2019. She had the position of school principal for 4 years. As a school nurse, she was a responsible authority in matters of health education and health promotion and she was invited to play an important role in increasing awareness of the school population through health education and health promotion programs. These programs, among other things, had the aim of providing knowledge, forming attitudes, and modifying behaviors that contribute to the creation of safe and healthy teaching conditions. Since 02/2019 she has been working as a Laboratory Teaching Staff at the University of Thessaly (Department of Physical Education and Sport Science) and she teaches the course "Safe Exercise and First Aid" and the new course "Public Health and Exercise". Since 2004, as a School Nurse, she worked in the development of programs, policies, and environments that enable school health. She was a coordinator of health education programs in schools. She also participated in a number of conferences and workshops, as well as a speaker in several educational programs for teachers and students, especially about school safety and hygiene, nutrition, physical activity, and other public health issues (about 60 lectures/presentations). Her writing concerns the publication of articles in scientific journals and refereed conferences and the creation of educational material in "school safety and hygiene", approved in 2016, 2017, 2018, 2019, and 2020 by the Institute of Educational Policy (IEP) and by the Ministry of Education and Religious Affairs for its pedagogical appropriateness. She has the role of the evaluator and writer in the scientific journals "Nursing and Research" and "International Journal of Educational Innovation". She is also an educator at the Institute of Educational Policy (IEP) and at the Scientific Association for the Promotion of Educational Innovation (EEPEK). She is a Research Associate and Lab Officer at the Laboratory of Exercise Biochemistry, Physiology and Nutrition (SmArT Lab) - University of Thessaly - Greece since February 2019.

Hasime Terziqi, Medical Doctor, Medical Faculty, Medical Faculty, " Hasan Prishtina" University -Prishtina Specialist in Plastic,Reconstructive and Aesthetic Surgery,, " Hasan Prishtina" University -Prishtina and Tirana and Medical Faculty. Master of Medical Sciences,Medical Faculty, " Hasan Prishtina" University - Prishtinë PHD (Doctor of Sciences), UMHATEM" NI PIROGOV "EAD. DEPARTMENT OF BURNS AND PLASTIC SURGERY. SOFIA, BULLGARI. Prof.ass. dr. in Medical Faculty, "Fehmi Agani" University - Gjakovë, Vice/ Dean in Medical Faculty, "Fehmi Agani" University - Gjakovë, Publication of the Monograph "Burn Care" 2023, co-author of the University Book "Diabetes Mellitus TIP 2, prevention and treatment through nursing care" with chapter- "Reconstruction of soft tissues of the diabetic foot " in 2024, reviewer of several medical Monographs and books in Kosovo, with more publication in different journals and lot of activities in management, education for students and healthcare in community.

V. Rajaram completed B.E. (Elec tronics and Communication) in the year 2007, M.E. in Commu nication Systems in the year 2010, and earned his Ph.D. in 2021. His areas of research include Wireless Sensor Net works, IoT (Internet of Things), and Networking. He has pub lished many papers in indexed journals. He has total of 15 years of teaching experience and has significance in teaching Digital Logic, Computer Organization and Architecture, IoT and Net working Protocols. Currently Working as Assistant Professor in Department of Networking and Communication, School of Computing, SRM Institute of Science and Technology, Kattankulathur, Chennai, India.

V. Pandimurugan is an Associate Professor in the Department of Computer Science and Engineering at Acharya University, Uzbekistan. He obtained his Ph.D. in Computer Science & Engineering from Manonmaniam Sundaranar University (MSU), Tirunelveli, in 2019. He earned his B.E. in Electrical and Electronics Engineering (EEE) from Anna University in 2005, followed by an M.E. in Computer Science & Engineering (CSE) in 2008. With 16 years of teaching experience, Dr. Pandimurugan has made significant contributions to research, publishing 42 papers in international journals and conferences. His expertise spans health monitoring, machine learning, networks, security, and IoT. Additionally, he has authored five Scopus-indexed book chapters, holds three international patents, and has two published Indian patents along with three granted Indian design patents.

Chunfang Zhou, Ph.D., Associate Professor, Leader of AI Learning Lab, Co-Director in STEM Education Research Center, Department of Mathematics and Computer Science, University of Southern Denmark (SDU), Denmark. Chunfang locates her research in a broad area of Science, Technology and Society (STS), with a particular focus on creativity studies, with relations to diverse domains including STEM education and science communication, AI and digital technologies, organisational learning, digitalisation, human-centered design, sustainability, group collaboration, knowledge management, Problem-Based Learning (PBL), and professional development.

Index

Symbols

3D printing 2, 8, 32, 227, 228, 229, 230, 231, 232, 233, 234, 235, 236, 237, 238, 239, 240, 241, 242, 243, 244, 245, 248, 249, 250, 251, 252, 253, 254, 255, 256, 257, 258, 259, 260, 261, 262, 263, 264, 265, 266, 267, 268, 269, 270, 271, 272, 273, 275, 276, 277, 278

A

Additive Manufacturing 227, 235, 245, 254, 260, 270, 272, 273, 275, 277
AI 2, 4, 12, 16, 17, 18, 19, 20, 28, 29, 31, 32, 37, 58, 60, 61, 63, 64, 65, 66, 67, 68, 69, 70, 71, 72, 73, 74, 75, 76, 77, 78, 79, 80, 81, 82, 83, 84, 85, 86, 87, 88, 89, 91, 92, 94, 95, 96, 97, 98, 99, 100, 101, 102, 103, 104, 105, 106, 107, 108, 109, 110, 111, 112, 113, 114, 115, 116, 117, 118, 119, 120, 121, 123, 125, 126, 127, 128, 129, 130, 131, 132, 133, 134, 135, 136, 137, 138, 139, 140, 141, 142, 143, 144, 146, 147, 148, 149, 150, 151, 153, 154, 155, 156, 164, 165, 168, 170, 172, 177, 179, 180, 181, 182, 183, 184, 187, 189, 199, 213, 227, 230, 237, 244, 247, 260, 263, 268, 269, 277, 279, 280, 283, 287, 288, 289, 290, 292, 293, 296, 298, 301, 303, 304, 305, 307, 309, 310, 312
artificial intelligence 2, 4, 5, 8, 12, 21, 24, 26, 28, 29, 30, 32, 34, 60, 63, 64, 70, 72, 83, 84, 85, 86, 87, 88, 89, 91, 94, 111, 112, 113, 114, 115, 116, 117, 118, 119, 120, 121, 123, 125, 146, 147, 148, 149, 150, 151, 152, 153, 154, 155, 156, 179, 180, 184, 187, 188, 189, 191, 193, 212, 217, 221, 222, 237, 244, 247, 248, 260, 263, 268, 276, 277, 279, 280, 283, 287, 288, 291, 292, 293, 294, 296, 298, 299, 300, 302, 303, 304, 305, 306, 308, 309, 312, 313
augmented reality 2, 8, 12, 14, 15, 23, 27, 32, 72, 124, 157, 159, 162, 164, 167, 170, 182, 185, 187, 188, 189, 194, 280, 286, 305
Automated Assessments 91, 96, 123

B

Blended Learning 13, 19, 35, 85, 195, 196, 198, 204, 208, 211, 214, 225, 285, 293, 311

C

CAD 3, 4, 5, 6, 11, 12, 15, 16, 17, 19, 21, 22, 25, 28, 31, 32, 228, 231, 232, 233, 236, 244, 248, 253, 262, 270, 272, 273, 274
Case-Based Learning 91, 96, 99, 110, 118, 129, 144, 166, 168
ChatGPT 28, 94, 95, 96, 102, 106, 107, 108, 109, 111, 112, 113, 114, 116, 117, 118, 119, 126, 146, 147, 150, 152, 153, 154, 155, 201, 223, 294, 297, 298, 299, 302, 304, 306, 307, 308, 310, 311, 313
Clinical Reasoning 63, 64, 65, 66, 81, 107, 124, 126, 131, 136, 137, 142, 143, 153, 155, 165, 168, 195, 196, 201, 204, 205, 214, 224
Content Development 91, 96, 98, 110, 126
curriculum 2, 4, 6, 8, 11, 12, 13, 16, 23, 26, 29, 30, 31, 46, 47, 60, 68, 69, 79, 80, 85, 86, 87, 92, 94, 98, 101, 107, 114, 115, 126, 129, 133, 139, 143, 182, 184, 196, 199, 200, 210, 214, 217, 221, 222, 225, 280, 287, 290, 296, 299, 309, 312, 313

D

Data privacy 4, 17, 34, 38, 64, 74, 75, 76, 77, 82, 89, 91, 104, 107, 109, 171,

183, 294
Decision-Making 6, 20, 34, 35, 39, 40, 53, 65, 66, 68, 69, 71, 73, 75, 79, 89, 91, 96, 101, 102, 105, 107, 110, 125, 126, 130, 132, 134, 135, 139, 141, 142, 143, 148, 150, 151, 161, 162, 163, 165, 166, 169, 170, 196, 199, 200, 201, 207, 211, 213, 214, 225, 244, 269, 279, 286, 289, 290, 305
dental education 1, 2, 3, 5, 6, 7, 8, 9, 11, 12, 13, 14, 15, 16, 17, 19, 21, 22, 23, 24, 25, 29, 30, 31, 32, 120, 236, 239, 240, 261, 267, 275, 276, 277
dentistry 1, 2, 3, 5, 7, 8, 9, 11, 12, 13, 14, 15, 16, 17, 18, 19, 20, 22, 24, 25, 26, 27, 28, 29, 30, 31, 32, 84, 86, 87, 113, 227, 228, 229, 230, 232, 233, 234, 235, 236, 237, 238, 240, 241, 242, 243, 244, 245, 247, 248, 249, 251, 252, 253, 254, 256, 257, 258, 259, 260, 261, 263, 264, 265, 266, 268, 270, 271, 272, 273, 274, 275, 276, 277, 311
Digital Dentistry 11, 13, 14, 16, 25, 26, 27, 28, 29, 30, 31, 86, 87, 228, 237, 244, 251, 260, 270
Digital Distractions 195, 196, 214, 288, 289, 311
Digital Innovations 17, 18, 23, 28, 37, 66, 238
Digital Technologies 3, 11, 13, 15, 16, 26, 28, 29, 32, 63, 65, 70, 82, 89, 146, 199, 294, 299
Digital transformation 2, 3, 26, 63, 66, 68, 89, 124, 277

E

educational technology 8, 32, 58, 116, 128, 152, 155, 180, 208, 220, 280, 294, 296, 304, 310, 311, 313
Ethical Implications 47, 107, 108, 118, 172, 177, 189, 253, 286, 287, 288, 300, 305, 306

F

Feedback 11, 12, 14, 15, 18, 21, 48, 69, 91, 96, 99, 100, 101, 123, 126, 128, 130, 131, 132, 134, 135, 139, 140, 141, 143, 144, 153, 158, 159, 160, 163, 164, 165, 168, 172, 173, 174, 175, 179, 181, 182, 183, 185, 186, 188, 202, 204, 264, 298

G

Generative AI 28, 65, 74, 75, 80, 111, 112, 113, 114, 116, 117, 118, 119, 120, 121, 126, 128, 129, 147, 149, 150, 153, 155, 156, 293

H

Healthcare 2, 3, 6, 7, 13, 19, 23, 26, 28, 29, 30, 34, 35, 37, 38, 39, 40, 46, 47, 48, 49, 52, 53, 55, 57, 58, 59, 64, 65, 66, 67, 68, 69, 70, 71, 72, 73, 75, 76, 77, 79, 80, 81, 82, 83, 85, 87, 88, 94, 101, 102, 103, 104, 105, 106, 107, 109, 111, 112, 115, 116, 118, 119, 120, 125, 126, 127, 132, 133, 136, 145, 146, 148, 149, 150, 151, 153, 154, 158, 160, 161, 162, 164, 168, 169, 170, 172, 177, 179, 180, 185, 186, 187, 189, 190, 191, 192, 193, 194, 195, 196, 200, 201, 205, 207, 209, 210, 211, 212, 213, 214, 222, 225, 227, 228, 230, 235, 241, 242, 247, 250, 252, 253, 254, 259, 260, 263, 265, 268, 269, 277, 280, 283, 289, 290, 291, 293, 294, 295, 296, 299, 302, 305, 312
Healthcare Professionals 40, 47, 48, 52, 59, 64, 65, 67, 68, 73, 76, 79, 81, 82, 85, 104, 125, 136, 170, 186, 214, 280, 290
Health informatics 119, 217, 308
Human Intelligence 32, 66, 89, 94, 95, 125, 155, 269, 279, 280

I

IoMT 157, 190, 310

L

Large Language Models 113, 114, 118, 120, 126, 130, 146, 147, 155, 156, 291, 299, 308, 313
Literature Review 26, 31, 35, 94, 96, 110, 117, 125, 128, 146, 248, 270, 281, 283, 295, 298, 300, 303, 311, 312

M

Medical education 3, 23, 25, 29, 39, 63, 64, 65, 66, 68, 69, 70, 71, 72, 73, 74, 75, 76, 77, 78, 79, 80, 81, 82, 83, 84, 85, 86, 87, 88, 91, 92, 94, 96, 99, 100, 101, 103, 104, 105, 106, 107, 109, 110, 111, 112, 113, 116, 117, 118, 119, 120, 121, 123, 124, 125, 126, 127, 128, 129, 130, 131, 133, 134, 136, 138, 140, 141, 142, 143, 145, 146, 147, 148, 149, 150, 151, 152, 153, 154, 155, 156, 157, 158, 159, 160, 161, 162, 163, 165, 166, 168, 170, 171, 172, 174, 175, 176, 177, 179, 180, 182, 183, 184, 185, 187, 188, 189, 190, 191, 192, 195, 196, 197, 199, 200, 201, 202, 203, 204, 205, 206, 207, 208, 209, 210, 211, 212, 213, 214, 216, 217, 218, 219, 220, 221, 222, 223, 224, 279, 280, 281, 283, 284, 285, 286, 287, 288, 289, 290, 291, 292, 293, 294, 295, 296, 297, 298, 299, 300, 301, 302, 304, 306, 307, 308, 310, 311, 312, 313
Medical Training 65, 66, 71, 73, 109, 123, 124, 125, 127, 129, 132, 134, 139, 140, 142, 144, 156, 159, 161, 163, 164, 165, 172, 178, 179, 180, 188, 189, 213, 280, 289
Medicine 63, 65, 72, 73, 74, 80, 83, 84, 85, 104, 105, 107, 111, 112, 115, 116, 117, 119, 120, 121, 123, 125, 126, 130, 138, 144, 147, 149, 150, 154, 156, 160, 162, 182, 188, 190, 191, 192, 193, 196, 208, 211, 214, 217, 218, 219, 220, 222, 224, 227, 230, 235, 270, 279, 280, 283, 292, 295, 296, 298, 299, 301, 303, 304, 310

O

Oral Health 5, 11, 15, 22, 24, 25, 29, 30, 204, 241, 243, 249, 251, 252, 255, 267, 275

P

Patient monitoring 157, 193
Professional Education 26, 33, 34, 35, 36, 55, 70, 280, 293

R

Reflective Practice-Based Learning 33, 35, 36, 42, 58
Risks and Ethical Considerations 91
Rural Dental Care 227, 232, 233, 252, 262, 263

S

Self-Directed Learning 65, 71, 100, 108, 126, 196, 199, 200, 202, 205, 214, 220
simulation training 8, 32, 189, 201

T

Technology Knowledge 54, 55
Technology Literacy 33, 34, 35, 36, 37, 38, 41, 42, 44, 45, 53, 54, 55, 58, 61
teledentistry 2, 3, 4, 8, 20, 22, 26, 32, 84
Tutoring 69, 81, 91, 96, 99, 108, 109, 110, 112, 121, 124, 126, 128, 136, 140, 141, 146, 147, 149, 151, 152, 154, 155

V

virtual reality 2, 3, 4, 5, 8, 11, 12, 14, 15, 21, 23, 25, 27, 32, 47, 69, 70, 71, 87, 124, 153, 159, 160, 163, 164, 165, 185,

186, 187, 188, 190, 191, 286, 293, 294, 303, 304, 308, 309, 312

W

Wearable technology 157, 158, 159, 160, 161, 162, 163, 164, 165, 166, 167, 168, 169, 170, 171, 172, 174, 175, 176, 177, 178, 179, 180, 181, 182, 183, 184, 188, 189, 194

www.ingramcontent.com/pod-product-compliance
Lightning Source LLC
LaVergne TN
LVHW062323300926
849161LV00007B/1544